T0205850

Herbal Treatment of Anxiety

Herbal Treatment of Anxiety: Clinical Studies in Western, Chinese and Ayurvedic Traditions explains the nature and types of anxiety, its neurobiology, the pathophysiology that exacerbates and perpetuates it, and the psychopharmacology of the chemical agents that relieve its manifestations. Throughout the text are discussions of Western, Chinese and Ayurvedic herbal treatments that have been clinically shown to be effective in relieving anxiety. The book also features a scientific discussion of the use of herbs and essential oils in aromatherapy and the mechanisms by which they may work. The book concludes by providing bases upon which herbs can be chosen to treat the anxiety of patients according to their individual needs.

Additional features include:

- Examines the increasingly popular subject of the use of herbs as a natural alternative treatment and provides a much-needed scientific basis for treatments often considered as merely "folk medicine."
- Discusses the psychoactive phytochemicals contained in herbs.
- Includes a chapter discussing the nature and mechanisms of action of adaptogens.
- Adds to the armamentarium of anxiolytics for providers who have become reluctant to prescribe benzodiazepines as treatment of anxiety, particularly in the context of the opiate crisis.
- Gives an introduction to herbal treatments of traditional Chinese and Ayurvedic medicine.
- Offers practical advice on initiating and managing herbal treatments.

Herbal Treatment of Anxiety is a valuable reference for psychiatrists, psychiatric nurse practitioners, primary care providers, naturopathic doctors and therapists interested in the most current scientific information on the effects of herbal treatments of anxiety disorders.

Scott D. Mendelson is a practicing psychiatrist in Roseburg, Oregon. He earned a Ph.D. in biopsychology at the University of British Columbia in Vancouver, Canada. He then worked for three years as a postdoctoral fellow at The Rockefeller University in the Laboratory of Neuroendocrinology under Bruce McEwen, Ph.D. During his doctoral work and as a postdoctoral fellow, he published 24 papers on the subjects of serotonergic and hormonal regulation of sexual behavior and the effects of stress on serotonin receptor subtypes in the brain. He then attended medical school at the University of Illinois and, after graduating in 1996, he did his residency in psychiatry at the University of Virginia. In 2007, Elsevier published his first book, *Metabolic Syndrome and Psychiatric Illness: Interactions, Pathophysiology, Assessment and Treatment*. In 2009, M. Evans published his second book, *Beyond Alzheimer's: How to Avoid the Modern Epidemic of Dementia*.

Clinical Pharmacognosy Series

Series Editors
Navindra P. Seeram and Luigi Antonio Morrone

Botanical medicines are rapidly increasing in global recognition with significant public health and economic implications. For instance, in developing countries, a vast majority of the indigenous populations use medicinal plants as a major form of healthcare. Also, in industrialized nations, including Europe and North America, consumers are increasingly using herbs and botanical dietary supplements as part of integrative health and complementary and alternative therapies. Moreover, the paradigm shifts occurring in modern medicine, from mono-drug to multi-drug and poly-pharmaceutical therapies, has led to renewed interest in botanical medicines and botanical drugs.

Natural Products and Cardiovascular Health
Catherina C. Caballero George

Aromatherapy: Basic Mechanisms and Evidence-Based Clinical Use
Giacinto Bagetta, Marco Cosentino, and Tsukasa Sakurada

Herbal Medicines: Development and Validation of Plant-Derived Medicines for Human Health
Giacinto Bagetta, Marco Cosentino, Marie Tiziana Corasaniti, and Shinobu Sakurada

Natural Products Interactions on Genomes
Siva G. Somasundaram

Principles and Practice of Botanicals as an Integrative Therapy
Anne Hume and Katherine Kelly Orr

Herbal Treatment of Major Depression: Scientific Basis and Practical Use
Scott Mendelson

Herbal Treatment of Anxiety: Clinical Studies in Western, Chinese and Ayurvedic Traditions
Scott D. Mendelson

Herbal Treatment of Anxiety

Clinical Studies in Western, Chinese and Ayurvedic Traditions

Scott D. Mendelson

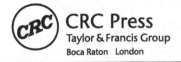

CRC Press
Taylor & Francis Group
Boca Raton   London

CRC Press is an imprint of the
Taylor & Francis Group, an **informa** business

Cover image: Shutterstock

First edition published 2023
by CRC Press
6000 Broken Sound Parkway NW, Suite 300, Boca Raton, FL 33487–2742

and by CRC Press
4 Park Square, Milton Park, Abingdon, Oxon, OX14 4RN

CRC Press is an imprint of Taylor & Francis Group, LLC

Library of Congress Cataloging-in-Publication Data
Names: Mendelson, Scott D., author.
Title: Herbal treatment of anxiety : clinical studies in Western, Chinese and ayurvedic traditions / Scott D. Mendelson, M.D. Ph.D.
Description: First edition. I Boca Raton : CRC Press, 2022. I Includes bibliographical references and index.
Subjects: LCSH: Anxiety disorders—Alternative treatment. I Herbs—Therapeutic use.
Classification: LCC RC531 .M46 2022 I DDC 616.85/22—dc23/eng/20220322
LC record available at https://lccn.loc.gov/2022003084

ISBN: 978-1-032-29159-8 (hbk)
ISBN: 978-1-032-29160-4 (pbk)
ISBN: 978-1-003-30028-1 (ebk)

DOI: 10.1201/9781003300281

Typeset in Times New Roman
by Apex CoVantage, LLC

Contents

Preface.. xix

Chapter 1   What Is Anxiety? 1

References 4

Chapter 2   Non-Pharmacological Treatments of Anxiety 7

References 9

Chapter 3   The Neurobiology of Anxiety 11

3.1   Brain Circuitry of Anxiety.....................................11
3.2   Neurochemistry...12
        3.2.1   Gamma Amino Butyric Acid.....................12
        3.2.2   Glutamate 13
        3.2.3   Monoamines..13
        3.2.4   Acetylcholine..14
        3.2.5   Endocannabinoids 14
        3.2.6   Endorphins 14
        3.2.7   Histamine 15
        3.2.8   Glycine 15
3.3   Stress...15
3.4   Inflammation 16
3.5   Metabolic Syndrome 16
3.6   Summary 17
References 18

Chapter 4   Medications Commonly Used to Treat Anxiety 23

4.1   Benzodiazepines..23
4.2   Buspirone..25
4.3   Antidepressants 25
4.4   Gabapentin..26
4.5   Pregabalin...27
4.6   Hydroxyzine 27
4.7   Propranolol 27
4.8   Clonidine 28
4.9   Neurosteroids..28
4.10 Mechanisms of Anxiolytic Drug Action.............. 28
References 29

Chapter 5   Anxiolytic Phytochemicals 33

            5.1   Flavonoids...33
            5.2   Terpenes... 34
            5.3   Alkaloids 35
            5.4   Phytochemicals That Relieve Anxiety 36
                   5.4.1   Amentoflavone...37
                   5.4.2   Apigenin 37
                   5.4.3   Baicalein.. 38
                   5.4.4   β-Caryophyllene 38
                   5.4.5   Bisabolol.. 38
                   5.4.6   Caffeic Acid... 38
                   5.4.7   3-Carene 39
                   5.4.8   Carvacrol..39
                   5.4.9   Chrysin 39
                   5.4.10   7,8,Dihydroxyflavone 40
                   5.4.11   Ellagic Acid... 40
                   5.4.12   Epigallocatechin Gallate 40
                   5.4.13   Eugenol...41
                   5.4.14   Ferulic Acid..41
                   5.4.15   Hispidulin 42
                   5.4.16   Hyperoside..42
                   5.4.17   Icariin 42
                   5.4.18   Isopulegol 43
                   5.4.19   Kaempferol 43
                   5.4.20   Limonene..43
                   5.4.21   Linalool 43
                   5.4.22   Luteolin 44
                   5.4.23   Menthol 44
                   5.4.24   Mangiferin 44
                   5.4.25   Myricetin..45
                   5.4.26   Naringin 45
                   5.4.27   Nerolidol...45
                   5.4.28   Nobiletin...45
                   5.4.29   Pinene 46
                   5.4.30   Resveratrol... 46
                   5.4.31   Quercetin 46
                   5.4.32   Rosmarinic Acid..47
                   5.4.33   Ursolic Acid..47
                   5.4.34   Wogonin 47
            References 48

Chapter 6   Herbal Treatment of Anxiety 55

            6.1   *Acorus calamus* 55
                   6.1.1   Anxiolytic Effects 55

	6.1.2	Mechanism of Action	56
	6.1.3	Dosage	56
	6.1.4	Toxicity	56
	6.1.5	Safety in Pregnancy	56
	6.1.6	Drug Interaction	56
6.2	*Avena sativa*		57
	6.2.1	Anxiolytic Effects	57
	6.2.2	Mechanism of Action	57
	6.2.3	Dosage	57
	6.2.4	Toxicity	57
	6.2.5	Safety in Pregnancy	58
	6.2.6	Drug Interactions	58
6.3	*Bacopa monnieri*		58
	6.3.1	Anxiolytic Effects	58
	6.3.2	Mechanism of Action	58
	6.3.3	Dosage	59
	6.3.4	Toxicity	59
	6.3.5	Safety in Pregnancy	59
	6.3.6	Drug Interactions	59
6.4	*Camellia sinensis*		59
	6.4.1	Anxiolytic Effects	59
	6.4.2	Mechanism of Action	60
	6.4.3	Dosage	60
	6.4.4	Toxicity	61
	6.4.5	Safety in Pregnancy	61
	6.4.6	Drug Interactions	61
6.5	*Cannabis sativa*		61
	6.5.1	Anxiolytic Effects	62
	6.5.2	Mechanism of Action	62
	6.5.3	Dosage	63
	6.5.4	Toxicity	63
	6.5.5	Safety in Pregnancy	63
	6.5.6	Drug Interactions	64
6.6	*Centella asiatica*		64
	6.6.1	Anxiolytic Effects	64
	6.6.2	Mechanism of Action	65
	6.6.3	Dosage	65
	6.6.4	Toxicity	65
	6.6.5	Safety in Pregnancy	65
	6.6.6	Drug Interactions	65
6.7	*Cinnamomum spp*		66
	6.7.1	Anxiolytic Effects	66
	6.7.2	Mechanism of Action	66
	6.7.3	Dosage	67
	6.7.4	Toxicity	67

6.7.5   Safety in Pregnancy...67
6.7.6   Drug Interactions..67
6.8   *Citrus aurantium*...67
6.8.1   Anxiolytic Effects 68
6.8.2   Mechanism of Action 68
6.8.3   Dosage...68
6.8.4   Toxicity..68
6.8.5   Safety in Pregnancy..68
6.8.6   Drug Interaction 68
6.9   *Convolvulus pluricaulis* 69
6.9.1   Anxiolytic Effects 69
6.9.2   Mechanism of Action 69
6.9.3   Dosage...69
6.9.4   Toxicity..69
6.9.5   Safety in Pregnancy..70
6.9.6   Drug Interaction 70
6.10   *Crocus sativus* 70
6.10.1   Anxiolytic Effects 70
6.10.2   Mechanism of Action 70
6.10.3   Dosage...71
6.10.4   Toxicity..71
6.10.5   Safety in Pregnancy..71
6.10.6   Drug Interactions..71
6.11   *Curcuma longa* 71
6.11.1   Anxiolytic Effects 72
6.11.2   Mechanism of Action 72
6.11.3   Dosage...72
6.11.4   Toxicity..72
6.11.5   Safety in Pregnancy..73
6.11.6   Drug Interactions..73
6.12   *Echinacea angustifolia*...73
6.12.1   Anxiolytic Effects 73
6.12.2   Mechanism of Action 73
6.12.3   Dosage...74
6.12.4   Toxicity..74
6.12.5   Safety in Pregnancy..74
6.12.6   Drug Interaction 74
6.13   *Echium amoenum* 74
6.13.1   Anxiolytic Effects 74
6.13.2   Mechanism of Action 75
6.13.3   Dosage...76
6.13.4   Toxicity..76
6.13.5   Safety in Pregnancy..76
6.13.6   Drug Interactions..76

6.14   *Eleutherococcus senticosus*..76
    6.14.1   Anxiolytic Effects 76
    6.14.2   Mechanism of Action.. 77
    6.14.3   Dosage.. 77
    6.14.4   Toxicity...78
    6.14.5   Safety in Pregnancy...78
    6.14.6   Drug Interactions...78
6.15   *Eschscholzia californica* 78
    6.15.1   Anxiolytic Effects 78
    6.15.2   Mechanism of Action...78
    6.15.3   Dosage..79
    6.15.4   Toxicity...79
    6.15.5   Safety in Pregnancy...79
    6.15.6   Drug Interaction 79
6.16   Euphytose 79
    6.16.1   Anxiolytic Effects 80
    6.16.2   Mechanism of Action... 80
    6.16.3   Dosage.. 80
    6.16.4   Toxicity... 80
    6.16.5   Safety in Pregnancy... 80
    6.16.6   Drug Interactions...81
6.17   *Evolvulus alsinoides*...81
    6.17.1   Anxiolytic Effects 81
    6.17.2   Mechanism of Action..81
    6.17.3   Dosage.. 82
    6.17.4   Toxicity... 82
    6.17.5   Safety in Pregnancy... 82
    6.17.6   Drug Interaction 82
6.18   *Foeniculum vulgare*.. 82
    6.18.1   Anxiolytic Effects 82
    6.18.2   Mechanism of Action... 83
    6.18.3   Dosage.. 83
    6.18.4   Toxicity... 83
    6.18.5   Safety in Pregnancy... 83
    6.18.6   Drug Interactions... 84
6.19   *Galphimia glauca*... 84
    6.19.1   Anxiolytic Effects 84
    6.19.2   Mechanism of Action... 84
    6.19.3   Dosage.. 85
    6.19.4   Toxicity... 85
    6.19.5   Safety in Pregnancy... 85
    6.19.6   Drug Interaction 85
6.20   *Ganoderma lucidum*... 85
    6.20.1   Anxiolytic Effects 85

6.20.2   Mechanism of Action 86
6.20.3   Dosage 86
6.20.4   Toxicity 86
6.20.5   Safety in Pregnancy.. 86
6.20.6   Drug Interaction 86
6.21   Ginkgo biloba 87
6.21.1   Anxiolytic Effects 87
6.21.2   Mechanism of Action 87
6.21.3   Dosage 87
6.21.4   Toxicity 88
6.21.5   Safety in Pregnancy.. 88
6.21.6   Drug Interactions.. 88
6.22   Humulus lupulus... 88
6.22.1   Anxiolytic Effects 88
6.22.2   Mechanism of Action 89
6.22.3   Dosage 89
6.22.4   Toxicity 89
6.22.5   Safety in Pregnancy.. 89
6.22.6   Drug Interactions.. 89
6.23   Hypericum perforatum 89
6.23.1   Anxiolytic Effects 90
6.23.2   Mechanism of Action 90
6.23.3   Dosage 91
6.23.4   Toxicity 91
6.23.5   Safety in Pregnancy..91
6.23.6   Drug Interactions..91
6.24   Lavandula angustifolia 91
6.24.1   Anxiolytic Effects 92
6.24.2   Mechanism of Action 92
6.24.3   Dosage 92
6.24.4   Toxicity 92
6.24.5   Safety in Pregnancy.. 92
6.24.6   Drug Interactions.. 92
6.25   Leonurus cardiaca 93
6.25.1   Anxiolytic Effects 93
6.25.2   Mechanism of Action 93
6.25.3   Dosage 93
6.25.4   Toxicity 94
6.25.5   Safety in Pregnancy.. 94
6.25.6   Drug Interaction 94
6.26   Lepidium meyenii 94
6.26.1   Anxiolytic Effects 94
6.26.2   Mechanism of Action 95
6.26.3   Dosage 95
6.26.4   Toxicity 95

        6.26.5 Safety in Pregnancy 95
        6.26.6 Drug Interaction 95
    6.27 *Lilium brownii* 95
        6.27.1 Anxiolytic Effects 96
        6.27.2 Mechanism of Action 96
        6.27.3 Dosage 96
        6.27.4 Toxicity 96
        6.27.5 Safety in Pregnancy 96
        6.27.6 Drug Interaction 96
    6.28 *Lippia citriodora* 96
        6.28.1 Anxiolytic Effects 97
        6.28.2 Mechanism of Action 97
        6.28.3 Dosage 97
        6.28.4 Toxicity 98
        6.28.5 Safety in Pregnancy 98
        6.28.6 Drug Interactions 98
    6.29 *Magnolia officinalis* 98
        6.29.1 Anxiolytic Effects 98
        6.29.2 Mechanism of Action 99
        6.29.3 Dosage 99
        6.29.4 Toxicity 99
        6.29.5 Safety in Pregnancy 99
        6.29.6 Drug Interactions 99
    6.30 *Matricaria recutita* 99
        6.30.1 Anxiolytic Effects 100
        6.30.2 Mechanism of Action 100
        6.30.3 Dosage 100
        6.30.4 Toxicity 101
        6.30.5 Safety in Pregnancy 101
        6.30.6 Drug Interaction 101
    6.31 *Melissa officinalis* 101
        6.31.1 Anxiolytic Effects 101
        6.31.2 Mechanism of Action 102
        6.31.3 Dosage 102
        6.31.4 Toxicity 102
        6.31.5 Safety in Pregnancy 102
        6.31.6 Drug Interactions 102
    6.32 *Mentha piperita* 102
        6.32.1 Anxiolytic Effects 103
        6.32.2 Mechanism of Action 103
        6.32.3 Dosage 103
        6.32.4 Toxicity 103
        6.32.5 Safety in Pregnancy 104
        6.32.6 Drug Interaction 104

6.33   *Nardostachys jatamansi* 104
       6.33.1   Anxiolytic Effects 104
       6.33.2   Mechanism of Action 104
       6.33.3   Dosage 105
       6.33.4   Toxicity 105
       6.33.5   Safety in Pregnancy.......................................105
       6.33.6   Drug Interaction 105
6.34   *Ocimum sanctum* 105
       6.34.1   Anxiolytic Effects 105
       6.34.2   Mechanism of Action 106
       6.34.3   Dosage 106
       6.34.4   Toxicity 106
       6.34.5   Safety in Pregnancy.......................................106
       6.34.6   Drug Interactions..106
6.35   *Panax ginseng* 106
       6.35.1   Anxiolytic Effects 107
       6.35.2   Mechanism of Action 108
       6.35.3   Dosage 108
       6.35.4   Toxicity 108
       6.35.5   Safety in Pregnancy.......................................108
       6.35.6   Drug Interactions..108
6.36   *Passiflora incarnata* 108
       6.36.1   Anxiolytic Effects 109
       6.36.2   Mechanism of Action 109
       6.36.3   Dosage 109
       6.36.4   Toxicity 109
       6.36.5   Safety in Pregnancy.......................................109
       6.36.6   Drug Interactions..110
6.37   *Piper methysticum* 110
       6.37.1   Anxiolytic Effects 110
       6.37.2   Mechanism of Action 110
       6.37.3   Dosage 111
       6.37.4   Toxicity 111
       6.37.5   Safety in Pregnancy.......................................111
       6.37.6   Drug Interactions..111
6.38   *Poria cocos* 112
       6.38.1   Anxiolytic Effects 112
       6.38.2   Mechanism of Action 112
       6.38.3   Dosage 113
       6.38.4   Toxicity 113
       6.38.5   Safety in Pregnancy.......................................113
       6.38.6   Drug Interactions..113
6.39   *Psilocybe spp* 113
       6.39.1   Anxiolytic Effects 114
       6.39.2   Mechanism of Action 115
       6.39.3   Dosage 116

6.39.4   Toxicity...116
6.39.5   Safety in Pregnancy...117
6.39.6   Drug Interaction 117
6.40   *Rhodiola rosea* 117
6.40.1   Anxiolytic Effects 117
6.40.2   Mechanism of Action 118
6.40.3   Dosage 118
6.40.4   Toxicity...118
6.40.5   Safety in Pregnancy...118
6.40.6   Drug Interactions...119
6.41   *Rosmarinus officinalis*...119
6.41.1   Anxiolytic Effects 119
6.41.2   Mechanism of Action 119
6.41.3   Dosage 120
6.41.4   Toxicity...120
6.41.5   Safety in Pregnancy...120
6.41.6   Drug Interactions...120
6.42   *Salvia officinalis*...120
6.42.1   Anxiolytic Effects 121
6.42.2   Mechanism of Action 121
6.42.3   Dosage 122
6.42.4   Toxicity...122
6.42.5   Safety in Pregnancy...122
6.42.6   Drug Interaction 122
6.43   *Schisandra chinensis*...122
6.43.1   Anxiolytic Effects 122
6.43.2   Mechanism of Action 123
6.43.3   Dosage..123
6.43.4   Toxicity...123
6.43.5   Safety in Pregnancy...123
6.43.6   Drug Interactions...123
6.44   *Scutellaria baicalensis* 124
6.44.1   Anxiolytic Effects 124
6.44.2   Mechanism of Action 124
6.44.3   Dosage.. 124
6.44.4   Toxicity...125
6.44.5   Safety in Pregnancy...125
6.44.6   Drug Interactions...125
6.45   *Silybum marianum* 125
6.45.1   Anxiolytic Effects 125
6.45.2   Mechanism of Action 126
6.45.3   Dosage 126
6.45.4   Toxicity...126
6.45.5   Safety in Pregnancy...126
6.45.6   Drug Interactions...126

6.46 *Tinospora cordifolia*..126
    6.46.1 Anxiolytic Effects 127
    6.46.2 Mechanism of Action 127
    6.46.3 Dosage..127
    6.46.4 Toxicity..127
    6.46.5 Safety in Pregnancy....................................128
    6.46.6 Drug Interaction 128
6.47 *Trifolium pratense* 128
    6.47.1 Anxiolytic Effects 128
    6.47.2 Mechanism of Action 129
    6.47.3 Dosage..129
    6.47.4 Toxicity..129
    6.47.5 Safety in Pregnancy....................................129
    6.47.6 Drug Interaction 130
6.48 *Valeriana jatamansi*..130
    6.48.1 Anxiolytic Effects 130
    6.48.2 Mechanism of Action 130
    6.48.3 Dosage..130
    6.48.4 Toxicity..131
    6.48.5 Safety in Pregnancy....................................131
    6.48.6 Drug Interaction 131
6.49 *Valeriana officinalis*...131
    6.49.1 Anxiolytic Effects 131
    6.49.2 Mechanism of Action 132
    6.49.3 Dosage..132
    6.49.4 Toxicity..132
    6.49.5 Safety in Pregnancy....................................132
    6.49.6 Drug Interactions..132
6.50 *Vitex agnus-castus*...132
    6.50.1 Anxiolytic Effects 133
    6.50.2 Mechanism of Action 133
    6.50.3 Dosage..133
    6.50.4 Toxicity..134
    6.50.5 Safety in Pregnancy....................................134
    6.50.6 Drug Interactions..134
6.51 *Withania somnifera* 134
    6.51.1 Anxiolytic Effects 134
    6.51.2 Mechanism of Action 135
    6.51.3 Dosage..135
    6.51.4 Toxicity..135
    6.51.5 Safety in Pregnancy....................................136
    6.51.6 Drug Interactions..136
6.52 *Zizyphus jujuba* 136
    6.52.1 Anxiolytic Effects 136
    6.52.2 Mechanism of Action 136

                    6.52.3   Dosage 137
                    6.52.4   Toxicity 137
                    6.52.5   Safety in Pregnancy 137
                    6.52.6   Drug Interactions 137
          6.53   Anxiolytic Herbs Recommended by Experts That
                  Remain Untested 137
                    6.53.1   *Borago officinalis* 138
                    6.53.2   *Lactuca virosa* 138
                    6.53.3   *Mimosa pudica* 139
                    6.53.4   *Nepeta cataria* 139
                    6.53.5   *Piscidia piscipula* 140
                    6.53.6   *Taraxacum officinale* 140
                    6.53.7   *Tilia spp* 140
          References 141

Chapter 7   Chinese Herbal Treatment of Anxiety 175

          7.1   Traditional Chinese Treatments of Anxiety 177
          7.2   Herbal Treatment in Traditional Chinese Medicine 177
                    7.2.1   *Bai zi yang xin tang* with *Shu gan ning
                             shen san* 178
                    7.2.2   *Ban xia hou pu* 179
                    7.2.3   *Bao shen* 180
                    7.2.4   *Geng ni an chun* 180
                    7.2.5   *Gui pi tang* 180
                    7.2.6   *Jiu wei zhen xin* 181
                    7.2.7   *Kami-shoyo-san* and *Hange-koboku-to* 181
                    7.2.8   *Rikkunshinto* 182
                    7.2.9   *Shen qi wu wei zi* 182
                    7.2.10   *Shen song yang xin* 183
                    7.2.11   *Suan zao ren tang* in Combination with *Zhi
                             zi chi tang* 183
                    7.2.12   *Wen dan tang* 184
                    7.2.13   *Xiao yao san* 185
                    7.2.14   *Xin wei tang* 185
                    7.2.15   *Yang xin tang* 185
                    7.2.16   *Yi gan san* 186
                    7.2.17   *Yi qi yang xin* 187
                    7.2.18   *Yukgunja* and *Banhabakchulchunma*
                             Decoctions 187
          7.3   Traditional but Untested Anxiolytic Chinese Herbal
                  Formulas 188
          7.4   The Mainstays of Chinese Herbal Treatments 190
                    7.4.1   *Acorus gramineus* 191
                    7.4.2   *Albizzia julibrissin* 191

7.4.3   *Angelicae gigantis* 192
7.4.4   *Bupleurum chinense* 192
7.4.5   *Cnidium officinale* 193
7.4.6   *Coptis chinensis* 193
7.4.7   *Curcuma wenyujin* 194
7.4.8   *Cynomorium songaricum* 194
7.4.9   *Ganoderma lucidum* 194
7.4.10   *Glycyrrhiza uralensis* 194
7.4.11   *Paeonia lactiflora* 195
7.4.12   *Panax ginseng* 195
7.4.13   *Pinellia ternata* 196
7.4.14   *Polygala tenuifolia* 196
7.4.15   *Polygonum multiflorum* 197
7.4.16   *Poria cocos* 197
7.4.17   *Rehmannia glutinosa* 197
7.4.18   *Schisandra chinensis* 198
7.4.19   *Zizyphus jujuba* 198
References 198

Chapter 8   Ayurvedic Herbal Treatment of Anxiety 205

8.1   Herbal Treatment of Anxiety in Ayurvedic Medicine 207
       8.1.1   *Ashwagandha churna* 208
       8.1.2   *Ashwagandha* and *Mandookaparni* 208
       8.1.3   *Asparagus racemosus* and *Glycyrrhiza glabra* 209
       8.1.4   *Brahmi gritha* 209
       8.1.5   Geriforte 209
       8.1.6   *Guduchyadi medhya rasayana* 210
       8.1.7   *Kushmandadi ghrita* 210
       8.1.8   *Medhyarasayana ghrita* and *Vachadi ghrita
                nasya* 211
       8.1.9   Mentat 211
       8.1.10   OCTA 212
       8.1.11   *Sarasvata choorna* 212
       8.1.12   *Sarpagandha ghana vati* 213
       8.1.13   *Shankhapushpi panak* and *Shirodhara* with
                Mamsyadi kwatha 214
       8.1.14   *Shankhapushpyadi ghana vati* 215
       8.1.15   *Vacha brahmi ghan* 216
       8.1.16   Worry Free 216
8.2   Mainstays of Ayurvedic 216
       8.2.1   *Acorus calamus* 216
       8.2.2   *Albizzia lebbek* 217
       8.2.3   *Allium cepa* 217
       8.2.4   *Anacyclus pyrethrum* 217

        8.2.5   *Asparagus racemosus* 218
        8.2.6   *Bacopa monnieri* 218
        8.2.7   *Benincasa hispida* 218
        8.2.8   *Cannabis sativa* 219
        8.2.9   *Centella asiatica* 219
        8.2.10   *Convolvulus pluricaulis* 219
        8.2.11   *Cuscuta reflexa* 219
        8.2.12   *Cynodon dactylon* 220
        8.2.13   *Evolvulus alsinoides* 220
        8.2.14   *Ficus religiosa* 220
        8.2.15   *Glycyrrhiza glabra* 221
        8.2.16   *Hyoscyamus niger* 221
        8.2.17   *Juglans regia* 222
        8.2.18   *Lawsonia inermis* 222
        8.2.19   *Moringa oleifera* 223
        8.2.20   *Nardostachys jatamansi* 223
        8.2.21   *Piper nigrum* 223
        8.2.22   *Punica granatum* 224
        8.2.23   *Saussurea lappa* 224
        8.2.24   *Tinospora cordifolia* 224
        8.2.25   *Valeriana jatamansi* 225
        8.2.26   *Vitex negundo* 225
        8.2.27   *Withania somnifera* 225
        References 225

Chapter 9   Adaptogens 231
        References 234

Chapter 10   Aromatherapy 237
        10.1   Herbs Utilized in Aromatherapy 241
                10.1.1   *Boswellia carterii* 241
                10.1.2   *Citrus aurantium* 242
                10.1.3   *Citrus sinensis* 242
                10.1.4   *Cymbopogon citratus* 242
                10.1.5   *Eugenia aromaticum* 243
                10.1.6   *Jasminum officinale* 244
                10.1.7   *Lavandula spp* 244
                10.1.8   *Matricaria recutita* 245
                10.1.9   *Melissa officinalis* 245
                10.1.10 *Mentha piperita* 245
                10.1.11 *Nardostachys jatamansi* 246
                10.1.12 Neroli Oil 246
                10.1.13 *Pelargonium graveolens* 246

           10.1.14 *Rosa damascena*.. 247
           10.1.15 *Rosmarinus officinalis* 248
           10.1.16 *Salvia officinalis*.. 248
           10.1.17 *Santallum spp* 249
   10.2   Herbal Combinations in Aromatherapy 249
           10.2.1   *Cymbopogon citratus* and *Eucalyptus* Massage
                   with *Lavandula officinalis* Inhalation...................... 250
           10.2.2   *Lavandula officinalis, Cananga odorata*, and
                   Citrus bergamia 250
           10.2.3   *Lavandula officinalis, Chamaemelum nobile*,
                   and *Citrus aurantium* 250
           10.2.4   *Lavandula officinalis, Pelargonium graveolens*,
                   and *Citrus reticulata* 251
           10.2.5   *Lavandula officinalis* and *Rosa damascena* 251
           10.2.6   *Lavandula officinalis* and *Santalum album*..............251
   10.3   Aromatherapy and Sleep 251
   10.4   Some Final Thoughts about Aromatherapy 252
   References 253

Chapter 11   Choosing an Herbal Treatment for Anxiety.....................................259

   11.1   Efficacy...259
   11.2   What Type of Anxiety Is Being Treated?................................261
   11.3   Single Herbs or Combinations? 261
   11.4   Treatment of Chronic Anxiety Disorders.............................. 263
   11.5   Comorbidities 264
           11.5.1   Major Depression 264
           11.5.2   Insomnia.. 266
           11.5.3   Menopause and Dysmenorrhea 268
           11.5.4   Pain.. 269
           11.5.5   Inflammation 270
           11.5.6   Irritable Bowel Syndrome 271
           11.5.7   Diabetes...271
           11.5.8   Dementia 272
   11.6   Safety...273
   11.7   Final Considerations about the Practical Use of Herbs.........276
   References 277

Index.. 287

Preface

This book is about the use of herbs to treat anxiety. There are several reasons why I wrote it. Foremost, I hope to provide health, hope, and healing to my fellow human beings who are suffering. However, I also have a great personal interest in herbs as medicine. I am a psychiatrist and a medical doctor, and I am well trained in biological sciences and Western medicine. I studied physiology, neurochemistry, and pharmacology, and this knowledge continues to guide me. However, I am also a child of the 1960s. During that unique period of time, I gained a great affinity for the philosophy of going back to nature. What is simple and natural is often the best treatment of illness. Though I prescribe man-made medications for many of my patients, I also tell them that there are no better medicines than fresh air, friendship, having fun, wholesome food, exercise, and restorative sleep. I have often told my patients that nature and our bodies always tell us the truth. We can depend on them. Human beings evolved in nature. Our bodies share the same chemicals of life not only with other animals but also with plants. We depend on the chemicals made in plants—that is, phytochemicals—as sources of nutrition and optimal health.

I am fascinated with herbs not only because they are natural but because they have a magnificent complexity. Understanding how herbs and the phytochemicals they contain affect our moods and thoughts pushes at the boundaries of our understanding of the chemistry of the brain. Many substances in plants, such as vitamins, are essential for health, and without them we grow sick and die. However, other plant substances can optimize health and reverse illness in more subtle ways. The discoverer of Vitamin C—Nobel Prize winner Albert Szent-Györgyi—years ago invented the term *vitamin P* to describe the role of phytochemicals called flavonoids in optimizing health. At the time, he could not elaborate on what his theoretical vitamin P might do. However, we now know that flavonoids and other phytochemicals can mimic the chemical messengers in the human body and influence the ways those natural chemical messengers pass on their signals within cells. In these ways, phytochemicals can affect energy metabolism, alter stress responses, enhance the immune system, fight inflammation, stimulate growth factors in the body, and modify other fundamental processes in the cells of our bodies. These same processes occur in the cells of our brain—our neurons and glial cells—and by these means phytochemicals affect our mood, thinking, sleep, and general sense of well-being.

David Sinclair, a researcher and professor at Harvard Medical School, has more recently proposed a grander ecological theory of phytochemical action in our bodies. Plants stressed by drought or other adverse conditions are known to bolster their resiliency by producing certain types of phytochemicals. Sinclair theorized that animals evolved to respond to those stress-induced chemicals in plants to prepare themselves for those environmental changes. This theory, xenohormesis, was initially focused on how certain drought-induced stress chemicals in plants, such as resveratrol, cause changes in the energy metabolisms of animals. Indeed, supplementation with resveratrol produces changes in the body much like those that result during food restriction. Like fasting, consumption of resveratrol alters metabolic processes and increases longevity in many species of animals. This theory has been expanded to include evolutionary adaptation of the human body to react to other types of information that plants provide about changes in the environment. Our scientific appreciation of how humans are part of a larger, interconnected web of life continues to grow.

Another reason I wrote this book is a distressing trend in medicine involving restrictions in the use of certain medications. The opiate crisis is genuine and concerning. Overdoses and other misuses of opiates have taken many lives. Benzodiazepines, a class of medications prescribed to treat anxiety, can have dangerous interactions with opiate pain medications. These medications must be prescribed with great caution. However, a person who has adapted to those medications is in little danger as long as doses are not rapidly increased. Unfortunately, many doctors are refusing to continue to those medications, regardless of how long a patient may have taken them or how stable that patient may have been on them. This often forces patients to choose between relief from pain or relief from anxiety. I see it as important to provide people with safe and effective herbal treatments of anxiety as alternatives to the benzodiazepine medications that have been taken away from them. Going back to nature thereby allows us a greater degree of independence. We all have access to nature, and nature treats us all equally. We can rely less on experts, many with their own biases, blind spots, and agendas.

In the following pages, I describe anxiety and the various ways it can be treated. I next turn to plants and the healing phytochemicals they contain. Then I discuss the many herbs that have been found to help relieve anxiety. Although many different herbs have been used throughout history to relieve anxiety, I have included only those herbs that have been shown to be effective in clinical studies. Every herbal treatment I discuss is accompanied by a citation of the scientific source of that information. This is both to give the reader confidence in the veracity of the information and to provide the interested reader further information to pursue. I discuss single herbs, mostly from traditional Western herbal medicine, and then go on to discuss herbal treatments—often combinations of herbs—from traditional Chinese medicine and Ayurvedic medicine of India. I have also included a chapter on aromatherapy with a science-based discussion on how this treatment modality is likely to work. As with the other discussions of herbs, I present only reports on aromatherapy treatments that are published and clinically verified. In the last chapter of the book, I give readers a basis to help them decide what herbal treatment might be best for their patients or, perhaps, for themselves. Some herbs that relieve anxiety also relieve depression, lessen pain, improve diabetes, ease the discomfort of menopause, or calm the fear and agitation that can come with Alzheimer's dementia. Knowledge of the multiple uses of various herbs allows more to be done with less, which is always good practice when giving medicines of any kind. I also consider matters of safety. There is wisdom in the old saying that anything strong enough to help you is strong enough to hurt you. Regardless of the type of medicine employed, herbal or man-made, there is always a risk-to-benefit ratio that must be weighed before treatment begins. Finally, I have words of advice for those who feel at a loss on how to start and manage herbal treatment. In fact, there are more similarities than differences between standard pharmacological treatment and the use of herbal treatments. As I emphasize in several places in this text, herbs do not act through magic but through molecules. However, I must admit that molecules themselves possess and exert a great deal of magic. *Natura naturans.*

1 What Is Anxiety?

Everyone experiences anxiety. It is one of the most frequent complaints that physicians, especially psychiatrists, hear from patients. According to the Anxiety and Depression Association of America, more than 40 million Americans suffer from a clinically significant anxiety disorder each year. Although anxiety is common, it can be a difficult feeling to define. There have been many investigations of what takes place in the central and peripheral nervous system during anxiety, and the neurobiology of anxiety will be discussed in a subsequent chapter. Here we consider the experiential and clinical manifestations of anxiety.

Fear, a feeling related to anxiety, is far simpler to understand. If a person came upon a bear while walking in the woods, they would likely feel a sudden rush of body sensations. These sensations are the result of the nervous system switching into the fight-or-flight mode to prepare to fight the bear or run away.[1] Their heart would begin to pound and their breathing grow faster and deeper. They might begin to sweat and tremble. The blood in their body would shift from the gut to the skeletal muscles, where oxygen and nutrients would be better utilized for fighting or running. That shift might lead to feelings of "butterflies in the stomach" or even nausea or diarrhea. Intense fear can also bring shortness of breath, dizziness, chest pain, chills, and disorientation. Subjectively, the experience is aversive and can include alterations in focus and sense of self, time, and space.[2] Fear is a powerful and necessary emotion. Curiously, given the attraction of "scary" movies, roller coasters, and dangerous hobbies, it appears that certain controlled forms of fear can be exhilarating. Perhaps a sense of having mastered one's fears is empowering and therapeutic.

Anxiety is a set of feelings and changes in the body similar to those of fear. The difference between anxiety and fear is that anxiety occurs when an object of fear is no longer present, when an expected source of fear has not yet appeared, or if the danger of circumstances has been misinterpreted.[3] Again, as a simple example, after having come upon a bear in the woods, one might later feel anxiety when wondering, "Is the bear still here? Will the bear come back?" Anxiety may arise during subsequent walks in the woods when the bear is recalled and its return anticipated. Hearing the sound of a falling branch or seeing the movement of windblown leaves might trigger suspicions, uneasiness, and all the feelings of fear, despite the fact that the bear may no longer be a threat.

Anxiety can come in a variety of forms and degrees of persistence and severity. According to the *Diagnostic and Statistical Manual* of the American Psychiatric Association, the various types of anxiety disorders in adults are phobias, social anxiety disorder, panic disorder, agoraphobia, generalized anxiety disorder, substance- or medication-induced anxiety disorder, and anxiety disorder due to a medical condition. Posttraumatic stress disorder, or PTSD, was long considered a form of anxiety disorder. However, it has recently been placed in a new and separate category—that is, a "trauma and stressor-related disorder." There is, nonetheless, a significant

DOI: 10.1201/9781003300281-1

1

component of anxiety suffered by those with PTSD. While manifesting in somewhat different ways, and having different psychological origins, all the aforementioned disorders share the same core symptoms of anxiety. That is, they share self-perpetuating, unwarranted, often irrational, and at times disabling fear-like responses.

A phobia, an irrational fear of a specific thing, develops when fear persists long after a person should have learned that their fear is out of step with the degree of danger they actually face. Studies indicate that the lifetime prevalence of specific phobias around the world ranges from 3% to 15%.[4] People can develop phobias toward dangerous animals, such as bears, dogs, snakes, or spiders. Phobias can also develop toward flying in airplanes, riding motorcycles, or swimming in the ocean. Feelings of anxiety can even grow to include things only vaguely related to the original object of fear. Using the example of the bear, later seeing a large dog with thick, bear-like fur might produce a feeling of fear similar to that generated by seeing the bear. There may later grow a vague sense of discomfort and uneasy anticipation around furry animals of any kind. A fur coat might even come to trigger anxiety. Similarly, anxieties about swimming in the ocean, with sharks and jellyfish, can grow to anxieties about swimming pools or even bathtubs full of water. This phenomenon is called generalization.[5] The full list of phobias is astonishingly long and includes phobias toward clowns, high places, storms, certain numbers, sharp objects, cars, enclosed spaces, and countless other things that may have been perceived as threats early in life or are reminiscent of serious threats experienced as an adult.

More often than not, anxiety evolves from anticipating emotional pain, embarrassment, rejection, or loss rather than the physical danger of meeting a wild animal in the woods. For some people the fear of standing in front of a crowd to give a speech may be as severe as that of standing in front of a roaring carnivore. Social anxiety disorder is a type of anxiety that can cause intense and persistent discomfort in being around other people.[6] It is common and may affect up to 7% of the population. In this disorder, there is often a deep fear of being watched and judged by others. A person may feel symptoms of anxiety when meeting new people, going out on a date, interviewing for a job, answering a question in class, or having to talk to a cashier in a store. Doing everyday things in front of people, such as eating, drinking, or using a public restroom, can cause anxiety or fear. There is frequently intense fear of being humiliated, judged, and rejected. Social anxiety disorder can affect work, school, and other daily activities. It can make it hard to make friends and start romantic relationships. It is more than mere shyness. It can be exquisitely painful, and the risk of suicide in sufferers of social anxiety disorder may be as high as that in sufferers of major depression. Indeed, the deep sense of loss and failure can often lead to major depression.[7] Sometimes the exact source of anxiety is not clear. A person may feel anxious almost every day, perhaps all day, for no obvious reason. Along with anxiety itself, they may complain of persistent edginess or restlessness, fatigue, difficulty concentrating, irritability, difficulty sleeping, and even physical symptoms such as aching muscles, persistent nausea, and digestive upset. When these symptoms exist more often than not throughout the day for six months or more, then the condition is called generalized anxiety disorder, or GAD. According to epidemiologic surveys, the estimated prevalence of GAD in the general population of the United States is 3.1% in the previous year and 5.7% over a patient's lifetime. The prevalence is approximately twice as high among women as among men.[8] Although chronic anxiety can be as mild as simply "worrying too much," GAD can be severe and persistent enough to be disabling. Some experience their worst anxiety in the morning, when they consider obstacles and potential sources of failure and embarrassment in the day ahead. Others report their worst anxiety occurs at night, when their mind wanders to relive embarrassing moments in the day or anticipate disturbing future possibilities. The fear of not getting to sleep and not being able to function the next day makes the anxiety worse. This vicious cycle often leads to complaints of insomnia and depression.

Some people can experience sudden and intense episodes of anxiety referred to as panic attacks. Surveys have found that 15% of respondents reported the occurrence of a panic attack over their lifetimes, whereas 3% reported a panic attack in the preceding month. About 1% met the *Diagnostic and Statistical Manual of Mental Disorders*, third edition, revised (*DSM-III-R*) criteria for panic disorder in the month preceding the interview.[9] These episodes of panic are usually brief, lasting 10 to 20 minutes, but can be longer. The physical symptoms of these attacks often included heart pounding, chest pain, sweating, and dizziness. They can be severe enough to drive people to emergency departments of hospitals out of fear they are suffering a heart attack or stroke. These people are said to suffer from panic disorder. Panic attacks can arise in situations that have previously been anxiety provoking, such as a crowded store or an airplane. However, they can also occur for no obvious reason. In some individuals, these attacks are infrequent and separated by long periods of feeling fine. In other cases, the very fear of experiencing panic can itself become an ongoing source of anxiety. People may thus experience persisting GAD punctuated by panic attacks. A not uncommon feature of this type of panic disorder is agoraphobia, which is a fear of being away from safety, exposed and unable to hide.[10] Such people often report feeling afraid to leave the safety of their home. They often have severe anticipatory anxiety about being surrounded in a crowd of people. Curiously, other people have a fear of open spaces; they might feel they are losing their boundaries and sense of themselves as if evaporating.

Anxiety disorders may exist on their own. However, they may also be comorbid with other psychiatric illnesses, such as major depression, obsessive compulsive disorder, bipolar affective disorder, attention deficit hyperactivity disorder, PTSD, or other psychiatric illnesses.[11] The anxiety may be secondary to one of those disorders or may exist independently. When anxiety is secondary to another illness, successful treatment of the primary illness often results in the resolution of the anxiety.

Medical conditions can also cause feelings of anxiety.[12] This is important because not only can these anxieties be reversed with medical treatment, but the anxiety may serve as an early indication that something is seriously wrong. For example, anxiety often accompanies overactivity of the thyroid gland or bouts of low blood sugar. Some rare conditions such as pheochromocytoma, a tumor of the adrenal gland, can produce the sweating, trembling, and pounding heart that occurs with severe anxiety.[13] Abnormal heart rhythms themselves can cause a very disturbing fluttery feeling in the chest that is quite anxiety provoking. There has long been a curious and controversial association between mitral valve prolapse and panic disorder. A quite recent meta-analysis has lent support to that connection, though it does not attempt to determine how the two conditions might be associated.[14] Certainly, nothing is more anxiety provoking than not being able to breathe. Anxiety is often associated with asthma and COPD. Unfortunately, whereas asthma and COPD can be anxiety provoking, anxiety, in turn, can exacerbate those conditions.[15–16]

Certain medications can cause feelings of anxiety. The triptan class of medications, used to treat migraine headache, have been known to induce states of anxiety.[17] The 5-alpha-reductase inhibitor finasteride, used to treat benign prostatic hypertrophy and baldness, is reported to cause anxiety and mood disorder. This is likely due to blocking the synthesis of anxiolytic neurosteroids in the brain.[18] Certain antibiotics, such as clarithromycin, can cause states of anxiety and mania, ostensibly due to antagonism of gamma amino butyric (GABA) activity.[19] Yohimbine, an alpha-2-receptor antagonist, is not prescribed but often purchased over the counter to treat erectile dysfunction. It is well known to precipitate panic states.[20]

The antidepressant bupropion has acquired a reputation for causing anxiety in some patients. However, there is not sufficient data to support describing it as anxiogenic.[21] Akathisia, a distressing sense of inner restlessness that resembles anxiety, can sometimes be provoked by antipsychotic medications, even when prescribed as augmentation for treatment of major depression or bipolar disorder.[22] Although rare, akathisia can also be provoked by certain antidepressants.[23]

It should be recognized that genetics can play a role in the development of anxiety disorders.[24] There is compelling evidence that certain types of anxiety disorders, including GAD, phobias, panic disorder, and simply "anxious temperament," run in families. It is not yet known which specific genes contribute to those disorders. Research has suggested that variations in genes coding for glutamic acid decarboxylase, the enzyme responsible for the synthesis of GABA from glutamate, and diazepam binding inhibitor, a protein that modulates GABA receptor activity, can affect risk for anxiety disorder. Links have also been made between anxiety and polymorphisms of genes affecting serotonergic and dopaminergic activities.[25] There are even suggestions that aberrations in mitochondrial DNA might predispose individuals to anxiety disorders and depression.[26] Curiously, none of the genes coding for GABA receptors have been strongly linked with any tendency toward anxiety disorder.[27] Although much remains to be determined, simply knowing that one can be biologically predisposed to anxiety can sometimes relieve the unnecessary but not uncommon sense of weakness and personal failure these disorders can cause.

REFERENCES

1. McCarty R. Chapter 4 — The fight-or-flight response: A cornerstone of stress research. In: G Fink (Ed.), *Stress: Concepts, Cognition, Emotion, and Behavior.* San Diego, CA: Academic Press; 2016. pp. 33–37.
2. LeDoux JE. Coming to terms with fear. *Proc Natl Acad Sci USA.* 2014;111:2871–2878.
3. Tovote P, Fadok JP, Lüthi A. Neuronal circuits for fear and anxiety. *Nat Rev Neurosci.* 2015;16:317–331.
4. Eaton WW, Bienvenu OJ, Miloyan B. Specific phobias. *Lancet Psychiat.* 2018;5(8): 678–686.
5. Agras WS, Chapin HN, Oliveau DC. The natural history of phobia: Course and prognosis. *Arch Gen Psychiatry.* 1972;26(4):315–317.

6. Stein MB, Stein DJ. Social anxiety disorder. *Lancet.* 2008;371(9618):1115–1125.
7. Arditte KA, Morabito DM, Shaw AM, et al. Interpersonal risk for suicide in social anxiety: The roles of shame and depression. *Psychiatry Res.* 2016;239:139–144.
8. Kessler RC, Wang PS. The descriptive epidemiology of commonly occurring mental disorders in the United States. *Annu Rev Public Health.* 2008;29:115–129.
9. Eaton WW, Kessler RC, Wittchen HU, et al. Panic and panic disorder in the United States. *Am J Psychiat.* 1994;151(3):413–420.
10. Wittchen H-U, Nocon A, Beesdo K, et al. Agoraphobia and Panic. *Psychother Psychosom.* 2008;77:147–157.
11. Brown TA, Campbell LA, Lehman CL, et al. Current and lifetime comorbidity of the DSM-IV anxiety and mood disorders in a large clinical sample. *J Abnorm Psychol.* 2001;110:585–599.
12. Shri R. Anxiety: Causes and management. *J Behav Sci.* 2010;5(1):100–118.
13. Crede RH, Kerr WJ. Pheochromocytoma: Report of a case with symptoms simulating acute anxiety attacks. *Postgrad Med.* 1952;11(4):288–293.
14. Tural U, Iosifescu DV. The prevalence of mitral valve prolapse in panic disorder: A meta-analysis. *Psychosomatics.* 2019;60(4):393–401.
15. Thoren CT, Petermann F. Reviewing asthma and anxiety. *Resp Med.* 2000;94:409–415.
16. Eisner MD, Blanc PD, Yelin EH, et al. Influence of anxiety on health outcomes in COPD. *Thorax.* 2010;65:229–234.
17. Amital D, Fostick L, Sasson Y, et al. Anxiogenic effects of sumatriptan in panic disorder: A double-blind, placebo-controlled study. *Eur Neuropsychopharmacol.* 2005;15(3):279–282.
18. Fertig R, Shapiro J, Bergfeld W, et al. Investigation of the plausibility of 5-alpha-reductase inhibitor syndrome. *Skin Appendage Disord.* 2016;2:120–129.
19. Ortiz-Dominguez A, Berlanga C, Gutierrez-Mora D. A case of clarithromycin-induced manic episode (antibiomania). *Int J Neuropsychopharmacol.* 2004;7:99–100.
20. Albus M, Zahn TP, Breier A. Anxiogenic properties of yohimbine. *Eur Arch Psychiatry Clin Neurosci.* 1992;241:337–344.
21. Wiseman CN. Does bupropion exacerbate anxiety? *Curr Psychiat.* 2012;11(6):E3–E4.
22. Blanchet P. Antipsychotic drug-induced movement disorders. *Can J Neurol Sci.* 2003;30(S1):S101–S107.
23. Lane RM. SSRI-induced extrapyramidal side-effects and akathisia: Implications for treatment. *J Psychopharmacol.* 1998;12:192–214.
24. Arnold PD, Zai G, Richter MA. Genetics of anxiety disorders. *Curr Psychiatry Rep.* 2004;6:243–254.
25. Lacerda-Pinheiro S-F, Pinheiro RFF, de Lima MAP, et al. Are there depression and anxiety genetic markers and mutations? A systematic review. *J Affec Disorders.* 2014;168:387–398.
26. Boles RG, Burnett BB, Gleditsch K, et al. A high predisposition to depression and anxiety in mothers and other matrilineal relatives of children with presumed maternally inherited mitochondrial disorders. *Neuropsych Gen.* 2005;137B(1):20–24.
27. Pham X, Sun C, Chen X, et al. Association study between GABA receptor genes and anxiety spectrum disorders. *Depress Anxiety.* 2009;26(11):998–1003.

2 Non-Pharmacological Treatments of Anxiety

Treatment for anxiety disorders includes medications, psychotherapy, and what are often referred to as "alternative" treatment methods, such as herbs, meditation, spiritual paths, yoga, breathing, exercise, dietary control, and a multitude of methods of lifestyle management and improvement. Ironically, while the later approaches may be seen as alternative or merely complimentary, they predate mainstream medical methods and have been relied upon for thousands of years as the products of shared human experiences. Indeed, there is basis to suggest that the modern medical models of medication and structured psychotherapy are themselves alternatives to more time-honored methods.

In-depth discussions of treatment of anxiety with medications and herbal preparations are given in the following chapters. The mechanisms of action of herbal treatments are simply the actions of the psychoactive phytochemicals they contain. Thus, discussions of the neurobiology of anxiety and the effects of anxiolytic medications set the stage for the in-depth coverage of herbal treatments of anxiety. First, however, it is worthwhile to discuss non-pharmacological approaches to the treatment of anxiety.

Psychotherapy is often referred to as talk therapy. However, that description trivializes this important form of treatment. A well-trained psychotherapist does far more than simply talk and listen, though those do form essential parts of therapy. The therapist's office should be the place where anything can be discussed without fear of judgment or ridicule. That in itself is healing. A good therapist also answers back to let the patient know they are being heard and understood. Feeling unheard and misunderstood is a common source of anguish, anxiety, and emotional pain. However, therapy is not all comfort and support. A skillful therapist will also encourage patients to explore the frightening, painful places they might not be willing to go on their own.

There are many different schools and styles of psychotherapy.[1] These include cognitive behavioral, Rogerian, gestalt, psychodynamic, rational-emotive, transactional analysis, and group therapy. Some explore childhood and the dynamics of old repressed feelings, whereas others focus on the here and now. All forms can be helpful. For example, a paper published in the *Journal of the American Psychiatric Association* showed that patients suffering from GAD responded equally well to two very different forms of psychotherapy: cognitive behavioral therapy and psychodynamic therapy.[2] Both cognitive behavioral therapy and psychodynamic therapy were also effective in treating social anxiety disorder, though there was a slight advantage seen with cognitive behavioral therapy.[3] Certain types of anxiety disorders—such as phobias or anxiety-ridden PTSD, in which the trigger is very specific—do tend to

DOI: 10.1201/9781003300281-2

respond well to specific types of psychotherapy, such as desensitization or flooding.[4] It is important to note that individual therapists—the way they interact and present themselves—may be even more important than the type of psychotherapy they perform.[5] Overall, studies suggest that treatment of anxiety disorders with various psychotherapeutic methods gives recovery rates of about 40%. Recovery is generally meant to be when an individual's complaints of anxiety and worry are no different than those of individuals without diagnoses of anxiety disorders.

Yoga has been a popular alternative method to treat anxiety and stress. Although sometimes dismissed as unscientific, the benefits of yoga have been demonstrated in clinical studies.[6] Yoga is also more comprehensive and wide ranging in technique than many people appreciate. Many recognize yoga as being only the challenging physical positions, called asanas, that stretch, strengthen, and relax the body. However, yoga also includes dietary, breathing, and meditation techniques that complement and enhance the more physical aspects. Some studies have suggested that while borrowing bits and pieces of yoga is helpful, it is not as effective as following the "yogic lifestyle" in its entirety. Nonetheless, the daily practice of asanas, even after a few weeks, has been shown to relieve anxiety and improve stress tolerance. This is particularly the case for those suffering physical complaints such as low-back pain or fibromyalgia. A recent study published in the journal *JAMA Psychiatry* found that Kundalini yoga relived anxiety in just over half of participants.[7] This was more effective than mere "stress education" but less effective than cognitive behavioral therapy. Of course, there is no reason why yoga cannot be combined with cognitive behavioral therapy.

Regulating one's breathing, through yogic or other techniques, can be a powerful method to relieve anxiety. Many Western therapists teach methods of slow, deep, abdominal breathing to relieve bouts of anxiety and panic. Daily practice of the more sophisticated yogic techniques of breath control, called pranayama, has been shown to improve anxiety and sense of well-being.[8] Interestingly, whereas some pranayama techniques are calming, others may be used to invigorate and strengthen the mind and body to build resistance to anxiety states.

Techniques to reach deep states of physical, emotional, and mental relaxation have also been used to relieve anxiety. One limb of yogic practice, yoga nidra, is devoted to the attainment of deep relaxation. Scientific studies have shown yoga nidra techniques to significantly alter brain waves, reduce blood pressure, and even alter measurements of blood chemistry, such as cholesterol and stress hormones in patients with heart diseases.[9] The Western technique of progressive relaxation,[10] first formalized in 1908 by Edmund Jacobson, guides the practitioner to tense then release parts of the body, step by step, until the entire body has been felt to alternately tighten and relax. This allows the individual to feel, by contrast, the impact of the state of full relaxation. This technique of progressive relaxation was expanded upon by American cardiologist Herbert Benson to include meditative and spiritual aspects such as prayer. The therapeutic methods of F. Matthias Alexander and Moshe Feldenkrais— the Alexander Technique[11] and Awareness Through Movement,[12] respectively—also bring awareness to unnecessary tension in movement and the way one uses one's body. The result is reduction of tension, stress, anxiety, and pain and improvement in body function and performance.

Studies have shown that physical exercise can be helpful to reduce panic disorder, GAD, and social anxiety.[13] It has been suggested that exercise helps by enhancing one's sense of self-reliance and personal strength, by distracting from thinking and worrying, and likely by changing certain aspects of brain chemistry. It has also been found that regular, strenuous exercise dampens overactivity of the sympathetic nervous system that mediates the fight-or-flight response. It is known, for example, that physically well-conditioned people have lower resting heart rates and lower blood pressures than sedentary individuals. Surprisingly, some studies have shown that the most strenuous forms of exercise—aerobic exercise, in which heart and respiratory rates increase for minutes at a time—may have no significant advantage over milder forms, such as simply going for a walk every day.

Many forms of meditation, both spiritual and secular, have been found to help relieve anxiety and stress. Meditation has often been described as "letting the mind go," then experiencing what it does without guidance, judgment, or restraint. This is often referred to as mindfulness.[14] Mindfulness-based meditation techniques have been shown to be at least as effective as standard stress management education methods in reducing symptoms of anxiety. Giving up control can be anxiety provoking, but learning that it is safe to do so can bring peace and release from anxiety. Allowing thoughts to go where they will can also help a person learn that thoughts once feared are harmless and without consequence. When embedded in a religious tradition, such as Buddhism, this experience of the peaceful mind is seen as experiencing the true nature of man and God. On the other hand, some forms of meditation, such as meditative prayer, may aim to focus the mind on God, love, mercy, or light to free the mind of trivial, painful, or anxiety-provoking thoughts. Honest, soul-searching prayer offers a similar relief from anxiety and a sense of belonging in the universe. Some forms of meditation allow people to lose themselves in purposeful action, eliminating unnecessary, interfering thoughts and extraneous body movements and tensions. The Japanese tea ceremony, tai chi, walking Zen meditation, Feldenkrais movement, or even the feel of the "perfect golf swing" can provide such sense of freedom, completeness, unity, and relief from anxiety and stress.

REFERENCES

1. Smith ML, Glass GV. Meta-analysis of psychotherapy outcome studies. *Am Psychol.* 1977;32(9):752–760.
2. Leichsenring F, Salzer S, Jaeger U, et al. Short-term psychodynamic psychotherapy and cognitive-behavioral therapy in generalized anxiety disorder: A randomized, controlled trial. *Am J Psychiat.* 2009;166:875–881.
3. Leichsenring F, Salzer S, Beutel ME, et al. Psychodynamic therapy and cognitive-behavioral therapy in social anxiety disorder: A multicenter randomized controlled trial. *Am J Psychiatry.* 2013;170:1–9.
4. Hussain MZ. Desensitization and flooding (implosion) in treatment of phobias. *Am J Psychiat.* 1971;127:1509–1514.
5. Blow AJ, Sprenkle DH, Davis SD. Is who delivers the treatment more important than the treatment itself? The role of the therapist in common factors. *J Mar Fam Ther.* 2007;33(3):298–317.
6. Gupta N, Shveta K, Vempati R, et al. Effect of yoga based lifestyle intervention on state and trail anxiety. *Indian J Physiol Pharmacol.* 2006;50:41–47.

7. Simon NM, Hofmann SG, Rosenfield D, et al. Efficacy of yoga vs cognitive behavioral therapy vs stress education for the treatment of generalized anxiety disorder: A randomized clinical trial. *JAMA Psychiat.* 2021;78(1):13–20.

8. Novaes MM, Palhano-Fontes F, Onias H, et al. Effects of yoga respiratory practice (Bhastrika pranayama) on anxiety, affect, and brain functional connectivity and activity: A randomized controlled trial. *Front Psychiat.* 2020;11:467.

9. Kumar K. A study on the impact on stress and anxiety through yoga Nidra. *Indian J Tradit Know.* 2008;7(3):401–404.

10. Bernstein DA, Carlson CR. Progressive relaxation: Abbreviated methods. In: P Lehrer, RL Woolfolk (Eds.), *Principles and Practice of Stress Management.* New York: Guilford Press; 1993. pp. 53–85.

11. Gelb M. *Body Learning: The Alexander Technique.* New York: Delilah Books; 1981.

12. Feldenkrais M. *Awareness Through Movement.* New York: Harper & Row, 1972.

13. Petruzzello SJ, Landers DM, Hatfield BD, et al. A meta-analysis on the anxiety-reducing effects of acute and chronic exercise. *Sports Med.* 1991;11:143–182.

14. Krisanaprakornkit T, Sriraj W, Piyavhatkul N, et al. Meditation therapy for anxiety disorders. *Cochrane DB Syst Rev.* 2006; (1). Art. No.: CD004998. DOI: 10.1002/14651858. CD004998.pub2.

3 The Neurobiology of Anxiety

Fear, the fight-or-flight response, and anticipatory anxiety to prepare for future threats are life-preserving activities of the central nervous system. They are evolutionarily ancient and deeply rooted in the mammalian brain. These responses can be initiated by activity in multiple neural pathways and are mediated by a variety of neurotransmitter systems. It has only recently become evident that persisting pathophysiological states, such as stress, inflammation, metabolic disturbance, and failures of cell maintenance, also contribute to anxiety disorders. To understand the pharmacological and, in turn, herbal treatment of anxiety, it is necessary to review its neurobiology.

3.1 BRAIN CIRCUITRY OF ANXIETY

The limbic system of the brain is largely responsible for generating the emotions experienced as anxiety. The limbic system is also responsible for laying down and retrieving memories, as well as comparing the current state with previous situations, which lends it to participating in anticipatory and reactive anxieties. The notion of the limbic system has grown over time, and there has yet to be universal agreement on which structures in the brain constitute the system. Nonetheless, a common list of limbic system structures includes the cingulate and parahippocampal gyri, hippocampus, amygdala, septum, and hypothalamus.[1] These ancient brain structures interact with the phylogenetically newer neocortical executive areas of the frontal cortex. The prefrontal, orbitofrontal, and ventromedial areas of the frontal cortex process and regulate the emotional responses of the limbic system through inhibitory, so-called top-down control. It is thought that overactivity of limbic areas and loss of inhibitory control by the executive areas of the brain result in various affective disorders, including the anxiety disorders and major depression.[2]

Overactivity of the amygdala is a hallmark of anxiety disorders. However, fMRI studies have shown various abnormalities in the neural circuitry including the amygdala, hippocampal and parahippocampal gyri, posterior insula, dorsal anterior cingulate cortex, ventrolateral prefrontal cortex, and temporal gyrus.[3] For example, when compared with their age-matched counterpart groups, anxious adults exhibited reduced activation in the ventromedial prefrontal cortex when appraising threat, which suggests disinhibition of the amygdala and other parts of the limbic system.[4] Another fMRI study similarly showed diminished ability of the ventromedial prefrontal cortex to inhibit activity in the amygdala in "clinically anxious" individuals.[5]

DOI: 10.1201/9781003300281-3

3.2 NEUROCHEMISTRY

The activities in the pathways of the brain that mediate anxiety are in turn mediated and modified by the interplay of a wide variety of neurochemicals. Gamma amino butyric acid and its various allosteric regulators, such as neurosteroids, play important roles in mediating anxiety and fear. Also involved are glutamate, serotonin, norepinephrine, dopamine; acetylcholine, endocannabinoids, endorphins, histamine, and glycine. Various neuropeptides, including cholecystokinin, galanin, neuropeptide Y, vasopressin, oxytocin, and corticotropin-releasing factor, interact with neurotransmitters to further modulate the anxiety and fear responses.[6]

3.2.1 GAMMA AMINO BUTYRIC ACID

Gamma amino butyric acid, commonly abbreviated as GABA, is the primary inhibitory neurotransmitter in the mammalian brain. It is ubiquitous in distribution, and it is thought to act in up to half of all synapses in the central nervous system.[7] GABA receptors are widely distributed in the mammalian brain and are found in high concentrations in areas of the brain that process fear and anxiety, including the cerebral cortex, hippocampus, amygdala, and other parts of the limbic system.[8]

Changes in overall GABAergic activity produce concomitant changes in anxiety and fear-like behaviors in mammals. Thus, infusions of GABA or GABA receptor agonists into the amygdala decrease fear- and anxiety-like behaviors, whereas depletion of GABA or infusions of GABA antagonists generate such behaviors.[9–11]

There are two main subtypes of GABA receptors in the brain, GABA-A and GABA-B.[12] Anxiolytic effects are attributed to activation of either type of GABA receptor. However, enhancement of activity at the GABA-A receptor is the mechanism of action of many anxiolytic medications. In addition, subtypes of GABA-A receptor contribute somewhat differently to the overall effect of increasing GABAergic activity. Indeed, it has been suggested that there may be 100 or more different GABA-A receptor subtypes.[13] Nonetheless, a simplified categorization is made by identifying GABA-A receptors that carry certain alpha subunits numbered 1 through 6.[14] Benzodiazepines, as a class, bind to GABA-A types 1, 2, 3, and 5 but not to types 4 or 6. More selective medications, such as zolpidem and eszopiclone, help induce sleep by selective activation of the GABA-A1 receptor.[15] On the other hand, they are less able to relieve anxiety, relax muscles, or counteract alcohol withdrawal than more fully acting benzodiazepines. The role of each subtype of GABA-A receptors in the experience of anxiety remains to be elucidated. It is safe to say that one of the holy grails of psychopharmacology is to find a benzodiazepine-like substance selective for certain subtypes of GABA-A receptors that relieves anxiety without undue sedation or risk of addiction.

Finally, the GABA-A receptor is large and complicated enough to be referred to as the GABA receptor complex. Aside from responding to GABA itself, these receptors have distinct binding sites for a variety of different ligands. Those ligands include the aforementioned benzodiazepines, as well as barbiturates, ethanol, anticonvulsants, muscimol, bicuculline, and various volatile general anesthetics.[16] Thus, many and differing molecules, including phytochemicals of various types, are able to interact with the GABA-A receptor complex to enhance or, on their own, produce anxiolytic effects.

Neurosteroids, including cortisone, allopregnanolone, pregnanolone, allopregnanolone, pregnenolone, and dehydroepiandrosterone, are important in acute and chronic anxiety. Steroid actions as manifestations of activity of the hypothalamic-pituitary-adrenal axis are often long term in nature and intended to allow adaptation to persistent challenges to the organism—that is, persistent stress. In this adaptive role, steroids have broad effects upon neurotransmitter systems in the brain, such as modulating synthesis of neurotransmitters and altering densities of receptors for those neurotransmitters in the brain.[17] However, acute effects of neurosteroids, which can either diminish or enhance anxiety, are mediated by the rapid action of neurosteroids directly on GABA-A receptors and glutamate receptors.[18] As discussed later, many plants produce terpenes with steroid-like structures that are likely to have both acute and chronic effects.

3.2.2 GLUTAMATE

Glutamate is the primary excitatory neurotransmitter in the brain. Like GABA, glutamate acts upon a wide variety of receptors, both ionotropic and metabotropic. Glutamate receptors are found in abundance in many of the areas of the brain known to process emotional responses, including fear and anxiety. Those areas include the amygdala, hippocampus, anterior cingulate cortex, orbitofrontal cortex, medial prefrontal cortex, and insular cortex. All those areas are richly innervated by glutamatergic neurons.[19]

In keeping with its role as an excitatory neurotransmitter, there may be glutamate-driven overactivity of certain neural circuits that mediate anxiety. For example, 1H-MRI studies have found increases in glutamate in the frontal cortex of healthy subjects with high versus low state-trait anxiety.[20] Similar studies have found increased glutamatergic activity in the anterior cingulate in individuals suffering social anxiety disorder.[21] Abnormally high levels of glutamate have also been found in the rostral anterior cingulate cortex of individuals suffering social phobia when shown frightening photographs.[22]

3.2.3 MONOAMINES

Serotonin is well known to play a role in anxiety. Indeed, in certain animal models, serotonergic drugs can be as effective as benzodiazepines in relieving anxiety-like behaviors. However, the role serotonin plays in anxiety is not as simple as is often suggested. Serotonin appears able to either increase or reduce anxiety, depending on where in the brain and upon which subtypes of serotonin receptors it is acting.[23] Similarly, while major depression is often described as a syndrome of depleted serotonin, both agonists and antagonists of serotonin can be used to treat that illness.[24]

The monoamine neurotransmitter norepinephrine also plays a role in mediating anxiety and fear responses. However, like serotonin, it can have either anxiogenic or anxiolytic effects, depending on whether a stressor is acute or chronic, whether it is predictable or unpredictable, and where in the brain the norepinephrine is acting.[25]

The third major monoamine neurotransmitter in the brain, dopamine, is also important in anxiety disorders. For example, it has been found that individuals with higher baseline levels of dopamine release in the amygdala and rostral anterior cingulate cortex tend to self-report lower degrees of trait anxiety.[26] On the other hand, animal studies suggest that certain types of dopaminergic activity, for example activation of the dopamine type 3 receptor, may enhance anxiety-like behavior.[27] Thus, it is clear that the effects of the monoamine neurotransmitters on anxiety are complex and multifaceted.

3.2.4 ACETYLCHOLINE

Acetylcholine is yet another central neurotransmitter with a significant role in the manifestation of anxiety. Some of the effects of acetylcholine may depend on the chronicity of stress, which subtypes of acetylcholine receptors are activated, and in which areas of the brain. The role played by nicotinic receptors is evident in the vast number of people who self-medicate symptoms of anxiety by inhaling cigarette smoke laden with nicotine.[28] Injection of either nicotinic or muscarinic antagonists into the dorsal hippocampi of mice produces anxiety-like behaviors.[29] On the other hand, activation of muscarinic receptors in the ventral hippocampus of chronically stressed mice also produces anxiety-like behavior.[30]

3.2.5 ENDOCANNABINOIDS

The limbic system is richly supplied with both endocannabinoids and cannabinoid receptors.[31] Thus, there is a basis for endocannabinoid participation in anxiety disorders. In animal studies, injection of cannabinoid agonists into the central gray inhibits panic-like behavior.[32] Although many individuals use cannabis to relax, a quite common response to cannabis intoxication is anxiety and panic.[33] Studies have shown high blood levels of endocannabinoids in patients with panic disorder compared to healthy controls.[34] However, it is not clear if this increase is a cause or an effect.

Despite evidence that cannabis can cause anxiety or panic, there is seemingly paradoxical evidence that blocking cannabis receptor with the cannabinoid antagonist rimonabant can precipitate severe anxiety. In fact, rimonabant was blocked from being marketed as a weight loss drug in the United States because of its severe psychiatric side effects.[35] Apparently, either over- or understimulation of cannabinoid receptors in the brain can disturb mood.

3.2.6 ENDORPHINS

Endorphins and the various receptors that mediate their effects are found throughout the mammalian limbic system.[36] Endorphins have substantial effects on mood, including anxiety and fear responses.[37] It has been suggested that increases in endorphin activity mediate some of the anxiolytic and mood-elevating effects of strenuous exercise.[38] It is known that many fall into opioid addiction out of a desire to self-medicate anxiety,[39] and the anxiety and general distress suffered by those experiencing opioid withdrawal is well known.[40] Blockade of endorphin activity may also exacerbate panic in otherwise normal individuals.[41]

3.2.7 HISTAMINE

The minor neurotransmitter histamine plays a role in anxiety. Animal studies have suggested that histamine may have differential effects on anxiety depending on which subtypes of histamine receptors are activated.[42] However, overall reduction of histamine levels in the brain may increase anxiety-like behavior.[43] Histamine also plays an important role in the regulation of sleep and wakefulness, which can be disturbed in anxiety disorders.[44]

3.2.8 GLYCINE

Glycine, a minor inhibitory neurotransmitter not generally thought of as being involved in affective disorders, may play role in anxiety. Blocking the glycine receptor is anxiogenic, and stimulating the receptor can help relieve anxiety, at least in animal models. Of importance in the current context, there are many phytochemicals that act at glycine receptors. Strychnine, a glycine antagonist extracted from *Nux vomica*, is perhaps the best-known example. A recent paper showed that methanolic extract of *Pericarpium zanthoxyli* stimulates the glycine receptor with anxiolytic effects.[45]

3.3 STRESS

Stress is any condition in which the body must adapt to threat. The neural circuitry within the brain that determines what is threatening includes the hippocampus, amygdala, and areas of the prefrontal cortex.[46] Thus, the stress response shares some of the same circuitry that is involved in the experience of anxiety. However, while anxiety is the affective experience endured, the stress response is the physiological process that enables the body to meet the challenge that is threatening and anxiety provoking. The acute stress response involves activation of the hypothalamic-pituitary-adrenal axis, resulting in stimulation of the sympathetic nervous system and release of adrenalin from the adrenal glands. The response also includes release of cortisol from the adrenal cortex, though this is cut short by negative feedback mechanisms. Beyond the fight-or-flight response to acute stress, there are events in daily life that produce a type of chronic stress and lead over time to wear and tear on the body that has been referred to allostatic load.[47]

Chronic stress results in changes in the brain, including hypertrophy and hyperexcitability of the amygdala[48] and dendritic shortening in neurons in the medial prefrontal cortex.[49] Each of those effects would be expected to exacerbate anxiety disorders. Chronic stress, with the persistent release of cortisol, also leads to impairment of the feedback system that protects against overactivation of the hypothalamic-pituitary-adrenal axis, thus perpetuating the problem.[50] Chronic stress attenuates the effectiveness of GABA in the hypothalamus[51] and amygdala, thus contributing to hyperactivity.[52] In the prefrontal cortex, GABAergic activity may be enhanced, thus reducing the ability of that area to control the runaway limbic system that can occur in anxiety disorders.[53] Along with GABA, chronic stress also adversely affects serotonergic, noradrenergic, and dopaminergic activity.[54]

3.4 INFLAMMATION

Aulus Cornelius Celsus's famous tetrad of inflammation—*calor* (warmth), *dolor* (pain), *tumor* (swelling), and *rubor* (redness)—remains valid 2,000 years after he described them. What has changed in our modern understanding is that inflammation is seen as a process propagated by cells and mediated by a variety of chemical messengers referred to as cytokines. These various chemical mediators of inflammation, whether produced in the brain itself or taken up by the brain from the bloodstream, can have effects on neural activity and, in turn, on affective disorders.[55] Indeed, there is evidence that cytokines can have neuromodulatory functions in neurons and glia that are different from those induced by these same chemicals in leukocytes during the inflammatory response to infection.[56] For example, the concerted actions of the inflammatory cytokines, interleukin 1β, tumor necrosis factor, interleukin 6, complement and prostaglandins, can alter the sensitivity of central GABA and glutamate receptors and decrease seizure threshold.[57] Yet another study has shown that interleukin 1β antagonizes GABAergic activity in cultured hippocampal cells.[58] Those effects would tend to exacerbate anxiety.

In some studies, increased concentrations of inflammatory signals, including tumor necrosis factor, interleukin 1β, interleukin 6, and C-reactive protein, have been found in blood samples of sufferers of GAD, panic disorder, agoraphobia, social phobia, and posttraumatic stress disorder.[59] Emotional stress can initiate the inflammatory cascade, as can oxidative stress and disorders of energy metabolism, such as metabolic syndrome. Persisting states of inflammation can then exacerbate those original pathophysiologies.[60] Breaking these self-perpetuating cycles can be an essential step in treating chronic affective disorders.

3.5 METABOLIC SYNDROME

Inflammation and stress can all alter brain activity and predispose people to affective disorders, including anxiety. Insulin resistance, and the damage and metabolic aberrations it generates in the brain and periphery, also predisposes sufferers of anxiety and stress to anxiety. The brain is not dependent on insulin to utilize glucose. Nonetheless, insulin plays many important roles in brain physiology. Mice deprived of insulin's central nervous system effects through a brain-specific knockout of the insulin receptor show a number of abnormalities including aberrant monoamine oxidase expression and increased dopamine turnover in the mesolimbic system. These animals also exhibit increases in anxiety-like behaviors.[61]

While inflammation, stress, and insulin resistance can occur independently of each other, the occurrence of one tends to induce and exacerbate the others. All three states occur in an overarching condition known as metabolic syndrome. The defining diagnostic signs of metabolic syndrome include hypertension, hypertriglyceridemia, low HDL, and high fasting glucose. However, metabolic syndrome also includes insulin resistance and increases in visceral fat. Visceral fat is a source of inflammatory cytokines, as well as chemical messengers that feed back to the brain and form a part of the so-called gut-brain axis.

In the context of metabolic syndrome, stress, inflammation, and insulin resistance combine to cause a cascade of downstream neural damage and aberrant function. Among those abnormalities are oxidative and nitrosative damage, abnormalities in neurotransmitter metabolism, mitochondrial dysfunction, and disturbances of cellular "housekeeping" processes, such as maintenance of normal levels of brain-derived neurotrophic factor and other such growth factors.[62]

In animal studies, genetic vulnerability to oxidative stress is associated with increased anxiety-like behaviors. Oxidative and nitrosative damage to the lipid-rich cell membranes of neurons results in decreases in membrane fluidity and damage membrane proteins that results in inactivation of receptors, enzymes, and ion channels. This in turn alters neurotransmission, neuronal function, and overall brain activity.[63] Oxidative stress also leads to diminished production of brain-derived neurotrophic factor (BDNF). For example, in human subjects suffering episodes of bipolar mania, blood levels of products of lipid peroxidation were in inverse correlation with levels of BDNF.[64] Decreased levels of BDNF are associated with anxiety as well as mood disorders.[65]

Mitochondria are both targets of stress and mediators of stress pathophysiology, including in the context of metabolic syndrome. Chronic stress manifests as decreased mitochondrial energy production capacity and altered mitochondrial morphology. Mitochondria in the brain lose mtDNA involved in maintaining proteins in the electron transport chain.[66] Abnormalities in mitochondrial function have been specifically linked to anxiety disorders. For example, anxiolytic neurosteroids that enhance GABAergic activity are produced in mitochondria. The outer mitochondrial translocator protein (TSPO) controls transport of cholesterol into the mitochondria to be turned into various neurosteroids. A defective polymorphism of the TSPO gene has been associated with anxiety-like disorders, likely by reducing rates of anxiolytic neurosteroid production.[67]

3.6 SUMMARY

Fear is a normal response to threats from the environment, and anxiety is a normal anticipation of and preparation for similar threats in the future. These responses are mediated by the limbic system, particularly the amygdala. Many neurochemical systems are involved in processing fear and anxiety responses, with GABA and glutamate being the most important. The monoamines, acetylcholine, histamine, glycine, endocannabinoids, and endorphins are also involved. There are also a variety of neurochemicals, including neurosteroids, that modulate activity at the GABA receptor complex. Anxiety disorders arise from the escape of components of the limbic system from executive control by the prefrontal cortex. Enhancing or diminishing activity in the neurotransmitter systems noted previously can alleviate or exacerbate anxiety. Although acute changes in neurotransmitter activity can alter anxiety responses, there are chronic conditions, such as stress, inflammation, and metabolic disturbances, that contribute to persistent states of anxiety. Thus, the most reasonable approach to pharmacological or herbal treatment of anxiety disorders is to provide acute relief from anxiety, as well as to correct the ongoing, chronic abnormalities that help perpetuate pathological anxiety.

REFERENCES

1. Rajmohan V, Mohandas E. The limbic system. *Indian J Psychiat.* 2007;49(2):132–139.
2. Martin EI, Ressler KJ, Binder E, et al. The neurobiology of anxiety disorders: Brain imaging, genetics, and psychoneuroendocrinology. *Psychiatr Clin North Am.* 2009;32(3):549–575.
3. Liao W, Qiu C, Gentili C, et al. Altered effective connectivity network of the amygdala in social anxiety disorder: A resting-state FMRI study. *PLoS One.* 2010;5(12):e15238.
4. Britton JC, Grillon C, Lissek S, et al. Response to learned threat: An fMRI study in adolescent and adult anxiety. *Am J Psychiat.* 2013;170:1195–1204.
5. Cha J, DeDora D, Nedic S, et al. Clinically anxious individuals show disrupted feedback between inferior frontal gyrus and prefrontal-limbic control circuit. *J Neurosci.* 2016;36(17):4708–4718.
6. Martin EI, Ressler KJ, Binder E, et al. The neurobiology of anxiety disorders: Brain imaging, genetics, and psychoneuroendocrinology. *Psychiatr Clin North Am.* 2009 Sep;32(3):549–575.
7. Young AB, Chu D. Distribution of GABA-A, and GABA-B, receptors in mammalian brain: Potential targets for drug development. *Drug Develop Res.* 1990;21:161–167.
8. Esmaeili A, Lynch JW, Sah P. GABAA receptors containing gammal subunits contribute to inhibitory transmission in the central amygdala. *J Neurophysiol.* 2009;101:341–349.
9. Sanders SK, Shekhar A. Regulation of anxiety by GABAA receptors in the rat amygdala. *Pharmacol Biochem Behav.* 1995;52(4):701–706.
10. Barbalho CA, Nunes-de-Souza RL, Canto-de-Souza A. Similar anxiolytic-like effects following intra-amygdala infusions of benzodiazepine receptor agonist and antagonist: Evidence for the release of an endogenous benzodiazepine inverse agonist in mice exposed to elevated plus-maze test. *Brain Res.* 2009;1267:65–76.
11. Heldt SA, Mou L, Ressler KJ. In vivo knockdown of GAD67 in the amygdala disrupts fear extinction and the anxiolytic-like effect of diazepam in mice. *Transl Psychiat.* 2012;2:e181.
12. Kardos J. Recent advances in GABA research. *Neurochem Int.* 1999;34(5):353–358.
13. Sieghart W, Sperk G. Subunit composition, distribution and function of GABAA receptors. *Curr Top Med Chem.* 2002;2:795–816.
14. Sigel E. Mapping of the benzodiazepine recognition site on GABA(A) receptors. *Curr Top Med Chem.* 2002;2(8):833–839.
15. Che Has AT, Absalom N, van Nieuwenhuijzen PS, et al. Zolpidem is a potent stoichiometry-selective modulator of $\alpha 1\beta 3$ GABAA receptors: Evidence of a novel benzodiazepine site in the $\alpha 1$-$\alpha 1$ interface. *Sci Rep.* 2016;6:28674.
16. Brambilla P, Perez J, Barale F, et al. GABAergic dysfunction in mood disorders. *Mol Psychiatr.* 2003;8:721–737.
17. McEwen BS. The brain on stress: Toward an integrative approach to brain, body and behaviour. *Perspect Psychol Sci.* 2013;8:673–675.
18. Mòdol L, Darbra S, Pallarès M. Neurosteroids infusion into the CA1 hippocampal region on exploration, anxiety-like behaviour and aversive learning. *Behav Brain Res.* 2011;222:223–229.
19. Cortese BM, Phan KL. The role of glutamate in anxiety and related disorders. *CNS Spectr.* 2005;10:820–830.

20. Grachev ID, Apkarian AV. Chemical mapping of anxiety in the brain of healthy humans: An in vivo 1H-MRS study on the effects of sex, age, and brain region. *Hum Brain Mapp.* 2000;11:261–272.

21. Phan KL, Fitzgerald DA, Cortese BM, et al. Anterior cingulate neurochemistry in social anxiety disorder: 1H-MRS at 4 Tesla. *Neuroreport.* 2005;16:183–186.

22. Phan KL, Fitzgerald DA, Cortese BM, et al. Response to emotionally salient faces and glutamate concentrations in the rostral anterior cingulate cortex in social phobia: Preliminary combined spectroscopic and functional magnetic resonance imaging studies at 4 Telsa. *Neuropsychopharmacology.* 2004;29:S193.

23. Graeff FG, On serotonin and experimental anxiety. *Psychopharmacology.* 2002; 163:467–476.

24. Carr GV, Lucki I. The role of serotonin receptor subtypes in treating depression: A review of animal studies. *Psychopharmacology.* 2011;213:265–287.

25. Goddard AW, Ball SG, Martinez J, et al. Current perspectives of the roles of the central norepinephrine system in anxiety and depression. *Depress Anxiety.* 2010;27:339–350.

26. Berry AS, White RL, Furman DJ, et al. Dopaminergic mechanisms underlying normal variation in trait anxiety. *J Neurosci.* 2019;39(14):2735–2744.

27. Steiner H, Fuchs S, Accili D. D3 dopamine receptor-deficient mouse: Evidence for reduced anxiety. *Physiol Behav.* 1997;63(1):137–141.

28. Picciotto MR, Lewis AS, van Schalkwyk GI, et al. Mood and anxiety regulation by nicotinic acetylcholine receptors: A potential pathway to modulate aggression and related behavioral states. *Neuropharmacology.* 2015;96:235–243.

29. File SE, Gonzalez LE, Andrews N. Endogenous acetylcholine in the dorsal hippocampus reduces anxiety through actions on nicotinic and muscarinic$_1$ receptors. *Behav Neurosci.* 1998;112(2):352–359.

30. Mei L, Zhou Y, Sun Y, et al. Acetylcholine muscarinic receptors in ventral Hippocampus Modulate stress-induced anxiety-like behaviors in mice. *Front Mol Neurosci.* 2020;13:1–12.

31. Heinbockel T, Wang ZJ, Brown EA, et al. Endocannabinoid signaling in neural circuits of the olfactory and limbic system. In R Meccariello, R Chianese (Eds.), *Cannabinoids in Health and Disease.* Rijeka: InTech Publisher; 2016. pp. 11–37.

32. Batista LA, Bastos JR, Moreira FA. Role of endocannabinoid signaling in the dorsolateral periaqueductal grey in the modulation of distinct panic-like responses. *J Psychopharmacol.* 2015;29:335–343.

33. Crippa JA, Zuardi AW, Martín-Santos R. Cannabis and anxiety: A critical review of the evidence. *Hum Psychopharm Clin.* 2009;24(7):515–523.

34. Petrowski K, Kirschbaum C, Gao W. Blood endocannabinoid levels in patients with panic disorder. *Psychoneuroendocrinology.* 2020;122:104905.

35. Mitchell PB, Morris MJ. Depression and anxiety with rimonabant. *Lancet.* 2007;370(9600):1671–1672.

36. Gackenheimer SL, Suter TM, Pintar JE, et al. Localization of opioid receptor antagonist [3H]-LY255582 binding sites in mouse brain: Comparison with the distribution of mu, delta and kappa binding sites. *Neuropeptides.* 2005;39(6):559–567.

37. Bodnar RJ, Klein GE. Endogenous opiates and behavior: 2004. *Peptides.* 2005;26, 2629–2711.

38. Anderson E, Shivakumar G. Effects of exercise and physical activity on anxiety. *Front Psychiat.* 2013;4:27.

39. Lejueza CW, Paulsona A, Daughters SB, et al. The association between heroin use and anxiety sensitivity among inner-city individuals in residential drug use treatment. *Behav Res Ther.* 2006;44(5):667–677.

40. Howe RC, Hegge FW, Phillips JL. Acute heroin abstinence in man: I. Changes in behavior and sleep. *Drug Alcohol Depend.* 1980;5(5):341–356.
41. Esquivel G, Fernández-Torre O, Schruers KRJ. The effects of opioid receptor blockade on experimental panic provocation with CO 2. *J Psychopharmacol.* 2009;23:975–978.
42. Yuzurihara M, Ikarashi Y, Ishige A. Effects of drugs acting as histamine releasers or histamine receptor blockers on an experimental anxiety model in mice. *Pharmacol Biochem Behav.* 2000;67(1):145–150.
43. Yoshikawa T, Nakamura T, Shibakusa T, et al. Insufficient intake of L-histidine reduces brain histamine and causes anxiety-like behaviors in male mice. *J Nutrit.* 2014;144(10):1637–1641.
44. Thakkar MM. Histamine in the regulation of wakefulness. *Sleep Med Rev.* 2001;15(1):65–74.
45. Kim TE, Jung JH, Yoon S, et al. Antianxiety effect of methanol extract of *Pericarpium zanthoxyli* using a strychnine-sensitive glycine receptor model. *Trop J Pharm Res.* 2016;15:951–957.
46. McEwen BS. Physiology and neurobiology of stress and adaptation: Central role of the brain. *Physiol Rev.* 2007;87(3):873–904.
47. McEwen BS, Eiland L, Hunter RG, et al. Stress and anxiety: Structural plasticity and epigenetic regulation as a consequence of stress. *Neuropharmacol.* 2012;62(1):3–12.
48. Rosenkranz JA, Venheim ER, Padival M. Chronic stress causes amygdala hyperexcitability in rodents. *Biol Psychiat.* 2010;67(12):1128–1136.
49. Wellman CL. Dendritic reorganization in pyramidal neurons in medial prefrontal cortex after chronic corticosterone administration. *J Neurobiol.* 2001;49(3):245–253.
50. McEwen BS. Plasticity of the hippocampus: Adaptation to chronic stress and allostatic load. *Ann NY Acad Sci.* 2001;933(1):265–277.
51. Verkuyl JM, Hemby SE, Joëls M. Chronic stress attenuates GABAergic inhibition and alters gene expression of parvocellular neurons in rat hypothalamus. *EJN.* 2004;20(6):1665–1673.
52. Liu Z-P, Song C, Wang M, et al. Chronic stress impairs GABAergic control of amygdala through suppressing the tonic GABAA receptor currents. *Mol Brain.* 2014;7:32.
53. McKlveen JM, Morano RL, Fitzgerald M, et al. Chronic stress increases prefrontal inhibition: A mechanism for stress-induced prefrontal dysfunction. *Biol Psychiat.* 2016;80(10):754–764.
54. Favoretto CA, Nunes YC, Macedo GC, et al. Chronic social defeat stress: Impacts on ethanol-induced stimulation, corticosterone response and brain monoamine levels. *J Psychopharmacol.* 2020;34:412–419.
55. Majda M, Saunders EFH, Engeland CG. Inflammation and the dimensions of depression: A review. *Front Neuroendocrinol.* 2019;56:100800.
56. Wilcox KS, Vezzani A. Does brain inflammation mediate pathological outcomes in epilepsy? *Adv Exp Med Biol.* 2014;813:169–183.
57. Vezzani A, Maroso M, Balosso S. Review IL-1 receptor/Toll-like receptor signaling in infection, inflammation, stress and neurodegeneration couples hyperexcitability and seizures. *Brain Behav Immun.* 2011;25(7):1281–1289.
58. Wang S, Cheng Q, Malik S, Yang J. Interleukin-1β inhibits gamma-aminobutyric acid type A (GABA(A)) receptor current in cultured hippocampal neurons. *J Pharmacol Exp Ther.* 2000;292(2):497–504.
59. Michopoulos V, Powers A, Gillespie CF, et al. Inflammation in fear- and anxiety-based disorders: PTSD, GAD, and beyond. *Neuropsychopharmacol.* 2017;42:254–270.
60. Mendelson SD. *Metabolic Syndrome and Psychiatric Illness: Interactions, Pathophysiology, Assessment and Treatment.* London, UK: Academic Press; 2008.

61. Kleinridders A, Cai W, Cappellucci L, et al. Insulin resistance in brain alters dopamine turnover and causes behavioral disorders. *PNAS*. 2015;112(11):3463–3468.

62. Mendelson SD. *Herbal Treatment of Major Depression: Scientific Basis and Practical Use*. CRC Press; 2020. pp. 19–30.

63. Bouayed J, Rammal H, Soulimani R. Oxidative stress and anxiety: Relationship and cellular pathways. *Oxid Med Cell Longev*. 2009;2(2):63–67.

64. Kapczinski F, Frey BN, Andreazza A, et al. Increased oxidative stress as a mechanism for decreased BDNF levels in acute manic episodes. *Rev Bras Psiquiatr*.2008;30:243–245.

65. Martinowich K, Manji H, Lu B. New insights into BDNF function in depression and anxiety. *Nature Neurosci*. 2007;10:1089–1093.

66. Picard M, McEwen BS. Psychological stress and mitochondria: A systematic review. *Psychosom Med*. 2018;80(2):141–153.

67. Da Pozzo E, Costa B, Martini C. Translocator protein (TSPO) and neurosteroids: Implications in psychiatric disorders. *Curr Mol Med*. 2012;12:426–442.

4 Medications Commonly Used to Treat Anxiety

Even psychiatrists who regularly prescribe psychoactive medications would not disagree with the growing notion that non-pharmacological treatment is the best initial treatment of anxiety disorders. However, while some patients may benefit from psychotherapy, their anxiety may be too severe to be treated by that method alone. Others are not "psychologically minded" and not good candidates for successful psychotherapy. Some may feel that non-pharmacological approaches such as yoga or meditation do not fit their lifestyles or worldviews. Some patients may suffer anxiety so severe that it interferes with any non-pharmacological effort to relieve it. In such cases, it may be most kind and expeditious to simply bypass that individual's active participation in treatment and allow a medication to do the work. Non-pharmacological methods can always be introduced after stabilization.

A variety of medications are used to treat anxiety. Most prominent among them are benzodiazepines, buspirone, antidepressants of various types, gabapentin, pregabalin, hydroxyzine, propranolol, clonidine, and medications that mimic or affect neurosteroids. In the current context, discussion of the types of medications used to treat anxiety and their mechanisms of action may further our understanding of the use of herbs to treat anxiety, as their mechanisms of action are generally quite similar.

4.1 BENZODIAZEPINES

Perhaps the most effective and commonly prescribed anxiolytic medications are the benzodiazepines. Benzodiazepines are now prescribed about 66 million times a year in the US, according to a report by the US National Center for Health Statistics.[1] More than one in eight US adults uses a benzodiazepine each year.

In 1955, Hoffmann-La Roche chemist Leo Sternbach serendipitously identified the first benzodiazepine, chlordiazepoxide. In 1960, it was marketed under the name Librium. Over the years, pharmacologists have pursued molecular modifications for enhanced activity, and a cadre of structurally related medications have come into being.[2] By and large, all benzodiazepines work the same way in the brain. The various benzodiazepines differ only in how quickly and how long they act. Rapidly acting benzodiazepines, such as alprazolam, can be useful for taking as needed for occasional panic attacks. Slow but long-acting benzodiazepines, such as clonazepam, are useful for use on a scheduled basis for treating those with persistent and severe anxiety.

Although benzodiazepines became available in 1960, it took 15 more years to determine their mechanism of action.[3] Benzodiazepines act by enhancing GABA

DOI: 10.1201/9781003300281-4

activity. Benzodiazepines act at a specific type of GABA receptor called the GABA-A receptor. To be precise, benzodiazepines act at four of the six subtypes of GABA-A receptors. There is a specific site on the GABA-A receptor where benzodiazepines bind, and it has been labeled as the benzodiazepine receptor. However, an interesting and ongoing controversy in neuroscience is whether or not there is a natural or endogenous benzodiazepine made by the body to activate the benzodiazepine receptor. A great deal of research over the last 30 years has not revealed any clear candidates. Diazepam binding inhibitor (DBI) is a peptide that displaces benzodiazepines from binding their sites on the GABA-A receptor complex. However, it is not an endogenous anxiolytic. Rather, it appears to act as an endogenous negative modulator of the GABA-A receptor complex.[4] Indeed, administration of DBI tends to induce anxiety-like states in laboratory studies of rodents.[5] There are many substances, such as vitamins, that the body needs but does not make and thus depends upon the environment and diet to provide. Might that be the case with the natural activator of the benzodiazepine receptor? In the current context, it is tempting to speculate that flavonoids or other phytochemicals in the "natural" human diet—that is, Albert Szent-Györgyi's vitamin P—might fill that role. Indeed, in his Nobel lecture from 1937, Szent-Györgyi proposed the flavanone hesperidin to be one such vitamin P candidate.[6] As discussed later, flavonoids bind with significant affinity to benzodiazepine receptors and other sites on the GABA-A receptor.

The ability of benzodiazepines to reduce anxiety of almost every kind is indisputable. These medications quite clearly provide relief for sufferers of GAD, social anxiety disorder, and panic disorder. There have been, however, controversies about long-term use of these medications. It has been recommended that treatment with benzodiazepines not continue beyond 6 to 8 weeks. Unfortunately, many anxiety disorders, particularly GAD, tend to be chronic conditions. Much of the controversy over benzodiazepines arises out of concern for adverse effects and abuse, and uncertainties as to whether chronic administration continues to provide meaningful relief from anxiety. All benzodiazepines have some tendency to produce tolerance, abuse, and addiction. Nonetheless, the risk of misuse of and addiction to benzodiazepines is not terribly high, and it can be cruel and unwise to withhold benzodiazepines simply out of fear for such risk. Harvard psychiatrist Carl Salzman has written extensively on this subject.[7] He has noted that about 6% of individuals prescribed benzodiazepines go on to abuse them. Many patients can be maintained on modest doses of benzodiazepines for many years without adverse effects, loss of efficacy, or the need to continually adjust dosage. Certainly, some individuals are higher risks than others, and patients should be screened. Those who have had serious issues with alcohol may not be good candidates for benzodiazepine therapy.

Another issue with benzodiazepines is that when taken in combination with certain other substances or medications, including alcohol or opiate pain medications, they can contribute to decreases in respiratory drive. This can be fatal. In the midst of the opiate overdose epidemic, many doctors have simply refused to prescribe benzodiazepines and opiates together.[8] This degree of caution is hard to blame, though studies have shown that individuals who have adapted to combined benzodiazepines and opiates after long use are at less risk and do not generally need to be taken off either medication as a mere matter of course.[9]

Finally, a recent concern has been reports that use of benzodiazepines is associated with increased risk for dementia.[10] It must firmly be stated that there is no clear cause and effect for this relationship. It is well known that benzodiazepines can disrupt the laying down of memories. However, that phenomenon is reversible and not indicative of the presence of dementia. There is also no relationship between when in life benzodiazepines were prescribed, for how long, or in what dose in relation to the development of dementia. On the other hand, it has been noted that severe anxiety and insomnia, which were the main reasons these people were prescribed benzodiazepines in the first place, are themselves major risk factors for developing dementia. In the end, the prescription of benzodiazepines, like every medication, must be seen in the light of its risks versus its benefits.

4.2 BUSPIRONE

Buspirone was first synthesized in 1968 and approved for use in the United States in 1986. It is a medication frequently prescribed by primary care physicians to treat anxiety disorders. The primary attraction of buspirone is that it has none of the dangerous side effects or potential for abuse seen with benzodiazepines. It is not related to benzodiazepines in either structure or mechanism of action. Rather, buspirone acts at a subtype of serotonin receptor in the brain, the 5-HT1A receptor. Indeed, it was initially seen as a potential antidepressant, but those results did not bear fruit.[11] The drug also mildly blocks dopamine receptors in the brain and was for a time thought to be a possible new approach to treating schizophrenia. Again, results were not positive.[12]

The primary targets of buspirone treatment have been GAD and social phobia. Initial reports suggested that while there were no acute anxiolytic effects of buspirone, ongoing treatment for those conditions might be as effective as treatment with benzodiazepines.[13] Unfortunately, the anxiolytic effects of buspirone have been rather lackluster.[14] While bestowing some benefits, it is not as effective as benzodiazepines in the treatment of GAD, and effects in social phobia are quite mixed. Certainly those who have previously benefitted from benzodiazepines rarely describe any benefit from being switched to buspirone. Indeed, the main attraction to buspirone is not its efficacy but rather the fact that it is not a benzodiazepine.

4.3 ANTIDEPRESSANTS

Antidepressants are another class of medications commonly used to treat anxiety disorders. Whereas there are several distinct classes of antidepressants and multiple members of each class, the primary mechanism of action of these medications is to enhance monoaminergic activity. Curiously, there do not appear to be significant differences among antidepressants in their abilities to treat GAD. Thus, there is no compelling reason to consider each individual antidepressant. For a more complete discussion, see the review by J.M. Gorman.[15]

Certainly, antidepressants are an obvious choice when anxiety is a component of a more general affective disorder, such as major depression, obsessive compulsive disorder, or PTSD, for which these medicines are first-line treatments. It has been found that roughly 50% of individuals who present to the primary care physician with complaints of major depression or an anxiety disorder will actually be found to suffer both conditions at the same time. Thus, by treating individuals complaining of anxiety with an antidepressant, it is reasonable to suspect that comorbid symptoms of depression will be helped and the patient will feel better. However, studies have shown that in patients suffering GAD without major depression or other psychiatric illnesses, antidepressants can be helpful in relieving symptoms of anxiety. In analyzing the anxiolytic effects of antidepressants, it was calculated that the number of patients needed to be treated to observe a successful outcome was 5.54. This degree of efficacy is deemed to be on the edge of being a reasonable choice of treatment.[16] Although effects of the various antidepressants on anxiety are quite similar, there may yet be some advantage in the use of monoamine oxidase inhibitors to treat panic disorder and social phobia.[17] Unfortunately, the dangers and inconveniences of those medications makes their use problematic.

The most attractive aspect of using antidepressants to treat anxiety is not efficacy but rather that benzodiazepines can be avoided. It must be remembered that even in the treatment of major depression, the ostensible raison d'être for this class of medications, antidepressants bring only about 40% of patients into full remission of symptoms.[18] They are even less effective when used specifically for anxiety.[19]

The length of time required for antidepressants to produce an anxiolytic effect is both troublesome and difficult to explain. Selective serotonin reuptake inhibitors (SSRIs) and serotonin/norepinephrine reuptake inhibitors (SNRIs) usually take between 2 and 6 weeks to produce an initial "partial" response, which is typically defined as at least 25% improvement in symptom severity from baseline. Full benefit may not be seen for another 4–6 weeks.[20] Given the fact that antidepressants almost immediately enhance monoaminergic activity, it prompts the question as to what the mechanism of anxiolytic action might actually be. For an in-depth discussion of how antidepressants work but often do not, see the discussion by Scott D. Mendelson.[21]

Antidepressants can also have troubling side effects. Indeed, it has been reported that 28% of patients stop taking antidepressants in the first month of treatment and 44% discontinue by the third month, largely due to side effects. One of the most common complaints is loss of sex drive and difficulty achieving orgasm. Nausea, diarrhea, headache, drowsiness, insomnia, nervousness, or weight gain lead others to stop treatment.[22]

4.4   GABAPENTIN

The drug gabapentin is prescribed for treatment of neuropathic pain and as an additive in the treatment of certain seizure disorders. Its structure is similar to that of GABA, and that—along with its highly suggestive name—has led people to assume that its effects in the brain are due to it mimicking GABA. However, this is not likely the case. The molecule has no direct effects on the GABA receptor, and it does not affect GABA uptake or metabolism.[23] Possible mechanisms of action include effects at calcium channels or N-methyl-D-aspartate (NMDA) receptors. There are case reports of gabapentin being useful in the treatment of panic, social anxiety disorder, and GAD.[24] An advantage of gabapentin is a low risk of abuse and even a potential to reduce abuse of alcohol in some patients.[25]

4.5 PREGABALIN

Pregabalin is a medication with many similarities to gabapentin. It is commonly used in the United States for the treatment of partial seizures and neuropathic pain. Like gabapentin, its likely mechanism of action is at calcium channels.[26] However, it has been approved in Europe for the treatment of GAD in adults, and it is used off label for this purpose in the United States as well.[27] There are also reports that pregabalin may be useful in the treatment of social anxiety disorder.[28] Side effects such as sedation, mental cloudiness, weight gain, and even possibility of abuse can make its use problematic for some.[29]

4.6 HYDROXYZINE

Hydroxyzine is an antihistamine medication that in recent years has become an increasingly popular treatment for anxiety. Like buspirone, it has no similarities to benzodiazepines and is thus safer and more palatable for primary care physicians to prescribe. Hydroxyzine is not a new medication. There was a report as early as 1959 showing that hydroxyzine provided "good to excellent" relief from anxiety in some patients.[30] Over the following 10 years, there were more reports about the ability of hydroxyzine to reduce anxiety, hostility, insomnia, and even symptoms of major depression. About 41% of individuals reported at least a 50% decrease in symptoms of anxiety, with the major side effect being drowsiness.[31] More recent studies have been less supportive of clinically significant anxiolytic effects of hydroxyzine. A 2010 paper from the Cochrane Review library did not see it as prudent to recommend hydroxyzine as a first-line treatment of GAD.[32] Indeed, while some complain about drowsiness from hydroxyzine, most complain that it simply isn't strong enough to relieve severe anxiety.

4.7 PROPRANOLOL

In 1894, the great American psychologist William James posed the question, "Do we run from a bear because we are afraid or are we afraid because we run?" In all likelihood, the truth is a little of both. Nonetheless, a large part of our experience of fear and anxiety involves the physical feelings of a pounding heart, quickening breath, sweating, tensing of the muscles, and the other physical components of the fight-or-flight response. Propranolol, and other so-called beta-blockers that prevent some components of the body's fight-or-flight response, can blunt the anxiety-provoking feelings that the fight-or-flight response can arouse. It must be remembered, however, that propranolol is lipophilic and crosses the blood-brain barrier. Thus, the effects of the drug could be central as well as peripheral.

The first formal description of anxiolytic effects of propranolol were in 1965, five years after its discovery, when it was serendipitously discovered that attempts to relive the tachycardia of thyrotoxicosis were accompanied by reports of relief of acute anxiety.[33] Unfortunately, subsequent studies have not given strong support for the routine use of propranolol or other beta-blockers in treating either GAD, panic disorder, or persistent social anxiety disorder.[34] Nonetheless, propranolol and other beta-blockers can be helpful for those who suffer from stage fright, performance anxiety, or other sources of anxiety, such as giving a speech, that are specific and time limited.[35]

4.8 CLONIDINE

Clonidine is a noradrenergic agonist that primarily acts presynaptically to reduce release of norepinephrine. However, postsynaptic action is likely as well. It is used primarily as a blood pressure medication. However, it has also frequently been used to block the distressing and anxiety-laden effects of opiate withdrawal.[36] Like propranolol, it has also been reported to alleviate some symptoms of anxiety disorders. In an early study, clonidine was found to significantly reduce symptoms of GAD and panic disorder. Curiously, the main effects of clonidine were decreases of "psychic" symptoms, with somatic symptoms being less affected. Moreover, symptoms were worsened by clonidine in 17% of subjects.[37] Of concern is the fact that clonidine can cause or exacerbate depression.[38] Other drawbacks of treating anxiety with clonidine are the potent blood pressure lowering effects of the medication and the sedation that many feel.

4.9 NEUROSTEROIDS

Allopregnanolone is a natural neurosteroid and positive allosteric modulator at GABA-A receptors.[39] Brexanolone, an aqueous formulation of allopregnanolone, has been found to be effective in the treatment of postpartum depression. The primary target in postpartum depression is depression. However, this condition presents with a substantial component of anxiety. In one study,[40] intravenous infusion of brexanolone significantly reduced symptoms of both depression and anxiety. Another analogue of allopregnanolone, ganaxolone, is also being studied as a treatment for PTSD. The initial study was suggestive of benefits, but underdosing may have prevented a significant effect.[41] Mifepristone is a potent glucocorticoid and progesterone receptor antagonist that has been successfully used to treat psychotic depression. It has been noted to reduce both the severe depression and anxiety that manifest in this condition.[42] Most recently, mifepristone was tested in adults over 60 years of age suffering both anxiety disorder and cognitive dysfunction. Participants with higher baseline cortisol levels showed improvements in memory and executive function and decreases in severity of anxiety after treatment with mifepristone. Improvements persisted as long as 8 weeks after the medication was stopped. Individuals with low-to-normal baseline cortisol showed little to no improvement with the medication.[43] These finding demonstrate the role of stress and abnormal activity in the hypothalamic-pituitary-adrenal axis in anxiety and mood disorders. It is worth noting that alphaxolone, a synthetic steroid active at GABA-A receptors, has sedating effects sufficiently strong to be useful for surgical anesthesia.[44]

4.10 MECHANISMS OF ANXIOLYTIC DRUG ACTION

In considering the medications described prior, we can conclude that there are several mechanisms by which medications can relieve anxiety. The most direct way is by increasing activity of the GABA neurotransmitter system that calms the brain, which is how the benzodiazepines act. Medications can also help relieve depression and other comorbidities and thus improve overall mental health and increase emotional resiliency. Some medications sedate anxious individuals—that is, make them a little sleepy—to make them less agitated and more relaxed. Some medications block the so-called fight-or-flight response and thus diminish the reactions to stress and blunt bodily sensations of anxiety that tend to make these experiences worse. A compelling argument has also been made that dampening the stress response by modulation of the hypothalamic-pituitary-adrenal axis is a common feature of anxiolytic medications.[45] In the current context, the most salient question is, "Are there herbal remedies that produce effects similar to those produced by the various medications prescribed to relieve symptoms of anxiety, and might they act by similar mechanisms?"

REFERENCES

1. Santo L, Rui P, Ashman JJ. Physician office visits at which benzodiazepines were prescribed: Findings from 2014–2016 national ambulatory medical care survey. *Natl Health Stat Report*. 2020;137:1–15.
2. Wick J. The history of benzodiazepines. *Consult Pharmacist*. 2013;(9):538–548.
3. Hacfely W, Kulcsár A, Möhler H, et al. Possible involvement of GABA in the central actions of benzodiazepines. *Adv Biochem Psychopharmacol*. 1975;(14):131–151.
4. Barbaccia ML, Berkovich A, Guarneri P, et al. Diazepam binding inhibitor: The precursor of a family of endogenous modulators of GABAA receptor function. History, perspective, and clinical implications. *Neurochem Res*. 1990;15:161–168.
5. Guidotti A, Forchetti CM, Corda MG, et al. Isolation, characterization and purification to homogeneity of an endogenous polypeptide with agonistic action on benzodiazepine receptors. *Proc Natl Acad Sci USA*. 1983;80:3531–3535.
6. Szent-Györgyi A. Oxydation, energy transfer and vitamins. *Nobel Lecture*. 11 Dec 1937.
7. Salzman C, Shader R. Not again: Benzodiazepines once more under attack. *J Clin Psychopharmacol*. 2015;35(5):493–495.
8. Hwang CS, Kang EM, Kornegay CJ, et al. Trends in the concomitant prescribing of opioids and benzodiazepines, 2002–2014. *Am J Prevent Med*. 2016;51(2):151–160.
9. Zin CS, Ismail F. Co-prescription of opioids with benzodiazepine and other co-medications among opioid users: Differential in opioid doses. *J Pain Res*. 2017;10:249–257.
10. Islam M, Iqbal U, Walther B, et al. Benzodiazepine use and risk of dementia in the elderly population: A systematic review and meta-analysis. *Neuroepidemiology*. 2016;47:181–191.
11. Eison AS, Temple DL. Buspirone: Review of its pharmacology and current perspectives on its mechanism of action. *Am J Med*. 1986;80(3):1–9.
12. Wilson TK, Tripp J. *Buspirone*. Treasure Island, FL: StatPearls Publishing; 2018.
13. Loane C, Politis M. Buspirone: What is it all about? *Brain Res*. 2012;1461:111–118.
14. Gomez AF, Barthel AL, Hofmann SG. Comparing the efficacy of benzodiazepines and serotonergic anti-depressants for adults with generalized anxiety disorder: A meta-analytic review. *Expert Opin Pharmacother*. 2018;19(8):883–894.
15. Gorman JM. Treatment of generalized anxiety disorder. *J Clin Psychiatry*. 2002; 63:17–23.
16. Kapczinski F, Lima MS, Souza JS, et al. Antidepressants for generalized anxiety disorder. *Cochrane Database Syst Rev*. 2003;2(2):CD003592.
17. van Vliet IM, Westenberg HGM, Den Boer JA. MAO inhibitors in panic disorder: Clinical effects of treatment with brofaromine: A double blind placebo-controlled study. *Psychopharmacology*. 1993;112:483–489.

18. Mendlewicz J. Towards achieving remission in the treatment of depression. *Dialogues Clin Neurosci.* 2008;10(4):371–375.
19. Schmitt R, Gazalle FK, Lima MS, et al. The efficacy of antidepressants for generalized anxiety disorder: A systematic review and meta-analysis. *Rev Bras Psiquiatr.* 2005;27(1):18–24.
20. Farach FJ, Pruitt LD, Jun JJ, et al. Pharmacological treatment of anxiety disorders: Current treatments and future directions *J Anxiety Disord.* 2012;26(8):833–843.
21. Mendelson SD. *Herbal Treatment of Major Depression: Scientific Basis and Practical Use.* Boca Raton, FL: CRC Press; 2020. pp. 7–10.
22. Khawam EA, Laurencic G, Malone DA. Side effects of antidepressants: An overview. *Clev Clin J Med.* 2006;73(4):351–361.
23. Rose MA, Kam PCA. Gabapentin: Pharmacology and its use in pain management. *Anaesthesia.* 2002;57(5):451–462.
24. Pollack MH, Matthews J, Scott EL. Gabapentin as a potential treatment for anxiety disorders. *Am J Psychiat.* 1998;155:992–993.
25. Leung JG, Hall-Flavin D, Nelson S, et al. The role of gabapentin in the management of alcohol withdrawal and dependence. *Ann Pharmacother.* 2015;49(8):897–906.
26. Ben-Menachem E. Pregabalin pharmacology and its relevance to clinical practice. *Epilepsia.* 2004;45(6):13–18.
27. Frampton JE. Pregabalin: A review of its use in adults with generalized anxiety disorder. *CNS Drugs.* 2014;28:835–854.
28. Pande AC, Feltner DE, Jefferson JW, et al. Efficacy of the novel anxiolytic pregabalin in social anxiety disorder—a placebo-controlled, multicenter study. *J Clin Psychopharmacol.* 2004;24:141–149.
29. Toth C. Drug safety evaluation of pregabalin. *Expert Opin Drug Saf.* 2012;11:487–502.
30. Middlefell R, Edwards KCS. Hydroxyzine (Atarax) in the relief of tension associated with anxiety neurosis and mild depressive states. *J Ment Sci.* 1959;105(440):792–794.
31. Darcis T, Ferreri M, Natens J, et al. The French GP study group for hydroxyzine. A multicenter double-blind placebo-controlled study investigating the anxiolytic efficacy of hydroxyzine in patients with generalized anxiety. *Hum Psychopharmacol.* 1995;10(3):181–187.
32. Guaiana G, Barbui C, Cipriani A. Hydroxyzine for generalized anxiety disorder. *Cochrane Database Syst Rev.* 2010;12:CD006815.
33. Turner P, Granville-Grossman KL. Effect of adrenergic receptor blockade of the tachycardia of thyrotoxicosis and anxiety state. *Lancet.* 1965;2:1316–1318.
34. Steenen SA, van Wijk AJ, van der Heijden GJ, et al. Propranolol for the treatment of anxiety disorders: Systematic review and meta-analysis. *J Psychopharmacol (Oxford).* 2016;30:128–139.
35. Bourgeois JA. The management of performance anxiety with beta-adrenergic blocking agents. *Jefferson J Psychiat.* 1991;9(2):13–28.
36. Gold MS, Redmond DE, Kleber HD. Clonidine blocks acute opiate-withdrawal symptoms. *Lancet.* 1978;312(8090):599–602.
37. Hoehn-Saric R, Merchant AF, Keyser ML, et al. Effects of clonidine on anxiety disorders. *Arch Gen Psychiatry.* 1981;38(11):1278–1282.
38. Prasad A, Shotliff K. Depression and chronic clonidine therapy. *Postgrad Med J.* 1993;69:327–328.
39. Walton N, Maguire J. Allopregnanolone-based treatments for postpartum depression: Why/how do they work? *Neurobiol Stress.* 2019;11:100198.
40. Kanes SJ, Colquhoun H, Doherty J, et al. Open-label, proof-of-concept study of brexanolone in the treatment of severe postpartum depression. *Hum Psychopharmacol.* 2017;32(2):e2576.

41. Rasmusson AM, Marx CE, Jain S, et al. A randomized controlled trial of ganaxolone in posttraumatic stress disorder. *Psychopharmacology.* 2017;234:2245–2257.
42. DeBattista C, Belanoff J. The use of mifepristone in the treatment of neuropsychiatric disorders. *Trends Endocrin Met.* 2006;17(3):117–121.
43. Lenze EJ, Hershey T, Newcomer JW, et al. Antiglucocorticoid therapy for older adults with anxiety and co-occurring cognitive dysfunction: Results from a pilot study with mifepristone. *Geri Psychiat.* 2014;29(9):962–969.
44. Cottrell GA, Lambert JJ, Peters JA. Modulation of GABAA receptor activity by alphaxalone. *BJP.* 1987;90(3):491–500.
45. Tafet GE, Nemeroff CB. Pharmacological treatment of anxiety disorders: The role of the HPA axis. *Front Psychiatry.* 2020;11:443.

5 Anxiolytic Phytochemicals

The experts at the Royal Botanic Garden at Kew estimate there to be about 390,000 different species of plants in the world. They have further estimated that of those plant species, about 18,000 have significant medicinal value. Some physicians dismiss the value of herbal medicines. Certainly the pharmaceutical companies would prefer to have people believe that plants have no benefits to offer. However, for centuries, healers—both folk and formal—have used plants now known to contain powerful medicinal substances. Among those derived directly from plants are morphine, quinine, pseudoephedrine, cocaine, colchicine, digoxin, atropine, galantamine, cannabidiol, salicylate, reserpine, sennosides, and other common medications that have been proven to relieve various forms of human suffering. The modern pharmaceutical industry has often looked to the plant world as a source for new medications. The Center for Biological Diversity, in Tucson, Arizona, has stated that of the top 150 prescribed medications in the United States, at least 118 were originally derived from plant sources.

Some proponents of herbal medicine speak of herbs with undue reverence, as if being "natural" lends them special, spiritual, even magical properties. However, the medicinal substances in plants are not miracles—they are molecules. These molecules, like those of synthesized pharmaceuticals, have medicinal properties related to their chemical structures. The molecules in plants, phytochemicals, are classified into the general categories of carbohydrates; lipids, which includes fatty acids, terpenes, and steroids; phenolics, which includes flavonoids, phenolic acids, and chalcones; and alkaloids. Among those types of molecules, flavonoids, terpenes, steroids, and alkaloids may hold the most promise for treatment of anxiety.

5.1 FLAVONOIDS

Flavonoids are a subclass of plant molecules known as polyphenols. The large, multi-ringed polyphenol molecules lend color to the leaves, fruits, and flowers of plants. The deep colors of the polyphenols attract pollinators, protect the plant's tissues from the sun's radiation, and, in some cases, help fight off bacterial infection. About half of plant polyphenols are classified as flavonoids, and the Linus Pauling Institute at Oregon State University has noted over 5,000 different variations of flavonoid molecules. The flavonoids are themselves categorized into six different subclasses, including: flavonols, such as catechin and epigallocatechin gallate, found in *Camellia sinensis* and *Theobroma cacao*; deeply blue and purple anthocyanidins, such as cyanidin and malvidin, from various berries and *Vitis vinifera*; flavanols, such as kaempferol and quercetin, found in many herbs and cruciferous vegetables;

DOI: 10.1201/9781003300281-5

flavones, such as apigenin and luteolin found in *Matricaria chamomilla* and *Apium graveolens*; flavanones, including hesperidin and naringenin from citrus; and isoflavones, such as daidzein and genistein, from *Glycine max*.

Flavonoids are particularly important in the discussion of herbal treatment of anxiety. Many readily cross from the bloodstream into brain tissue, where they are able act to reduce the symptoms of anxiety.[1] Of particular significance, many have been found to be active at GABA-A receptors.[2] This is similar to the activity of the premier anxiolytic medications, the benzodiazepines. Some flavonoids and flavonoid derivatives bind with high affinity to the benzodiazepine site of the GABA-A receptor complex. For example, amentoflavone, a biflavonoid derivative of apigenin, was found in binding studies to have a Ki as high as 7nm at the benzodiazepine site.[3] Such high binding affinity rivals that of many benzodiazepines themselves.[4] Whereas benzodiazepines as a class tend to affect the GABA-A1, 2, 3, and 5 subtypes, there is evidence that some flavonoids may exhibit selectivity for subtypes of GABA-A receptors. For example, the naturally occurring flavonoid 6-hydroxyflavone appears to selectively affect the A2 and A3 subtypes of GABA receptors.[5]

Flavonoids may also bind at sites on the GABA-A complex other than the benzodiazepine binding site. Thus, they have pharmacological properties distinct from benzodiazepines. At least two different sites have been elucidated, a high-affinity flumazenil-sensitive site and a low-affinity, flumazenil-insensitive site. Flavonoids can exert either positive or negative allosteric effects on the GABA receptor complex, and some may even stimulate the receptor in the absence of GABA.[6] An interesting example of the complexities that can occur among flavonoids is the activities of epigallocatechin gallate, or EGCG. EGCG acts as a negative modulator of GABAA receptors in high concentrations. At low concentrations it has no direct effect on the action of GABA on GABA-A receptors, yet it potentiates the positive modulation by diazepam.[7]

Along with anti-anxiety actions at GABA receptors, some flavonoids act as inhibitors of monoamine oxidases in the manner of some antidepressants. Quercetin and apigenin act at quite low nanomolar and micromolar concentrations to inhibit those enzymes. Flavonoids can also act deep within the chemical machinery of cells— for example, through interaction with the mitogen-activated protein kinase (MAPK) cascades[8]—to affect the ways cells respond to stress and inflammation and to help maintain their systems of self-repair. Such actions in neurons in the brain produce antidepressant effects that can indirectly relieve anxiety. Chalcones are molecular precursors in the biosynthesis of flavonoids. Some chalcones have been identified as possessing anxiolytic effects.[9]

5.2 TERPENES

Terpenes are another common class of molecules found in plants. There are about 20,000 different terpenes known to exist in the natural world. They can be simple in structure, such as isovaleric acid, a branched chain of five carbon atoms. They can also be multi-ringed, steroid-like molecules. They are often aromatic and are responsible for the pleasant fragrances of pine and citrus fruits, the floral aroma of *Lavandula angustifolia*, and the pungent odors of *Cannabis sativa*.

Essential oils extracted from plants are often touted as offering calming, anxiolytic effects. There are many studies supporting those impressions.[10] Most essential oils are rich in monoterpenes and sesquiterpenes, and many of those have been found to enhance activity at GABA receptors.[11]

An interesting group of terpene-derived molecules are the cannabinoids. Cannabinoids from *Cannabis sativa*, including cannabidiol and tetrahydrocannabinol, contain phenolic and terpene components that are enzymatically melded into hybrid molecules.[12] These molecules are well known to have psychotropic effects, including anxiolytic properties. However, some people can experience disorientation and panic after consuming cannabis containing high levels of tetrahydrocannabinol. It is likely that specific action at cannabinoid receptors in the brain mediates those effects, with interactions among other phytochemical components of *Cannabis sativa*—cannabinoids, terpenes, and flavonoids—altering the overall effect. This is known as the "entourage effect."[13] Surprisingly, not all cannabinoids come from cannabis. The common liverwort, *Marchantia polymorpha*, contains perrottetinene, a mildly psychoactive cannabinoid very similar in structure to tetrahydrocannabinol.[14] Cannabidiol that occurs in *Cannabis sativa* can also be found in the genetically related *Humulus* species of plants, of which hops is a member.[15] Cannabidiol is also found in common flax, *Linum usitatissimum*. Cannabigerol found in *Cannabis sativa* is also found in some plants of the genus *Helichrysum*. Conversely, some plants produce molecules that affect cannabinoid receptors in the brain but do not have the structure of cannabinoids from cannabis. For example, some species of *Echinacea* contain alkylamides that are similar in structure to the so-called endocannabinoids the body itself makes to stimulate cannabinoid receptors.[16]

Animals also produce terpenes, many of which, such as cholesterol and other steroids, are essential to life. This may explain how various steroid-like tri- and tetraterpenes of plant origin can affect human health, as they may mimic or block the effects of substances natural to the human body. Many of the so-called adaptogen herbs, such as *Withania somnifera* and *Panax ginseng*, contain triterpene sterols, saponins, and steroids that buffer activity in the hypothalamic-pituitary-adrenal axis.[17] Other plant-derived steroids are pharmacologically active in humans. Glycyrrhetic acid, a steroid triterpene from licorice, or *Glycyrrhiza glabra*, binds to mineralocorticoid and glucocorticoid receptors. It can act as an anti-inflammatory agent but may also cause severe hypertension due to salt retention.[18] Diosgenin, a triterpene phytosteroid extracted from *Dioscorea villosa*, was once used as an inexpensive starting point in the manufacturing of contraceptive steroids.[19]

5.3 ALKALOIDS

Alkaloids are nitrogen-containing molecules produced by about a quarter of plants. Generally, the nitrogen occurs within a ring of the alkaloid molecule.[20] Many alkaloids are toxic to animals, and it is likely that alkaloids serve to protect the plants from animal and insect predators. For example, the human LD50 of nicotine, an alkaloid contained in tobacco, *Nicotiana tabacum*, may be as low as 60mg/kg.[21] Milligram for milligram, that would make nicotine as toxic as cyanide.

The nitrogen groups in alkaloids make them similar to nitrogen-containing neu-rotransmitters and other molecules active in the brain. Indeed, many well-known psychedelic and hallucinogenic plant substances are alkaloids.[22] Many of the psychedelic alkaloids, including psilocybin from *Psilocybe* mushrooms, mescaline from *Lophophora williamsii*, lysergic acid from *Claviceps purpurea*, and dimethyl-tryptamine from the *Banisteriopsis caapi* vine, derive their unique effects on con-sciousness by stimulating the serotonin 2A receptor in the brain. These types of alkaloids can be used by experienced therapists at psychedelic doses to treat intrac-table depression.[23] Other psychoactive alkaloids derived from plants are scopolamine from *Datura stramonium*, morphine from *Papaver somniferum*, and ephedrine from *Ephedra sinica*. Galantamine, a cholinesterase-inhibiting medication approved by the FDA to treat Alzheimer's disease, is an alkaloid originally obtained from bulbs of *Galanthus caucasicus*, the Caucasian snowdrop flower.

The neurotransmitter GABA that is so important in calming the brain and ner-vous system is itself a nitrogen-containing molecule with an alkaloid-like structure. Thus, it is not surprising that many plant-derived alkaloids can mimic the activity of GABA in the brain. The sanjoinine alkaloids extracted from the *Zizyphus jujuba*, a staple in traditional Chinese medicine, produce anxiolytic effects by stimulating the GABA system.[24] In fact, sanjoinine is one of many large molecule alkaloids cat-egorized as cyclopeptide alkaloids. These alkaloids have been found in a variety of plants of the *Acanthaceae*, *Malvaceae*, *Phyllanthaceae*, and *Rubiaceae* families. Extracts of some of those plants have been found to exhibit anticonvulsant and anx-iolytic effects, possibly mediated by GABA receptors.[25] Neurotransmitters other than GABA can also be involved in the anxiolytic effects of plant alkaloids. For example, the antipsychotic alkaloid alstonine, extracted from *Littorina littorea* and the Nigerian tree *Alstonia scholaris*, produces anxiolytic effects in animals by stimu-lating serotonin receptors and reducing activity of the stimulating neurotransmitter, glutamate.[26] Finally, some alkaloids have antidepressant effects that, in turn, can help alleviate anxiety in some individuals. Harmala alkaloids from *Passiflora incarnata* would be in that category.[27]

5.4 PHYTOCHEMICALS THAT RELIEVE ANXIETY

It is the phytochemicals contained in an herb that give it the ability to relieve anxiety. Some anxiolytic herbs contain quite unique phytochemicals. These chemicals are often named using variations of the scientific names of those herbs, reflecting that they were first discovered while investigating the properties of those specific plants. For example, a variety of so-called eleutherosides have been isolated from Siberian ginseng, which has the scientific name *Eleutherococcus senticosus*. The eleuthero-sides are a family of steroid-like triterpenes that do not exert immediate anxiolytic effects. However, they are likely responsible for the gradual onset of adaptogenic effects of this herb.[28] Those effects build resiliency that, with time, lessens both anxi-ety and depression. The flavone baicalein can be extracted from skullcap, known scientifically as *Scutellaria baicalensis*. Baicalein relieves anxiety-like behaviors in animal studies, and while this appears due to effects on the GABA-A receptor, it is not through action at the benzodiazepine site.[29] Rosavin can be extracted from the herb *Rhodiola rosea*. Rosavin is a terpene derivative categorized as a cinnamyl alcohol glycoside. It has both anxiolytic and antidepressant effects in animals and is thought to be a major contributor to those same effects in humans.[30] However, it is never the case that an herb contains an entirely unique set of phytochemicals. All plants share a basic, underlying chemistry of life. They need to grow; build roots, stems and leaves; synthesize sugar from sunlight; metabolize that sugar; attract pollinating insects; pollinate; produce seeds; ward off predators; and protect themselves from oxidation and ultraviolet light. All plants engage in these same biochemical processes, and many utilize some of the same—or at least similar—phytochemicals to do so. A surprisingly large number of phytochemicals are shared among plants with anxiolytic properties, and many of these phytochemicals have been found on their own to exert anxiolytic effects.

5.4.1 AMENTOFLAVONE

Amentoflavone is a biflavonoid—that is, bis-apigenin. It is found in over 120 plants, perhaps most notably *Ginkgo biloba*, *Hypericum perforatum*, *Chamaecyparis obtusa*, and *Xerophyta* species. At least one study has demonstrated anxiolytic-like effects of amentoflavone in mice. These effects were attenuated with flumazenil, suggesting mediation by benzodiazepine receptors. Other of its effects were blocked by serotonin and noradrenaline antagonists, indicating ability to affect monoamines.[31] Amentoflavone acts as an allosteric modulator at GABA-A receptors[32] and may act as an antagonist at the κ-opioid receptor.[33] K-opioid antagonists are thought to exert anxiolytic effects.[34]

5.4.2 APIGENIN

Apigenin is the most prominent flavonoid in *Matricaria chamomilla*. However, it is also found in *Ocimum basilicum*, *Apium graveolens*, *Vitex agnus-castus*, various citrus of the *Rutaceae* family, *Ginkgo biloba*, *Zizyphus jujuba*, *Melissa officinalis*, *Scutellaria baicalensis*, *Hypericum perforatum*, and other medicinal herbs. Chemically, it is 4',5,7-trihydroxyflavone, and it has been found to exert a variety of beneficial biological effects.[35]

Apigenin has shown anxiolytic effects in tests of rodents in the elevated plus maze.[36] It also has sedative effects in mice that can be blocked by the benzodiazepine antagonist flumazenil. This suggests that the anxiolytic effects of the flavonoid are due at least in part to action at the benzodiazepine receptor.[37] Vitexin, the glucoside of apigenin, also produces anxiolytic and anticonvulsant effects in mice through a GABAergic mechanism.[38] Vitexin has been found to inhibit activity at the NMDA receptor,[39] suggesting other possible mechanisms of action of herbs that contain apigenin and its derivatives. This effect is interesting because ketamine, a medication with newly discovered, rapid antidepressant effects, acts largely by blocking the NMDA receptor. Indeed, apigenin also exhibits antidepressant-like effects in animals.[40]

5.4.3 BAICALEIN

Baicalein, a flavone, is found in *Scutellaria* species and *Oroxylum indicum* as used in Ayurvedic medicine. Baicalein has been found to have anxiolytic effects in mice in the elevated plus maze. Pentylenetetrazol and the natural human steroid, dehydroepiandrosterone sulfate (DHEAS), antagonized those anxiolytic-like effects, but flumazenil and dl-p-chlorophenilalanine ethyl ester did not. Those findings suggest action at GABAergic but non-benzodiazepine sites.[41] It is worth noting that in one study, the glycoside of baicalein, baicalin, was more potent in producing an antidepressant effect.[42] This is likely due to differences in bioavailability.

5.4.4 β-CARYOPHYLLENE

β-caryophyllene is a ringed molecule categorized as a bicyclic sesquiterpene. It is found in *Cannabis sativa*, *Syzygium aromaticum*, *Echinacea purpurea*, *Ocimum tenuiflorum*, *Mentha piperita*, various species of *Salvia*, and other plants.[43] β-caryophyllene has anxiolytic, antidepressant, and pain-relieving effects in mice that can be reversed by administration of the CB2 antagonist AM630, suggesting involvement of cannabinoid receptors in the brain.[44] However, other studies suggest GABAergic, serotonergic, and nitrergic activities, as the anxiolytic effects in mice could also be attenuated by pretreatment with flumazenil, bicuculline, or l-arginine.[45]

5.4.5 BISABOLOL

Bisabolol (α-(−)-bisabolol) is a sesquiterpene present in a variety of plants, including *Betonica officinalis*, *Laserpitium latifolium*, and various species of the genus *Scrophularia*. However, its most common source is *Matricaria chamomilla*. Bisabolol produced anxiolytic-like effects in mice in the elevated plus maze. Pretreatment with flumazenil was able to reverse the effect of bisabolol, suggesting mediation by the benzodiazepine receptor.[46] The sesquiterpene also exhibits significant antiinflammatory and antinociceptive effects.[47]

5.4.6 CAFFEIC ACID

Caffeic acid and its quinic acid ester, chlorogenic acid, are found in *Evolvulus alsinoides*, *Echinacea angustifolia*, *Camellia sinensis*, *Melissa officinalis*, *Leonurus cardiaca*, *Passiflora incarnata*, *Ganoderma lingzhi*, *Rosmarinus officinalis*, *Salvia officinalis*, and *Schisandra chinensis*. Indeed, these related phenolic compounds are nearly ubiquitous, as they are intermediates in lignin biosynthesis, which occurs in all woody plants.[48] Caffeic acid exerts an anxiolytic effect in mice than can be overcome by treatment with NMDA, suggesting action at that receptor.[49] In another study, anxiolytic effects of caffeic acid on mice in the elevated plus maze and open field were partially reversed by flumazenil, suggesting involvement of benzodiazepine receptors.[50]

5.4.7 3-CARENE

3-carene is a bicyclic monoterpene that occurs in species of pine trees but also in *Cannabis sativa*, *Rosmarinus officinalis*, *Ocimum basilicum*, and *Piper nigrum*. Although there is little information in specific regard to anxiety, this phytochemical is known to enhance sleep in experimental animals through interaction with GABA-A receptors. Oral administration of 3-carene increases sleep duration and reduces sleep latency in pentobarbital-induced sleep test in mice. These effects were reversed by flumazenil.[51]

Extracts of the aerial parts of the *Pinaceae* species, *Abies pindrow*, are rich in 3-carene as well as the related monoterpenes pinene and limonene (discussed later). The tree has long been used in the Himalaya region of India and Nepal as a treatment for anxiety. However, it has never been tested clinically. That prompted a recent study in which the ethyl acetate fraction of the extract of *Abies pindrow*, which was rich in flavonoids and terpenes, produced an anxiolytic effect in mice in the elevated plus maze. Its potency was similar to that of diazepam.[52]

5.4.8 CARVACROL

Carvacrol (5-isopropyl-2-methylphenol) is a monoterpenic phenol present in the essential oil of many plants, including *Origanum vulgare*, *Thymus vulgaris*, *Origanum majorana*, *Lepidium sativum*, and *Lavandula angustifolia*. Carvacrol produced an anxiolytic-like effect in mice in elevated plus maze and open field tests. Those effects were attenuated by flumazenil, suggesting that they were mediated by activating benzodiazepine receptors.[53]

In another study, sub-chronic administration of carvacrol over 5 days was found to produce similar anxiolytic-like effects in rats subjected to lipopolysaccharide-induced neuroinflammation. In this case, other mechanisms of action were explored. The anxiolytic effect of carvacrol weas accompanied by attenuation of the lipopolysaccharide-induced increases in cyclooxygenase, tumor necrosis factor-alpha, and c-Jun N-terminal kinase. Those effects, in turn, were determined to be the result of modulation of the antioxidant gene Nrf2, a master regulator of the antioxidant pathway.[54] Those data suggest that ongoing treatment with carvacrol has a potent anti-inflammatory effect that can reduce inflammation-induced anxiety-like behaviors.

5.4.9 CHRYSIN

Chrysin, also called 5,7-dihydroxyflavone, is a flavone found in *Passiflora incarnata*, as well as *Matricaria chamomilla*, *Scutellaria baicalensis*, *Daucus carota*, *Oroxylum indicum*, and several species of mushroom. Studies have shown chrysin to possess significant anxiolytic effects in laboratory animals. A study showed chrysin to have an anxiolytic-like effect in rats in the elevated plus maze. This effect was reversed by flumazenil, suggesting mediation by benzodiazepine receptors.[55] One study was cautionary in that while acute treatment with chrysin produced an anxiolytic effect in rats in the elevated plus maze, diminished effects were seen with chronic treatment. That suggested the development of tolerance as might occur with benzodiazepine treatment.[56] However, chrysin may act by mechanisms other than enhancing GABA activity. For example, a study showed antidepressant-like effects of chronic chrysin treatment in rats. Those effects were accompanied by changes in receptor densities of 5-HT1A and 5-HT2A receptors in the raphe nuclei and hippocampus, which were similar to those produced by treatment with fluoxetine.[57]

5.4.10   7,8,Dihydroxyflavone

7,8,dihydroxyflavone is a flavonoid found in a variety of herbs, including *Godmania aesculifolia*, *Tridax procumbens*, and *Primula vulgaris*. It has been the subject of intense research after reports that it acts as a centrally active, small-molecule, selective tropomyosin receptor kinase B (TrkB) agonist.[58] The TrkB receptor is ordinarily stimulated by brain-derived neurotrophic factor. Although most animal studies have focused on antidepressant effects, at least one study has found evidence of anxiolytic effects of this flavonoid.[59] In that case, rats were chronically treated with alcohol, then subjected to acute alcohol withdrawal. Treatment with 7,8,dihydroxyflavone significantly reduced anxiety-like behaviors in the open field and elevated plus maze assays. Furthermore, 7,8-DHF prevented alcohol withdrawal and enhanced glutamatergic transmission in the amygdala of those animals, but it had no effect on GABAergic transmission in that area of the brain. Interestingly, microinjection of K252a, a TrkB antagonist, into the amygdala blocked the effects of 7,8-DHF on anxiety-like behavior. Thus, the effects appear to have been due to activation of the TrkB receptor.

5.4.11   Ellagic Acid

Ellagic acid is a polyphenolic compound found in oak leaves and a variety of mushrooms, fruits, and vegetables. It offers significant antioxidant, anti-inflammatory, and neuroprotective effects.[60] Several studies have also demonstrated anxiolytic-like effects in laboratory animals.

Ellagic acid significantly increased the percentage of time mice spent in the open arms of the elevated plus maze. This effect was comparable to that of diazepam. Moreover, this anxiolytic-like effect of ellagic acid was antagonized by pretreatment with either picrotoxin, a non-competitive GABA-A receptor antagonist, or flumazenil, a specific benzodiazepine antagonist. Thus, its effects were clearly mediated by action at GABA-A receptors.[61] It also produces antidepressant-like effects in rodents, which may contribute to any anxiolytic effects it can offer.[62]

5.4.12   Epigallocatechin Gallate

Epigallocatechin gallate, often abbreviated as EGCG, is the ester of epigallocatechin and gallic acid. Its primary source in human consumption is green tea, *Camellia sinensis*. However, it is also found in trace amounts in apple skin, plums, onions, hazelnuts, pecans, and carob powder.

Animal studies have found ECCG to exert anxiolytic, anti-inflammatory, and stress-reducing effects. Chronic administration of EGCG reduced anxiety provoked in a rat model of myocardial infarction. At the same time, it reduced levels of the inflammatory cytokine IL-6 in the hippocampi of those animals, as well as reduced general markers of neuroinflammation.[63] Chronic administration of EGCG also significantly attenuated the freezing response of rats after contextual fear conditioning. At the same time, treatment increased levels of brain-derived neurotrophic factor and the anxiolytic neurosteroid allopregnanolone.[64] Acute administration of EGCG counteracted the anxiogenic effects of caffeine in rats.[65]

Of particular interest is that EGCG is one of the few phytochemicals to be evaluated in humans for anxiolytic effects. Acute intake of EGCG produced increases in self-rated calmness and reductions in self-rated levels of stress in otherwise normal human subjects. These self-reports tended to be supported by EEG data gathered at the time. Tracings revealed significant overall increases in alpha, beta, and theta activity. Together, those results suggest states of relaxation and attentiveness.[66] In patients diagnosed with multiple sclerosis, chronic EGCG combined with daily intake of ketogenic coconut oil significantly lowered anxiety scores in the State-Trait Anxiety Inventory while lowering serum IL-6 levels. However, none of these patients was formally diagnosed as suffering an anxiety disorder.[67]

While anti-inflammatory effects may mediate effects of chronic treatment with EGCG, it is not clear what might mediate its acute anxiolytic effects. EGCG affects GABA-A receptors, but the interaction is complex. In cultured neurons, ECGC inhibited GABA activation yet also enhanced diazepam-induced increases in GABA-A receptor response.[68]

5.4.13 EUGENOL

The phenolic molecule eugenol lends clove, *Syzygium aromaticum*, its spicy aroma. But it is also in *Cinnamomum verum*, *Foeniculum vulgare*, *Ocimum basilicum*, *Melissa officinalis*, *Rosa* species, *Pelargonium graveolens*, and other aromatic herbs. Eugenol has anxiolytic effects in rodents, and these effects were associated with downregulation of brain neurokinin 1 receptors.[69] However, eugenol has also been found to enhance GABA-A receptor activity,[70] as well as to inhibit monoamine oxidase.[71]

5.4.14 FERULIC ACID

Ferulic acid is a phenolic molecule similar in structure to caffeic and chlorogenic acids mentioned previously. It is found in *Humulus lupulus*, *Leonurus cardiaca*, and *Ganoderma lingzhi*. It is particularly abundant in grains, including oats, *Avena sativa*. Ferulic acid reduced anxiety-like behavior of mice in alcohol withdrawal.[72] Ferulic acid also produces antidepressant-like effects in mice, along with increases in central activities of the neurotransmitters serotonin and norepinephrine. The latter was likely due to inhibition of monoamine oxidase.[73] Monoamine oxidase inhibitors are known to produce both antidepressant and anxiolytic effects in humans.

In yet another study,[74] ferulic acid exhibited anxiolytic-like effects in a mouse model of maternal separation stress. Those effects were eliminated by challenge with NMDA, and treatment also reduced the expression of NMDA receptor subunit genes in brain tissue. Those results suggested involvement of the NMDA receptor.

5.4.15 Hispidulin

Hispidulin is a flavone found in many medicinal herbs, including *Grindelia squarrosa*, *Fridericia chica*, *Saussurea involucrata*, *Crossostephium chinense*, and various species of *Artemisia* and *Salvia*. This flavonoid may have somewhat unique neuropharmacological effects. Although not specifically shown to exert anxiolytic effects, many of the herbs in which hispidulin is found have been used for this purpose, and animal studies have shown this flavone to exhibit benzodiazepine-like effects.

In binding studies, hispidulin binds to the benzodiazepine receptor and displaces flumazenil with an IC50—that is, the concentration needed to displace 50% of flumazenil—of about 1 micromolar.[75] That suggests a weak, but significant affinity for benzodiazepine receptors. On the other hand, hispidulin reduced methamphetamine-induced hyperlocomotion in rats, but not through any dopaminergic mechanism. Moreover, the flavone was found to be acting at the α6GABA-A receptor, a GABA-A subtype that is acted upon by alcohol but not benzodiazepines.[76] Hispidulin crosses the blood-brain barrier and exerts anticonvulsant effects in a manner similar to that of diazepam.[77] Hispidulin also exhibits antidepressant-like effects in mice that were shown to be due in part to inhibition of the NMDA receptor.[78]

5.4.16 Hyperoside

Hyperoside is an anthocyanin glycoside in *Hypericum perforatum*, *Drosera rotundifolia*, *Lamiaceae Stachys*, *Prunella vulgaris*, *Rumex acetosella*, *Cuscuta chinensis*, *Camptotheca acuminate*, leaves of trees of the genus *Betula*, species of *Tagetes*, and *Camellia sinensis*. Hyperoside showed anxiolytic-like effects in mice that had undergone a series of severe stresses, a paradigm suggested to be a murine model of PTSD. Chronic administration of hyperoside over the following 2 weeks was found to alleviate anxiety-like behavior in a subsequent test in the elevated plus maze.[79] The mechanism of action was not explored, and there are no reports in the literature of activity at GABA-A receptors. However, hyperoside has been found to exert antidepressant-like effects in both rats and mice, and those effects were thought to be mediated through protection against corticosterone-induced neurotoxicity.[80]

5.4.17 Icariin

Icariin is a flavonol glycoside from *Epimedium grandiflorum* and other species of *Epimedium*. It is one of the few isolated phytochemicals that has undergone study of anxiolytic effects in human subjects.[81] In that case, subjects suffering comorbid bipolar affective disorder and alcohol dependence were treated with 300mg of icariin per day for 8 weeks in an open-label pilot study. Scores on the Hamilton Anxiety Rating Scale before and after those 8 weeks of treatment showed significant decreases in anxiety. Significant decreases were also observed in symptoms of depression and in days of heavy drinking.

There are no clear indications from the literature that icariin might exert anxiolytic effects through action at GABA receptors, as do many other flavonoids and their glycosides. However, icariin also produces antidepressant effects—which in some cases themselves can produce anxiolytic effects—and those may be mediated by anti-inflammatory effects or enhancement of brain-derived neurotrophic factor.[82-83]

5.4.18 ISOPULEGOL

Isopulegol is a monoterpene found in a variety of aromatic plants, including *Cannabis sativa*, *Cymbopogon citratus*, species of *Pelargonium*, species of *Eucalyptus*, and *Mentha suaveolens*. The terpene produced an anxiolytic-like effect in mice in the open field and elevated plus maze tests. This effect was similar to that of diazepam, albeit without decreases in motor activity. Isopulegol also decreased sleep latency time and prolongation of the pentobarbital-induced sleeping time as was seen with diazepam.[84] Isopulegol also attenuated pentylenetetrazol-induced convulsions in mice. That effect was prevented by flumazenil, as would be expected if acting at benzodiazepine receptors.[85]

5.4.19 KAEMPFEROL

Kaempferol is a flavonol often contained in anxiolytic herbs. It is found in *Matricaria chamomilla*, *Hypericum perforatum*, *Salvia officinalis*, species of *Tilia*, *Lepidium meyenii*, *Mentha piperita*, *Trifolium pratense*, *Ginkgo biloba*, *Rosmarinus officinalis*, and many other herbs. It has been shown on its own to relieve anxiety-like symptoms. Kaempferol binds to GABA-A receptors in the brain. Intracerebroventricular microinjection of kaempferol reduced anxiety-like behavior of rats in the elevated plus maze test, and this effect was partially reversed by flumazenil. Thus, it was due in part to activation of benzodiazepine receptors.[86] In another study, kaempferol facilitated extinction learning in fear-conditioned rats in association with inhibition of fatty-acid amide hydrolase, suggesting interaction with endocannabinoid systems.[87]

5.4.20 LIMONENE

Limonene is a cyclic monoterpene and a major component of various citrus oils. However, it is also found in *Cannabis sativa*, *Vitex agnus-castus*, *Foeniculum vulgare*, *Boswellia sacra*, species of *Mentha*, species of *Rosa*, and *Salvia officinalis*. Several studies have shown limonene to have anxiolytic effects in rodents. In one study, limonene reduced stress-induced anxiety-like behavior in the elevated plus maze, though the mechanism of action was not determined.[88] In another study, limonene-induced anxiolytic activity and GABA release augmentation were blocked by an adenosine A2A receptor antagonist.[89] The stimulant, caffeine, is an example of an A2A receptor antagonist.

5.4.21 LINALOOL

Linalool is a fragrant and spicy terpene found in *Citrus aurantium*, *Cannabis sativa*, *Vitex agnus-castus*, *Cinnamomum verum*, *Foeniculum vulgare*, *Ocimum sanctum*, *Lavandula angustifolia*, *Melissa officinalis*, *Leonurus cardiaca*, *Rosmarinus officinalis*, *Rosa spp*, and many other fragrant herbs. Animal studies of anxiolytic effects of linalool have been inconsistent. Intraperitoneal administration appears to produce a sedative rather than an anxiolytic effect.[90] On the other hand, intraperitoneally administered linalool enhanced extinction of fear-induced learning, which is also an effect of benzodiazepines.[91] Perhaps most interesting are multiple reports showing anxiolytic effects of inhaled linalool, as might occur in use as aromatherapy. In one such example, inhaled linalool had anxiolytic effects in mice in the light/dark box and elevated plus maze assays. These effects were blocked by flumazenil, indicating mediation by benzodiazepine receptors. Remarkably, those anxiolytic effects were not seen in anosmic mice, suggesting odor to be the salient factor.[92]

There is also evidence that linalool may stimulate cannabinoid receptors.[93] The antinociceptive effects of linalool appear to be mediated by multiple systems in the brain, including actions at muscarinic, opioid, dopamine, adenosine, NO2, and NMDA receptors.[94]

5.4.22 LUTEOLIN

The flavonoid luteolin is found in *Matricaria chamomilla*, *Foeniculum vulgare*, *Ginkgo biloba*, *Ocimum sanctum*, *Zizyphus jujuba*, *Melissa officinalis*, *Avena sativa*, *Passiflora incarnata*, and other herbs. Luteolin, also notated as 3′,4′,5,7-tetrahydroxyflavone, significantly increased activity of mice in the novelty suppressed feeding and elevated plus maze tests.[95] Luteolin binds with only low affinity to benzodiazepine receptors, and its effects are not reversed by flumazenil. Thus, it does not appear to act at benzodiazepine receptors in the brain.[96]

5.4.23 MENTHOL

Menthol is a terpene alcohol found in many species of *Mentha*. Administration of menthol reduced anxiety-like behavior of mice in the elevated plus maze. It also reduced immobility time in the forced swimming test—an assay of antidepressant effect—and decreased the level of cortisol in the blood.[97] There is evidence that menthol modulated activities at both GABA-A and glycine receptors.[98] Interestingly, there is also a report that topically applied menthol can relieve pain, anxiety and catastrophizing in human colorectal cancer patients. Whether this was due to absorption or aromatherapy effects is unclear.[99]

5.4.24 MANGIFERIN

Mangiferin is a glucoside of the xanthoid norathyriol. The leaves and bark of *Mangifera indica*, the mango tree, are the primary sources. However, mangiferin is also found in many other herbs, including *Iris unguicularis*, *Anemarrhena asphodeloides*, *Bombax ceiba*, *Asplenium montanum*, *Coffea arabica*, and species of the genera *Salacia* and *Cyclopia*.[100] Among those herbs, *Anemarrhena asphodeloides* is of particular interest, as it appears in several herbal combinations traditionally used in Chinese medicine to treat anxiety.

In mice subjected to lipopolysaccharide-induced stress, mangiferin pretreatment significantly reduced anxiety-like behaviors in the elevated plus maze, light/dark box, and open field tests.[101] In that study, mangiferin was found to reduce markers of oxidative stress in brain tissues, as well as to reduce levels of the inflammatory cytokine interleukin-1β in hippocampus and prefrontal cortex. In a study using not pure mangiferin but a hydroethanolic extract of *Mangifera indica* rich in the substance, anxiety-like behaviors of mice were reversed by flumazenil or the 5-HT2 receptor antagonist metergoline.[102]

5.4.25 MYRICETIN

Myricetin is a flavonol from leaves of *Betula pendula, Scutellaria baicalensis, Allium sativum, Ginkgo biloba*, species of *Hibiscus*, species of *Tagetes, Allium cepa, Camellia sinensis*, and wine. This phytochemical exerts significant anxiolytic-like activity in mice in the elevated plus maze, light/dark box, open field, and hole board apparatus.[103]

Studies suggest that myricetin can increase GABAergic activity[104] and decrease release of glutamate,[105] both of which could contribute to anxiolytic effects. Myricetin has also attenuated depression-like behavior in mice subjected to a prolonged course of restraint stress. The flavonol also decreased serum levels of corticosterone in stressed animals. In the hippocampus, myricetin attenuated decreases in glutathione peroxidase but enhanced levels of BDNF.[106]

5.4.26 NARINGIN

Naringin is a flavanone-7-O-glycoside found in most citrus fruits, as well as *Prunus avium, Solanum lycopersicum, Theobroma cacao, Origanum vulgare, Mentha aquatica, Aglaomorpha quercifolia*, and various beans. Naringin demonstrated an anxiolytic-like effect in mice placed in the elevated plus maze.[107] It also reduced anxiety-like behaviors of rats exposed to the insecticide deltamethrin.[108] Aside from anxiolytic effects, naringin is thought to have antidepressant and memory-enhancing properties mediated in part by antioxidant, antinitrosative, and anticholinesterase activities.[109]

5.4.27 NEROLIDOL

Nerolidol is a sesquiterpene alcohol found in plants including *Citrus spp, Zingiber officinale, Jasminum spp, Lavandula angustifolia, Melaleuca alternifolia, Cannabis sativa, Cymbopogon citratus*, and some species of *Orchidaceae*. Nerolidol showed anxiolytic activity in mice in the elevated plus maze and open field tests. Those effects were not due to diminished motor activity.[110] This sesquiterpene also diminishes pentylenetetrazol-induced kindling in mice, which is also an effect seen with benzodiazepines.[111] Along with actions mediated by the GABA-A receptor, nerolidol acts to reduce oxidative stress and neuroinflammation in the brain.[112]

5.4.28 NOBILETIN

Nobiletin is an O-methylated flavone from the peel of various species of citrus. Like several other flavonoids from citrus, it has been found have anxiolytic-like effects.

Nobiletin has been found to reduce anxiety-like behavior of mice in the elevated plus maze in murine models of Alzheimer's[113] and Parkinson's[114] diseases, both of which are neurodegenerative conditions. The anxiolytic-like effect of nobiletin may be explained by a study of its effects in a mouse model of epilepsy. In that study, nobiletin exhibited an antiseizure effect through enhancing central GABA activity while buffering glutamate activity.[115]

5.4.29 PINENE

Pinene is a bicyclic monoterpene. It can be obtained from *Cannabis sativa, Vitex agnus-castus, Foeniculum vulgare, Lavandula angustifolia, Mentha piperita, Rosmarinus officinalis, Eleutherococcus senticosus*, and other herbs. Not surprisingly, it is prominent in the sap of various species of pine trees. Pinene has produced significant anxiolytic-like effects in rodents. In one such study, the effects were accompanied by substantial enhancement of antioxidant effects of glutathione in hippocampal tissue.[116] Some effects of pinene, including the induction of sleep, can be blocked by flumazenil and are thus mediated by benzodiazepine receptors.[117] There are also indications of monoaminergic enhancement.[118]

5.4.30 RESVERATROL

Resveratrol is a stilbenoid produced by a wide variety of plants in response to injury or when the plant is under attack by pathogens.[119] It has gained a reputation as an adaptogen and longevity agent, but definitive proof is lacking.[120] In a rat model of PTSD, resveratrol reversed stress-induced anxiety-like behaviors in the open field and elevated plus maze. Those effects were accompanied by decreases in corticotropin-releasing hormone levels and increases in phosphorylation of cyclic adenosine monophosphate response element binding protein and brain-derived neurotrophic factor levels.[121] Resveratrol also exhibited anxiolytic- and antidepressant-like effects in hypothyroid rats. Those effects were also accompanied by amelioration of hyperactivity of the hypothalamic-pituitary-adrenal axis.[122] However, a meta-analysis of 225 patients found no compelling evidence of effects of resveratrol on anxiety or other aspects of mood in humans.[123] It is possible that the notoriously low bioavailability of resveratrol played a role in those results.

5.4.31 QUERCETIN

Quercetin is one of the most common flavonoids. It is found in *Citrus spp, Matricaria chamomilla, Petroselinum crispum, Salvia officinalis, Camellia sinensis, Ginkgo biloba, Cymbopogon citratus, Trifolium pratense, Ganoderma lingzhi, Schisandra chinensis, Hypericum perforatum*, and many other medicinal herbs. Quercetin is also one of the most studied phytochemicals. It has been found to be neuroprotective through its anti-inflammatory, antioxidant, antiexcitotoxic, and anticholinesterase activities. It also exerts anxiolytic-like effects in a variety of circumstances across species.[124] For example, quercetin produced anxiolytic-like effects in mice in the open field and elevated plus maze tests.[125] Interestingly, these effects were only partially reversed by flumazenil. Others found that anxiolytic-like effects of quercetin in mice were not blocked by flumazenil but were decreased by treatment with the GABA agonist trans-4-aminocrotonic acid, suggesting an as of yet undefined interaction with GABA receptors.[126] In yet another study, anxiolytic effects of quercetin in mice were attributed to action at serotonin 1A receptors.[127] Quercetin does not readily cross the blood-brain barrier. Thus, various methods have been tried to increase its ability to affect the brain, such as enzymatic modification or nanoencapsulation.[128]

5.4.32 ROSMARINIC ACID

Rosmarinic acid, a phenolic compound and ester of caffeic acid, is contained in *Foeniculum vulgare*, *Ocimum sanctum*, *Echium amoenum*, *Melissa officinalis*, and *Rosmarinus officinalis*. Animal studies have shown anxiolytic-like effects. Rosmarinic acid reduced stress-induced freezing behavior in mice. Interestingly, this effect occurred without reductions in spontaneous motor behavior.[129] It also ameliorated stress-induced anxiety-like behavior in rats.[130] In this latter study, the effects of rosmarinic acid were inhibited by the blockage of the ERK (extracellular signal-regulated kinase) signaling. The ERK pathway communicates signals from a variety of receptor on the surface of the cell to the DNA in the nucleus of the cell. Rosmarinic acid does enhance activity at GABA-A receptors.[131] Thus, its anxiolytic effects are likely mediated, at least in part, by GABA-A receptors.

5.4.33 URSOLIC ACID

Ursolic acid is a large, steroid-like molecule classified as a pentacyclic triterpenoid carboxylic acid. It is found in *Boswellia sacra*, *Ocimum sanctum*, *Aloysia citrodora*, *Rosmarinus officinalis*, *Salvia officinalis*, *Nardostachys jatamansi*, and other medicinal herbs. Ursolic acid has both anxiolytic and antidepressant effects in rodents. Acutely administered ursolic acid exhibits anxiolytic-like effects in mice in the open field and elevated plus maze tests but not the light/dark box or marble burying tests.[132] In rats, acute treatment reduced anxiety in both the elevated plus maze and bright and dark arena. It did so in a manner similar to the effects of diazepam.[133] Ursolic acid enhances pentobarbital-induced sleep, and that effect was attenuated by the GABA-A receptor antagonist bicuculline. Thus, the anxiolytic effects of ursolic acid may be mediated at least in part by action at GABA-A receptors.[134] Ursolic acid also produces antidepressant effects in mice that have been attributed to enhancement of serotonergic and noradrenergic activities.[135]

5.4.34 WOGONIN

Wogonin, or 5,7-dihydroxy-8-methoxyflavone, is an O-methylated flavone found in *Scutellaria baicalensis*. This herb, known by the common English name skullcap, is commonly used in traditional Chinese medicine. This flavone is also found in other *Scutellaria* species, as well as in the Indian plant *Andrographis paniculata* and in stems of the Chinese herb *Anodendron affine*.[136] Wogonin produced an anxiolytic-like effect in mice in the elevated plus maze. That effect was blocked by the benzodiazepine antagonist Ro 15–1788, indicating mediation by benzodiazepine receptors.[137]

REFERENCES

1. Youdim KA, Dobbie MS, Kuhnle G, et al. Interaction between flavonoids and the blood-brain barrier: In vitro studies. *J Neurochem.* 2003;85:180–192.
2. Jäger AK, Saaby L. Flavonoids and the CNS. *Molecules.* 2011;16:1471–1485.
3. Medina JH, Viola H, Wolfman C, et al. Overview—Flavonoids: A new family of benzodiazepine receptor ligands. *Neurochem Res.* 1997;22:419–425.
4. Braestrup C, Nielsen M. Benzodiazepine receptors. *Arznei-forschung.* 1980;30 (5a):852–857.
5. Ren LH, Wang F, Xu ZW, et al. GABA(A) receptor subtype selectivity underlying anxiolytic effect of 6-hydroxyflavone. *Biochem Pharmacol.* 2010;79:1337–1344.
6. Hanrahan JR, Chebib M, Johnston GAR. Interactions of flavonoids with ionotropic GABA receptors. *Adv Pharmacol.* 2015;72:189–266.
7. Campbell EL, Chebib M, Johnston GAR. The dietary flavonoids apigenin and ([1])-epigallocatechin gallate enhance the positive modulation by diazepam of the activation by GABA of recombinant GABAA receptors. *Biochem Pharmacol.* 2004;68:1631–1638.
8. Schroeter H, Boyd C, Spencer JPE, et al. MAPK signaling in neurodegeneration: Influences of flavonoids and of nitric oxide. *Neurobiol Aging.* 2002;23:861–880.
9. Jamal H, Ansari WH, Rizvi SJ. Evaluation of chalcones—a flavonoid subclass, for their anxiolytic effects in rats using elevated plus maze and open field behaviour tests. *Fund Clin Pharmacol.* 2008;22(6):673–681.
10. Lee YL, Wu Y, Tsang HW, et al. A systematic review on the anxiolytic effects of aromatherapy in people with anxiety symptoms. *J Altern Complement Med.* 2011;17:101–108.
11. Wang Z-J, Heinbockel T. Essential oils and their constituents targeting the GABAergic system and sodium channels as treatment of neurological diseases. *Molecules.* 2018;23:1061.
12. Citti C, Braghiroli D, Vandelli MA, et al. Pharmaceutical and biomedical analysis of cannabinoids: A critical review. *J Pharmaceut Biomed.* 2018;147:565–579.
13. Ferber SG, Namdar D, Hen-Shoval D, et al. The "entourage effect": Terpenes coupled with cannabinoids for the treatment of mood disorders and anxiety disorders. *Curr Neuropharmacol.* 2020;18(2):87–96.
14. Toyota M, Shimamura T, Ishi H, et al. New bibenzyl cannabinoid from the New Zealand Liverwort *Radula marginata. Chem Pharm Bull.* 2002;50:1390–1392.
15. Cushing D, Kristipati S, Shastri R, et al. Measuring the bioactivity of phytocannabinoid cannabidiol from cannabis sources, and a novel non-cannabis source. *J Med Phyto Res.* 2018;1:8–23.
16 Raduner S, Majewska A, Chen JZ, et al. Alkylamides from Echinacea are a new class of cannabinomimetics. Cannabinoid type 2 receptor-dependent and -independent immunomodulatory effects. *J Biol Chem.* 2006;281:14192–14206.
17. Wagner H, Nörr H, Winterhoff H. Plant adaptogens. *Phytomedicine.* 1994;1(1):63–76.
18. Ulmann A, Menard J, Corvol P. Binding of glycyrrhetinic acid to kidney mineralocorticoid and glucocorticoid receptors. *Endocrinology.* 1975;97(1):46–51.
19. Djerassi C. Steroid research at Syntex: "the pill" and cortisone". *Steroids.* 1992;57(12):631–641.
20. Böttger A, Vothknecht U, Bolle C. Alkaloids. In: *Lessons on Caffeine, Cannabis & Co.* Berlin: Springer; 2018. pp. 179–203.
21. Mayer B. How much nicotine kills a human? Tracing back the generally accepted lethal dose to dubious self-experiments in the nineteenth century. *Arch Toxicol.* 2014;88(1):5–7.
22. Schultes RE. Indole alkaloids in plant hallucinogens. *J Psychedel Drug.* 1976;8(1):7–25.

23. Bouso JC, Ona G, dos Santos RG, et al. Psychedelic medicines in major depression: Progress and future challenges. In: YK Kim (Eds.), *Major Depressive Disorder: Current Research and Management Approaches.* Singapore: Springer Nature; 2021.
24. Han H, Ma Y, Eun JS, et al. Anxiolytic-like effects of sanjoinine A isolated from Zizyphi spinosi semen: Involvement of GABA receptors. *Planta Med.* 2008;74–PA99.
25. Tuenter E, Exarchou V, Apers S, et al. Cyclopeptide alkaloids. *Phytochem Rev.* 2017;16:623–637.
26. Elisabetsky E, Costa-Campos L. The alkaloid alstonine: A review of its pharmacological properties. *Evid-Base Compl Alt Med.* 2005;3:39–48.
27. Ingale AG, Hivrale AU. Pharmacological studies of *Passiflora sp.* And their bioactive compounds. *Afr J Plant Sci.* 2010;4:417–426.
28. Kimura Y, Sumiyoshi M. Effects of various *Eleutherococcus senticosus* cortex on swimming time, natural killer activity and corticosterone level in forced swimming stressed mice. *J Ethnopharmacol.* 2004;95:447–453.
29. Marques de Carvalho RS, Duarte FS, Monteiro de Lima TC. Involvement of GABAergic non-benzodiazepine sites in the anxiolytic-like and sedative effects of the flavonoid baicalein in mice. *Behav Brain Res.* 2011;221(1):75–82.
30. Perfumi M, Mattioli L. Adaptogenic and central nervous system effects of single doses of 3% rosavin and 1% salidroside *Rhodiola rosea* L. extract in mice. *Phytother Res.* 2007;21(1):37–43.
31. Ishola IO, Chatterjee M, Tota S, et al. Antidepressant and anxiolytic effects of amentoflavone isolated from *Cnestis ferruginea* in mice. *Pharmacol Biochem Behav.* 2012;103(2):322–331.
32. Hanrahan JR, Chebib M, Davucheron NL, et al. Semisynthetic preparation of amentoflavone: A negative modulator at GABA(A) receptors. *Bioorg Med Chem Lett.* 2003;13(14):2281–2284.
33. Katavic PL, Lamb K, Navarro H, et al. Flavonoids as opioid receptor ligands: Identification and preliminary structure-activity relationships. *J Nat Prod.* 2007;70(8):1278–1282.
34. Chavkin C. Kappa-opioid antagonists as stress resilience medications for the treatment of alcohol use disorders. *Neuropsychopharmacology.* 2018;43(9):1803–1804.
35. Zhou X, Wang F, Zhou R, et al. Apigenin: A current review on its beneficial biological activities. *J Food Biochem.* 2017;41(4):e12376.
36. Kumar S, Sharma A. Apigenin: The anxiolytic constituent of *Turnera aphrodisiaca.* *Pharm Biol.* 2006;44(2):84–90.
37. Gazola AC, Costa GM, Castellanos L, et al. Involvement of GABAergic pathway in the sedative activity of apigenin, the main flavonoid from *Passiflora quadrangularis* pericarp. *Rev Bras Farmacog.* 2015;25:158–163.
38. de Oliveira DD, da Silva CP, Iglesias BB, et al. Vitexin possesses anticonvulsant and anxiolytic-like effects in murine animal models. *Front Pharmacol.* 2020;11:1181.
39. Aseervathama GSB, Suryakalaa U, Doulethunisha, et al. Expression pattern of NMDA receptors reveals antiepileptic potential of apigenin 8-C-glucoside and chlorogenic acid in pilocarpine induced epileptic mice. *Biomed Pharmacother.* 2016;82:54–64.
40. Yi L-T, Li J-M, Li Y-C, et al. Antidepressant-like behavioral and neurochemical effects of the citrus-associated chemical apigenin. *Life Sci.* 2008;82(13–14):741–751.
41. de Carvalho RSM, Duarte FS, de Lima TCM. Involvement of GABAergic non-benzodiazepine sites in the anxiolytic-like and sedative effects of the flavonoid baicalein in mice. *Behav Brain Res.* 2011;221(1):75–82.
42. Li Y-C, Shen J-D, Liu Y-M, et al. Screening of antidepressant effects of four main flavonoids compounds from *Scutellaria baicalensis.* *Chinese J Exper Trad Med Form.* 2012;18:166–169.
43. Scandiffio R, Geddo F, Cottone E, et al. Protective effects of (E)-β-Caryophyllene (BCP) in chronic inflammation. *Nutrients.* 2020;12(11):3273.

44. Bahi A, Al Mansouri S, Al Memari E. β-Caryophyllene, a CB2 receptor agonist produces multiple behavioral changes relevant to anxiety and depression in mice. *Physiol Behav.* 2014;135:119–124.

45. da Silva Oliveira GL, da Silva JCC, dos Santos CL, et al. Anticonvulsant, anxiolytic and antidepressant properties of the β-caryophyllene in Swiss mice: Involvement of benzodiazepine-GABAAergic, serotonergic and nitrergic systems. *Curr Mol Pharmacol.* 2021;14:36–51.

46. Tabari MA, Tehrani MAB. Evidence for the involvement of the GABAergic, but not serotonergic transmission in the anxiolytic-like effect of bisabolol in the mouse elevated plus maze. *N-S Arch Pharmacol.* 2017;390:1041–1046.

47. Barreto RSS, Quintans JSS, Amarante RKL, et al. Evidence for the involvement of TNF-α and IL-1β in the antinociceptive and anti-inflammatory activity of *Stachys lavandulifolia* Vahl. (*Lamiaceae*) essential oil and (-)-α-bisabolol, its main compound, in mice. *J Ethnopharmacol.* 2016;191:9–18.

48. Boerjan W, Ralph J, Baucher M. Lignin biosynthesis. *Ann Rev Plant Biol.* 2003;54:519–546.

49. Lorigooini Z, Nasiri boroujeni S, Balali-Dehkordi S, et al. Possible involvement of NMDA receptor in the anxiolytic-like effect of caffeic acid in mice model of maternal separation stress. *Heliyon.* 2020;6(9):e04833.

50. Monteiro AB, de Souza Rodrigues CK, do Nascimento EP, et al. Anxiolytic and antidepressant-like effects of *Annona coriacea* (Mart.) and caffeic acid in mice. *Food Chem Toxicol.* 2020;136:111049.

51. Woo J, Yang H, Yoon M, et al. 3-Carene, a phytoncide from pine tree has a sleep-enhancing effect by targeting the GABAA-benzodiazepine receptors. *Exp Neurobiol.* 2019;28(5):593–601.

52. Kumar D, Kumar S. Screening of antianxiety activity of *Abies pindrow* Royle aerial parts. *Indian J Pharm Ed Res.* 2015;49(1):66–70.

53. Melo FHC, Venâncio ET, De Sousa DP. Anxiolytic-like effect of carvacrol (5-isopropyl-2-methylphenol) in mice: Involvement with GABAergic transmission. *Fundament Clin Pharmacol.* 2010;24(4):437–443.

54. Naeem K, Al Kury LT, Nasar F. Natural dietary supplement, carvacrol, alleviates LPS-induced oxidative stress, neurodegeneration, and depressive-like behaviors via the Nrf2/HO-1 pasthway. *J Inflamm Res.* 2021;14:1313–1329.

55. Brown E, Hurd NS, McCall S, et al. Evaluation of the anxiolytic effects of chrysin, a *Passiflora incarnate* extract in the laboratory rat. *AANA J.* 2007;75(5):333–337.

56. Germán-Ponciano LJ, Puga-Olguín A, Rovirosa-Hernández MJ, et al. Differential effects of acute and chronic treatment with the flavonoid chrysin on anxiety-like behavior and Fos immunoreactivity in the lateral septal nucleus in rats. *Acta Pharm.* 2020;70:387–397.

57. German-Ponciano LJ, Rosas-Sánchez GU, Ortiz-Guerra SI, et al. Effects of chrysin on mRNA expression of 5-HT1A and 5-HT2A receptors in the raphe nuclei and hippocampus. *Rev Bras Farmacogn.* 2021;31:353–360.

58. Jang SW, Liu X, Yepes M, et al. A selective TrkB agonist with potent neurotrophic activities by 7,8-dihydroxyflavone. *Proc Natl Acad Sci USA.* 2010;107(6):2687–2692.

59. Wang N, Liu X, Li XT, et al. 7,8-Dihydroxyflavone alleviates anxiety-like behavior induced by chronic alcohol exposure in mice involving tropomyosin-related kinase B in the amygdala. *Mol Neurobiol.* 2021;58:92–105.

60. Ríos J-L, Giner RM, Marín M, et al. A pharmacological update of ellagic acid. *Planta Med.* 2018;84(15):1068–1093.

61. Girish C, Raj V, Arya J, et al. Involvement of the GABAergic system in the anxiolytic-like effect of the flavonoid ellagic acid in mice. *Eur J Pharmacol.* 2013;710(1–3):49–58.

62. Huang X, Li W, You B, et al. Serum metabonomic study on the antidepressant-like effects of ellagic acid in a chronic unpredictable mild stress-induced mouse model. *J Agri Food Chem.* 2020;68(35):9546–9556.

63. Wang J, Li P, Qin T, et al. Protective effect of epigallocatechin-3-gallate against neuro-inflammation and anxiety-like behavior in a rat model of myocardial infarction. *Brain Behav.* 2020;10(6):e01633.

64. Lee B, Shim I, Lee H, et al. Effects of epigallocatechin gallate on behavioral and cognitive impairments, hypothalamic—pituitary—adrenal axis dysfunction, and alternations in hippocampal BDNF expression under single prolonged stress. *J Med Food.* 2018;21:979–989.

65. Park K-S, Oh JH, Yoo H-S, et al. (–)-Epigallocatechin-3-O-gallate (EGCG) reverses caffeine-induced anxiogenic-like effects. *Neurosci Let.* 2010;481(2):131–134.

66. Scholey A, Downey LA, Ciorciari J, et al. Acute neurocognitive effects of epigallocatechin gallate (EGCG). *Appetite.* 2012;58:767–770.

67. Platero JP, Cuerda-Ballester M, Ibáñez V, et al. The impact of coconut oil and epigallocatechin gallate on the levels of IL-6, anxiety and disability in multiple sclerosis patients. *Nutrients.* 2020;12(2):305.

68. Campbell EL, Chebib M, Johnston GAR. The dietary flavonoids apigenin and (–)-epigallocatechin gallate enhance the positive modulation by diazepam of the activation by GABA of recombinant GABAA receptors. *Biochem Pharmacol.* 2004;68(8):1631–1638.

69. Siyal FJ, Zahida Memon Z, Siddiqui RA. Eugenol and liposome-based nanocarriers loaded with eugenol protect against anxiolytic disorder via down regulation of neurokinin-1 receptors in mice. *Pak J Pharm Sci.* 2020;33(Suppl 5):2275–2284.

70. Sahin S, Eulenburg V, Heinlein A, et al. Identification of eugenol as the major determinant of GABA-A-receptor activation by aqueous *Syzygium aromaticum* L. (clove buds) extract. *J Funct Food.* 2017;37:641–649.

71. Tao G, Irie Y, Li D-J. Eugenol and its structural analogs inhibit monoamine oxidase A and exhibit antidepressant-like activity. *Bioorgan Med Chem.* 2005;13(15):4777–4788.

72. Kotwal S, Upaganlawar AB, Mahajan M, et al. Protective effects of ferulic acid in alcohol withdrawal induced anxiety and depression in mice. *Malays J Med Biol Res.* 2015;2:231–236.

73. Chen J, Lin D, Zhang C, et al. Antidepressant-like effects of ferulic acid: Involvement of serotonergic and norepinergic systems. *Metab Brain Dis.* 2015;30:129–136.

74. Lorigooini Z, Nouri A, Mottaghinia F, et al. Ferulic acid through mitigation of NMDA receptor pathway exerts anxiolytic-like effect in mouse model of maternal separation stress. *J Bas Clin Physiol Pharmacol.* 2021;32(1):20190263.

75. Kavvadias D, Abou-Mandour AA, Czygan F-C, et al. Identification of benzodiazepines in *Artemisia dracunculus* and *Solanum tuberosum* rationalizing their endogenous formation in plant tissue. *Biochem Biophys Res Commun.* 2000;269:290–295.

76. Liao Y-H, Lee H-J, Huang W-J, et al. Hispidulin alleviated methamphetamine-induced hyperlocomotion by acting at α6 subunit-containing GABAA receptors in the cerebellum. *Psychopharmacology.* 2016;233:3187–3199.

77. Kavvadias D, Sand P, Youdim KA. The flavone hispidulin, a benzodiazepine receptor ligand with positive allosteric properties, traverses the blood—brain barrier and exhibits anticonvulsive effects. *Br J Pharmacol.* 2004 Jul;142(5):811–820.

78. Abdelhalim A, Khan I, Karim N. The contribution of ionotropic gabaergic and N-methyl-D-aspartic acid receptors in the antidepressant-like effects of hispidulin. *Phcog Mag.* 2019;15(62):62–70.

79. Orzelska-Gorka J, Szewczyk K, Kedzierska E, et al. Hyperoside isolated from *Impatiens glandulifera* Royle alleviates depressive and anxiety-like responses in a mouse model of posttraumatic stress disorder. *Acta Neurobiol Exp.* 2019;79(Suppl 1).

80. Zheng M, Liu C, Pan F, et al. Antidepressant-like effect of hyperoside isolated from *Apocynum venetum* leaves: Possible cellular mechanisms. *Phytomedicine.* 2012;19(2):145–149.

81. Xiao H, Wignall N, Brown ES. An open-label pilot study of icariin for co-morbid bipolar and alcohol use disorder. *Am J Drug Alc Abuse.* 2016;42(2):162–167.

82. Liu B, Xu C, Wu X, et al. Icariin exerts an antidepressant effect in an unpredictable chronic mild stress model of depression in rats and is associated with the regulation of hippocampal neuroinflammation. *Neurosci.* 2015;294:193–205.

83. Gonga M-J, Han B, Wang S, et al. Icariin reverses corticosterone-induced depression-like behavior, decrease in hippocampal brain-derived neurotrophic factor (BDNF) and metabolic network disturbances revealed by NMR-based metabonomics in rats. *J Pharmaceut Biomed.* 2016;123:63–73.

84. Silva MIG, Neto MRA, Neto PFT, et al. Central nervous system activity of acute administration of isopulegol in mice. *Pharmacol Biochem Behav.* 2007;88(2):141–147.

85. Silva MIG, Silva MAG, Neto MRA, et al. Effects of isopulegol on pentylenetetrazol-induced convulsions in mice: Possible involvement of GABAergic system and antioxidant activity. *Fitoterapia.* 2009;80(8):506–513.

86. Zarei M, Sarihi A, Ahmadimoghaddam D, et al. Effects of intracerebroventricular micro-injection of kaempferol on anxiety: Possible GABAergic mechanism involved. *Avicenna J Neuro Psycho Physiol.* 2021;8(2):109–114.

87. Ahmad H, Rauf K, Zadas W et al. Kaempferol facilitated extinction learning in contextual fear conditioned rats via inhibition of fatty-acid amide hydrolase. *Molecules.* 2020;25(20):4683.

88. Bigdeli Y, Asle-Rousta M, Rahnema M. Effects of limonene on chronic restraint stress-induced memory impairment and anxiety in male rats. *Neurophysiology.* 2019;51:107–113.

89. Song Y, Seo S, Lamichhane S, et al. Limonene has anti-anxiety activity via adenosine A2A receptor-mediated regulation of dopaminergic and GABAergic neuronal function in the striatum. *Phytomedicine.* 2021;83:153474.

90. Cline M, Taylor J, Flores J, et al. Investigation of the anxiolytic effects of linalool, a lavender extract, in the male Sprague-Dawley rat. *AANA J.* 2008;76(1):47–52.

91. Shaw D, Norwood K, Kennedy P, et al. Effects of linalool on extinction of mouse operant behaviour. *Behav Pharmacol.* 2020;31(1):73–80.

92. Harada H, Kashiwadani H, Kanmura Y, et al. Linalool odor-induced anxiolytic effects in mice. *Front Behav Neurosci.* 2018;12:241.

93. Hecksel R, LaVigne J, Streicher JM. In defense of the "entourage effect": Terpenes found in cannabis sativa activate the cannabinoid receptor 1 in vitro. *FASEB.* 2020;34:1.

94. Guimarães AG, Quintans JSS, Quintans-Júnior LJ. Monoterpenes with analgesic activity—a systematic review. *Phytother. Res.* 2013;27:1–15.

95. Gadotti VM, Zamponi GW. Anxiolytic effects of the flavonoid luteolin in a mouse model of acute colitis. *Mol Brain.* 2019;12:114.

96. Coleta M, Campos MG, Cotrim MD, et al. Assessment of luteolin (3,4,5,7-tetrahydroxyflavone) neuropharmacological activity. *Behav Brain Res.* 2008;189:75–82.

97. Albishi FM, Albeshi SM, Alotaibi K, et al. The effect of menthol on anxiety and related behaviors in mice. *Bahrain Med Bull.* 2020;42(4):277–282.

98. Hall AC, Turcotte CM, Betts BA, et al. Modulation of human GABAA and glycine receptor currents by menthol and related monoterpenoids. *Eur J Pharmacol.* 2004;506(1):9–16.

99. Storey DJ, Colvin L, Boyle D, et al. A cool solution for colo-rectal cancer survivors? Topical menthol improved oxaliplatin chemotherapy induced peripheral neuropathy (OcCIPN) related pain, anxiety and catastrophizing. *Psycho-Oncology.* 2012;21(Suppl 2):9.

100. Walia V, Chaudhary SK, Sethiya NK. Therapeutic potential of mangiferin in the treatment of various neuropsychiatric and neurodegenerative disorders. *Neurochem Int.* 2021;143:104939.
101. Jangra A, Lukhi MM, Sulakhiya K, et al. Protective effect of mangiferin against lipopolysaccharide-induced depressive and anxiety-like behaviour in mice. *Eur J Pharmacol.* 2014;740:337–345.
102. Ishola IO, Awodele O, Eluogu CO. Potentials of *Mangifera indica* in the treatment of depressive-anxiety disorders: Possible mechanisms of action. *J Comp Integr Med.* 2016;13(3):275–287.
103. Mohan M, Jadhav SS, Kasture VS, et al. Effect of myricetin on behavioral paradigms of anxiety. *Pharm Biol.* 2009;47(10):927–931.
104. Zhang XH, Ma ZG, Rowlands DK, et al. Flavonoid myricetin modulates receptor activity through activation of channels and CaMK-II pathway. *eCAM.* 2012;2012:758097.
105. Chang Y, Chang C-Y, Wang S-J, et al. Myricetin inhibits the release of glutamate in rat cerebrocortical nerve terminals. *J Med Food.* 2014;18–15:516–523.
106. Ma Z, Wang G, Cui L, et al. Myricetin attenuates depressant-like behavior in mice subjected to repeated restraint stress. *Int J Mol Sci.* 2015;16(12):28377–28385.
107. Fernandez SP, Nguyen M, Yow TT, et al. The flavonoid glycosides, myricitrin, gossypin and naringin exert anxiolytic action in mice. *Neurochem Res.* 2009;34:1867–1875.
108. Mani VM, Sadiq AMM. Naringin modulates the impairment of memory, anxiety, locomotor, and emotionality behaviors in rats exposed to deltamethrin: A possible mechanism association with oxidative stress, acetylcholinesterase and ATPase. *Biomed Prev Nutr.* 2014;4(4):527–533.
109. Ben-Azu B, Nwoke EE, Aderibigbe AO, et al. Possible neuroprotective mechanisms of action involved in the neurobehavioral property of naringin in mice. *Biomed Pharmacother.* 2019;109:536–546.
110. Goel RK, Kaur D, Pahwa P. Assessment of anxiolytic effect of nerolidol in mice. *Indian J Pharmacol.* 2016;48(4):450–452.
111. Kaur D, Pahwa P, Goel RK. Protective effect of nerolidol against pentylenetetrazol-induced kindling, oxidative stress and associated behavioral comorbidities in mice. *Neurochem Res.* 2016;41:2859–2867.
112. Iqubala A, Sharma S, Najmi AK, et al. Nerolidol ameliorates cyclophosphamide-induced oxidative stress, neuroinflammation and cognitive dysfunction: Plausible role of Nrf2 and NF- κB. *Life Sci.* 2019;236:116867.
113. Fakour M, Kiasalari Z, Ghasemi R, et al. The effect of nobiletin on behavioral function in elevated plus maze and forced swimming tests in intrahippocampal amyloid beta-induced model of Alzheimer's disease in the rat. *Daneshvar Med.* 2019;27(2):51–58.
114. Khorasani M, Kiasalari Z, Ghasemi R, et al. The effect of nobiletin on performance of rats in forced swimming and elevated plus maze tests in intranigral lipopolysaccharide rat model of Parkinson's disease. *J Bas Clin Pathophysiol.* 2020;8(1):28–34.
115. Yang B, Wang J, Zhang N. Effect of nobiletin on experimental model of epilepsy. *Trans Neurosci.* 2018;9(1):211–219.
116. Saeedipour S, Rafieirad M. Anti-anxiety effect of Alpha-pinene in comparison with Diazepam in adult male rats. *Feyz.* 2020;24(3):253–245.
117. Yang H, Woo J, Pae AN, et al. α-Pinene, a major constituent of pine tree oils, enhances non-rapid eye movement sleep in mice through GABAA-benzodiazepine receptors. *Mol Pharmacol.* 2016;90(5):530–539.
118. Guzman-Gutierrez SL, Bonilla-Jaime H, Gomez-Cansino R, et al. Linalool and β-pinene exert their antidepressant-like activity through the monoaminergic pathway. *Life Sci.* 2015;128:24–29.
119. Fremont L. Biological effects of resveratrol. *Life Sci.* 2000;668:663–673.

120. Vang O, Ahmad N, Baile CA, et al. What is new for an old molecule? Systematic review and recommendations on the use of resveratrol. *PLOS One*. 2011;6(6):e19881.
121. Li G, Wang G, Shi J, et al. trans-Resveratrol ameliorates anxiety-like behaviors and fear memory deficits in a rat model of post-traumatic stress disorder. *Neuropharmacology*. 2018;133:181–188.
122. Ge J-F, Xu Y-Y, Qin G, et al. Resveratrol ameliorates the anxiety- and depression-like behavior of subclinical hypothyroidism rat: Possible involvement of the HPT Axis, HPA Axis, and Wnt/β-Catenin pathway. *Front Endocrinol*. 2016;7:44.
123. Farzaei MH, Rahimi R, Nikfar S, et al. Effect of resveratrol on cognitive and memory performance and mood: A meta-analysis of 225 patients. *Pharmacol Res*. 2018;128:338–344.
124. Islam MS, Quispe C, Hossain R, et al. Neuropharmacological effects of quercetin: A literature-based review. *Front Pharmacol*. 2021;12:665031.
125. Murade V, Waghmare A, Pakhare D, et al. A plausible involvement of GABAA/benzo-diazepine receptor in the anxiolytic-like effect of ethyl acetate fraction and quercetin isolated from Ricinus communis Linn. leaves in mice. *Phytomed Plus*. 2021;1(3):100041.
126. Jung JW, Lee S. Anxiolytic effects of quercetin: Involvement of GABAergic system. *J Life Sci*. 2014;24:290–296.
127. Li J, Liu QT, Chen Y, et al. Involvement of 5-HT1A receptors in the anxiolytic-like effects of quercitrin and evidence of the involvement of the monoaminergic system. *eCAM*. 2016:6530364.
128. Pateiro M, Gómez B, Munekata PES, et al. Nanoencapsulation of promising bioactive compounds to improve their absorption, stability, functionality and the appearance of the final food products. *Molecules*. 2021;26(6):1547.
129. Takeda H, Tsuji M, Miyamoto J, et al. Rosmarinic acid and caffeic acid reduce the defensive freezing behavior of mice exposed to conditioned fear stress. *Psychopharmacology*. 2002;164:233–235.
130. Nie H, Peng Z, Lao N, et al. Rosmarinic acid ameliorates PTSD-like symptoms in a rat model and promotes cell proliferation in the hippocampus. *Prog Neuro-Psychopharmacol Biol Psychiatry*. 2014;51:16–22.
131. Kwon YO, Hong JT, Oh K-W. Rosmarinic acid potentiates pentobarbital-induced sleep behaviors and non-rapid eye movement (NREM) sleep through the activation of GABAA-ergic systems. *Biomol Ther (Seoul)*. 2017;25(2):105–111.
132. Colla ARS, Rosa JM, Cunha MP, et al. Anxiolytic-like effects of ursolic acid in mice. *Eur J Pharmacol*. 2015;758:171–176.
133. Pemminati S, Gopalakrishna HN, Venkatesh V, et al. Anxiolytic effect of acute administration of ursolic acid in rats. *Res J Pharm Biol Chem Sci*. 2011;2:431–437.
134. Jeon SJ, Park HJ, Gao Q, et al. Ursolic acid enhances pentobarbital-induced sleeping behaviors via GABAergic neurotransmission in mice. *Eur J Pharmacol*. 2015;762:443–448.
135. Colla AR, Oliveira A, Pazini FL, et al. Serotonergic and noradrenergic systems are implicated in the antidepressant-like effect of ursolic acid in mice. *Pharmacol Biochem Behav*. 2014;124:108–116.
136. Tai MC, Tsang SY, Chang LYF, et al. Therapeutic potential of wogonin: A naturally occurring flavonoid. *CNS Drug Rev*. 2005;11(2):141–150.
137. Hui KM, Huen MS, Wang HY, et al. Anxiolytic effect of wogonin, a benzodiazepine receptor ligand isolated from *Scutellaria baicalensis* Georgi. *Biochem Pharmacol*. 2002;64:1415–1424.

6 Herbal Treatment of Anxiety

In this chapter are discussions of herbs that have been shown in clinical studies to be effective in the treatment of anxiety. These herbs are often used individually in Western herbalism. The use of combinations of herbs is also seen in Western practice but is the general rule in traditional Chinese and Indian Ayurvedic approaches to medicine. Herbal treatments of anxiety in those latter two traditions of healing are discussed in subsequent chapters.

All the herbs included in this chapter have either been tested in clinical studies or are at least discussed in case reports as having anxiolytic effects. Included are discussions of the primary phytochemicals that have been identified in the herbs, as well as the likely mechanisms of action of the herbs and their constituent phytochemicals. There are suggestions about dosage of the herbs and information on toxicity. Also included are recommendations about the use of herbs during pregnancy. Pregnancy is not always a carefree time, and many women seek relief from what can be significant anxiety. They might suspect that natural, herbal remedies must be safe remedies, but that is not always the case. Finally, there are notes about possible interactions of these herbs with drugs.

6.1 ACORUS CALAMUS

Acorus calamus is a plant is widely cultivated in different parts of temperate and subtemperate regions of the world and is native to India, Sri Lanka, Japan, China, Burma, Mongolia, southern Russia, Europe, and the northern US. It is known as sweet flag in Western herbalism and has been used for conditions as wide ranging as colic, diarrhea, diabetes, bronchitis, inflammation, and hemorrhoids. It has also been commonly used in psychiatric conditions, particularly anxiety and depression. It has long been used in Ayurvedic medicine, where is called *vacha* or *bach*, and it is a common ingredient in combinations used to treat *chittodvega*, a syndrome similar to GAD. Various species of *Acorus* are also common ingredients in traditional Chinese medicine, including in treatment of anxiety and depression.[1]

6.1.1 ANXIOLYTIC EFFECTS

Along with many studies of its anxiolytic effects in animals, there is at least one human trial of *Acorus calamus*. In an open study without a control group, subjects diagnosed with GAD were treated with 500mg of dried a hydroethanolic extract of *Acorus calamus* twice daily over a two-month period. Symptoms were assessed at

DOI: 10.1201/9781003300281-6

baseline and after two months of treatment using Hamilton's Brief Psychiatric Rating Scale. Treatment with *Acorus calamus* significantly attenuated symptoms of anxiety, as well as reports of symptoms suggestive of depression.[2]

6.1.2   MECHANISM OF ACTION

The α- and β-asarones are likely the most important active constituents of *Acorus calamus*. Both isoforms exert anxiolytic and antidepressant-like effects in animals.[3] Other phytochemicals identified in *Acorus calamus* are terpineol, 2-alyl-5-ethoxy-4-methoxyphenol, epieudesmin, spathulenol, borneol, eugenol, galgravin, retusin, geranylacetate, sakuranin, isoelemicin, ursolic acid, apigenin, linalool, and elemicin.[4] Several of those phytochemicals are noted in this text as possessing anxiolytic-like effects.

6.1.3   DOSAGE

In the study noted prior,[2] 500mg of dried hydroalcoholic extract of *Acorus calamus* was given twice daily. In another study using dried powdered rhizome, 500mg was given twice daily.[5]

6.1.4   TOXICITY

With so many other beneficial herbs available, *Acorus calamus* is best avoided. β-asarone contained in various amounts in the herb has been found to cause hepatocellular carcinoma in animals. This has led to *Acorus calamus* being banned in Europe and the United States.[6] The *Botanical Safety Handbook* offers a surprisingly benign impression of *Acorus calamus*. They note that *Acorus calamus* from India and other Asian locales contains the highest concentrations of β-asarone, whereas *Acorus calamus* from North America contains little if any β-asarone. Nonetheless, they also confirm that all varieties of *Acorus calamus* are prohibited in foodstuff in the United States. In a paper from India, written by Ayurvedic practitioners, the dangers of β-asarone are recognized, and an elaborate *shodhana*, or detoxification process of *vacha*, is described. However, there is no verification that this process spares the patient from liver toxicity.[7]

6.1.5   SAFETY IN PREGNANCY

Considering the toxicity of β-asarone and the status of *Acorus calamus*, it is advised to avoid it in pregnancy.

6.1.6   DRUG INTERACTION

Constituents of *Acorus calamus* are known to interact with CYP3A4 and CYP2D6. In one study, effective levels of valproate and carbamazepine were increased by co-administration of *Acorus calamus* extract.[8]

6.2 AVENA SATIVA

The common oat, or *Avena sativa*, is a member of the grass family. It is native to Europe, Asia, and Northwest Africa and has been cultivated for thousands of years as a food grain. It is the same oat as in oatmeal, though for medicinal purposes, it is harvested earlier when the seeds are green in the so-called milky stage. It may be too common and simple to be seen as a serious herbal treatment. However, it contains a variety of flavonoids, flavonolignans, triterpenoid saponins, sterols, and tocols, as well as the somewhat unique indole alkaloids called avenanthramides. Oat spikelets, sprouts, and grass are used for medicinal purposes. Unfortunately, references do not always discriminate. Traditionally, *Avena sativa* has been used as a stimulant, antispasmodic, antitumor, diuretic, and neurotonic.[9]

6.2.1 ANXIOLYTIC EFFECTS

Green oat has a reputation for having a soothing, calming effect. Oat grass is among the herbs most recommended by the American Herbalists Guild to treat anxiety. On the other hand, the well-regarded German Commission E has concluded that anxiolytic effects of *Avena sativa* have not been firmly established. One recent study of adult males and females found that daily consumption of green oat extracts improved cognitive performance and reduced physiological signs of stress. However, none of those individuals had been diagnosed with anxiety disorders.[10]

6.2.2 MECHANISM OF ACTION

Several phytochemicals in oat spikelets, including apiginen, caffeic acid, kaempferol, luteolin, and ferulic acid, are known to mimic effects of benzodiazepines at GABA-A receptors in the brain and would thus be expected to produce anxiolytic effects.[11-12] Extracts of green oats have also shown a significant inhibitory effect on monoamine oxidase B.[13] That enzyme breaks down the neurotransmitters dopamine and norepinephrine in the brain, and blocking its activity may be expected to have an antidepressant-like effect. That, in turn, might help alleviate anxiety with continued treatment.

6.2.3 DOSAGE

Pursell recommends 1–2 droppers of tincture one to three times a day. Alternatively, one may make an infusion using 1 to 2 teaspoons of oat straw per cup, then drinking 1 to 4 cups a day.[14]

6.2.4 TOXICITY

In one study, authors reported some difficulty in determining the LD50. None of the doses of dried methanolic extract of *Avena sativa* that they administered to mice, in doses up to 2,000mg/kg, had any obvious toxic effects.[15] That extrapolated LD50 dose (which was not actually lethal to mice) is roughly 150g for a 75kg human adult. That is far beyond the recommended dose.

6.2.5 SAFETY IN PREGNANCY

The *Botanical Safety Handbook* notes no evidence to confirm either safety or adverse effects of *Avena sativa* during pregnancy.[16]

6.2.6 DRUG INTERACTIONS

The *Botanical Safety Handbook* notes no known interactions with drugs.

6.3 BACOPA MONNIERI

Bacopa monnieri, also known as *brahmi* or water hyssop, is a creeping perennial plant native to the warm wetlands of India. It has small oblong leaves and purple flowers. *Bacopa monnieri* leaf has been used for over 3,000 years as an Ayurvedic treatment for a range of cognitive issues. In ancient Ayurvedic texts, it is placed among the *medhya rasayana*—a class of herb thought able to sharpen memory and intellect. However, it has also been thought to improve resiliency—that is, to act as an adaptogen—and to relieve anxiety.[17]

6.3.1 ANXIOLYTIC EFFECTS

Several studies have shown ability of *Bacopa monnieri* to reduce levels of anxiety. However, none have been performed in people diagnosed to be suffering a recognized anxiety disorder. In a double-blinded study of patients aged 65 years or older with mild cognitive impairment, 12 weeks of treatment with a standardized extract of *Bacopa monnieri* improved cognitive function and significantly reduced levels of anxiety as measured by the State-Trait Anxiety Inventory.[18] In a similar study of younger healthy adults, 12 weeks of extract of *Bacopa monnieri* both improved cognitive function and reduced anxiety.[19] However, in one study,[20] only a trend was found in the ability of *Bacopa monnieri* to reduce anxiety. In another, no anxiolytic effects were seen at all.[21]

6.3.2 MECHANISM OF ACTION

Bacopa monnieri contains a unique group of complex triterpenoid saponins called bacosides, as well as the triterpenoids jujubogenins and pseudojujubogenins and their glycosides. The latter triterpenoids are also found in the herb *Zizyphus jujuba*, which is frequently used in Chinese medicine. *Bacopa monnieri* also contains the steroid-like betulinic acid, stigmastanol, stigmasterol and β-sitosterol, and the alkaloids brahmine, nicotinine, and herpestine.[22] The most active phytochemicals in *Bacopa monnieri* are thought to be the bacosides, particularly bacoside A. Bacoside A has been shown to enhance activity at GABA receptors in the brain.[23] β-sitosterol, a steroid common among medicinal herbs, on its own has an anxiolytic effect that can synergize with such effects of other phytochemicals.[24] Studies in animals have also shown that extracts of *Bacopa monnieri* affect the activities of other neurotransmitters in the brain, including acetylcholine, dopamine, serotonin, and noradrenaline. The antidepressant effects of these activities are likely to contribute to anxiolytic effects of ongoing treatment with the herb.[25]

6.3.3 DOSAGE

Easley and Horne recommend dosage of 1 to 3ml of dried leaf tincture up to three times daily, or 400 to 500mh capsules of standardized extract two times a day.[26]

6.3.4 TOXICITY

The LD50 of dried ethanolic extract of *Bacopa monnieri* in mice has been reported to be 520mg/kg.[27] This would extrapolate to roughly 40g for a human adult weighing 75kg.

6.3.5 SAFETY IN PREGNANCY

The *Botanical Safety Handbook* noted no literature regarding the safety of *Bacopa monnieri* during pregnancy.[28]

6.3.6 DRUG INTERACTIONS

A study shows that *Bacopa monnieri* extract can inhibit the activities of the cytochrome P450 enzymes CYP1A2, CYP3A4, CYP2C9, and CYP2C19. Thus, use of the herb could increase blood levels of drugs metabolized by those enzymes.[29]

6.4 *CAMELLIA SINENSIS*

Tea is the most popular brewed beverage in the world. It is brewed from the leaves of the *Camellia sinensis* plant that is native to Asia. Due to its popularity, the plant is now cultivated in most tropical and subtropical regions of the world. There are many types of tea, and differences in how each tea is processed can alter the content of phytochemicals in the finished product. Green teas are steamed to inactivate oxidizing enzymes. The result is that in comparison with oolong, red, black, and other types of tea, they contain the highest amounts of certain beneficial polyphenols.[30] To differentiate with other forms, the common term *green tea* will hereafter be used.

6.4.1 ANXIOLYTIC EFFECTS

Two recent reviews of the effects of green tea on cognition, mood, and human brain function have shown that ongoing consumption of green tea, and several of the phytochemicals it contains, can offer significant anxiolytic effects.[31–32] Indeed, one study of elderly people showed that long-term consumption of any form of tea significantly reduces the likelihood of symptoms of anxiety or depression.[33] The processing of green tea, which spares many of the anxiolytic components of the herb, makes it particularly well suited for this purpose. Interestingly, the anxiolytic effects produced by green tea are somewhat different than those produced by most other herbs. Whereas many herbs can have a mildly sedating effect, and can even relieve insomnia in higher doses, green tea produces a state of alert calmness.

Particular interest has been shown toward L-theanine, the unique amino acid found in green tea. One of the reviews[31] noted prior specially concerns L-theanine, and the conclusion was that "supplementation of 200–400mg/day of L-theanine may assist in the reduction of stress and anxiety in people exposed to stressful conditions." A study showed that green tea with caffeine removed, leaving L-theanine as the main active ingredient, relieved anxiety and "excessive stress responses" in college students.[34] Another study showed that ingestion of L-theanine significantly increased alpha wave activity in the brain.[35] This activity, measured by an electroencephalogram, indicates a state of relaxation of the mind without inducing drowsiness. It must be mentioned that at least study found that daily doses of L-theanine over 10 weeks had no beneficial effects on anxiety or sleep.[36]

6.4.2 MECHANISM OF ACTION

Among the phytochemicals in the green form of *Camellia sinensis* are the galloylated catechin, epigallocatechin-3-gallate; the phenolic acids, chlorogenic acid and caffeic acid; and the flavonoids, kaempferol, myricetin, and quercetin.[37] All those phytochemicals may contribute anxiolytic effects by enhancing GABA activity in the brain. However, among the phytochemicals found in green tea, the amino acid analogue L-theanine may be the most important actor. Neurochemical studies have shown that L-theanine can enhance serotonin, dopamine, and GABA levels in the brain. Its structure is similar to that of the natural brain chemical glutamine, and it appears to regulate glutamate activity in the brain. Glutamate tends to excite the brain; thus, dampening glutamate may produce a calming effect.[38] Of course, all types of tea prepared from *Camellia sinensis* contain significant amounts of caffeine, and it is known that too much caffeine can cause restlessness, poor sleep, heart palpitations, and other symptoms of anxiety. However, there is evidence that caffeine works together with L-theanine to sharpen focus and enhance cognition.[39] The feeling of having focus and control in itself can have an anxiolytic effect. Indeed, many people with ADHD who are treated with stimulants report feeling less anxious because they are more focused and better organized. Caffeine may also have a mild antidepressant effect in humans.[40] Thus, daily use of green tea may improve mood and thus indirectly reduce anxiety.

6.4.3 DOSAGE

There are no dose recommendations for green tea. It is generally drunk ad libitum and can be tailored to individual tastes. Nonetheless, a recommendation of 4 cups a day would be reasonable.

6.4.4 TOXICITY

Green tea has quite low toxicity. For example, the essential oil of tea leaves, one of the more potent forms of the herbs, has been reported have an oral LD50 of 8,560mg/kg in rats. The oral LD50 of EGCG in rats was estimated to be between 186.8mg/kg and 1,868mg/kg. The LD50 of tea polysaccharides was reported to be 4.19g/kg.[41] There are reports of liver toxicity.

6.4.5 SAFETY IN PREGNANCY

The *Physician's Desk Reference for Nonprescription Drugs and Dietary Supplements* recommends that pregnant women limit their intake of green tea such that caffeine intake remains below 300mg daily.[42]

6.4.6 DRUG INTERACTIONS

In the *Botanical Safety Handbook*, the warning of potential drug interaction with various forms of *Camellia sinensis* involves concerns over the caffeine they contain. Caffeine is metabolized primarily by the CYP1A2 enzyme. Thus, there can be interactions with medications also metabolized by that enzyme. It was found, for example, that co-administration of fluvoxamine can substantially increase serum caffeine levels.[43] Other medications largely metabolized by CYP1A2 with potential for interactions with caffeine from intake of stronger brews of *Camellia sinensis* include mexiletine, clozapine, psoralens, idrocilamide, phenylpropanolamine, furafylline, theophylline, and quinolones.[44]

6.5 *CANNABIS SATIVA*

Cannabis, also known as marijuana, is a genus of plants in the family *Cannabaceae*. The genus includes three species, *sativa*, *indica*, and the lesser known *ruderalis*. Cannabis is thought to have originally come from central Asia, but it has been spread by humans throughout the temperate and tropical areas of the world. For thousands of years, it has been used for fiber, recreation, and spiritual quests. It has also been used for medicinal purposes. Hippocrates did not speak of using cannabis. However, his 5th-century BCE contemporary, Herodotus, described the use of cannabis seeds by the Scythians in their mourning rituals. The Scythians likely appreciated its mind-altering effects, as they were said to toss cannabis seeds onto red-hot rocks and inhale the vapors that were released, then howl. Pliny the Elder, the 1st-century Roman historian, catalogued some medical uses of cannabis that included the drying up of leaking semen, ridding the ears of vermin, easing the pain of gout and arthritis, and treating the bellies of farm animals.[45] The Chinese used hemp for rope, cloth, and bowstrings. However, as far back as 4000 BCE, references were also made to its use as an anesthetic for surgical procedures.[46]

Cannabis was valued in the Ayurvedic medicine of ancient India. In the 3,000-year-old Atharva Veda, the ancient Sanskrit repository of "knowledge for everyday life," cannabis was described as "one the five most sacred plants on Earth" and that "a guardian angel resides in its leaves." It was said to be a "source of happiness," a "joy-giver," and a "liberator."[47] The medical use of cannabis has persisted, and among its current applications are the treatment of chronic pain, muscle spasticity, cachexia, nausea, inflammation, and seizures.

6.5.1 ANXIOLYTIC EFFECTS

Cannabis has long been thought to reduce anxiety. On the other hand, one of the most common complaints about cannabis is panic attacks and feeling "paranoid."[48] Thus, it is clear that there are many different responses to the herb. Nonetheless, it is clear that many people use cannabis to relax and relieve anxiety, and one study has shown that approximately two-thirds of patients decreased their use of prescribed anti-anxiety medications—generally benzodiazepines—after starting to use cannabis for their anxiety. About the same percentage of people no longer needed sleep medications when using cannabis.[49]

The different effects of the cannabis plant on anxiety are almost certainly due to the fact that the herb contains a variety of phytochemicals that produce quite different effects in the brain. The substance delta-9-tetrahydrocannabinol, commonly known as THC, is not only the chemical in cannabis that causes the "high" but is also likely to be the chemical responsible for the acute anxiety and panic that some people experience while smoking cannabis. In one study, high doses of pure THC produced severe anxiety in some subjects, and this was largely blocked by the addition of 15mg to 60mg of cannabidiol.[50] Cannabidiol, perhaps better known as CBD, is another phytochemical found in cannabis that does not produce the cannabis high. Curiously, in that study, the CBD on its own did not have much effect on the baseline of anxiety. Even high doses have been found to have little effect on baseline levels of anxiety.[51] However, cannabidiol has been reported to reduce anxiety in patients diagnosed with social anxiety disorder during a public speaking exercise.[52] Public speaking is one of the most difficult tasks for such people. The dose of CBD given in that study was much larger than the doses seen in commercially available vials of "CBD oil." In this study subjects received 600mg of CBD, whereas 10mg or 20mg is the usual dose derived from a dropper full of the typical commercial product. In another study, administration of 400mg of CBD to subjects who had been diagnosed with GAD reduced anxiety during an anxiety-provoking brain scan procedure.[53] The brain scan also showed that changes in blood flow in the brain were consistent with what is typically seen when anxiety is reduced.

Studies have found that strains of cannabis with high contents of CBD in relation to their THC content are less likely to cause anxiety and panic and may be a good choice for people using cannabis to relax and ease anxiety.[54]

6.5.2 MECHANISM OF ACTION

Cannabis contains a variety of unique, structurally related phytochemicals collectively known as cannabinoids. The best known of these substances are THC and CBD. However, there are scores of other cannabinoids of varying importance and concentration in cannabis. Among those are tetrahydrocannabinolic acid, delta-8-tetra-hydrocannabinol, cannabigerol, cannabichromene, cannabinol, cannabicitran, cannabidiolic acid, cannabielsoin, cannflavin, and others. The plant also contains a wide variety of flavonoids and terpenes that may contribute medicinal effects. These include some phytochemicals that are found in other medicinal plants, such as borneol, camphor, β-caryophyllene, geraniol, humulene, linalool, myrcene, pinene, terpineol, and others.[55]

The THC in cannabis produces the high that many people enjoy. Thus, it is difficult to say that THC invariably has adverse effects. However, it can cause panic. Thankfully, CBD, especially in high doses, can relieve the THC-induced panic effect of cannabis and may help relieve other forms of anxiety as well.[56] This may be due to action at cannabinoid receptors. However, CBD may also produce anxiolytic effects through action at 5-HT1A receptors.[57] The terpenoids and flavonoids in cannabis are likely to act at GABA and possibly other receptors in the brain as well. The rather unique mechanisms by which cannabis can reduce anxiety suggests that it may be additive with other anxiety-relieving herbs.[58]

6.5.3 DOSAGE

Because of the variance of strength of cannabis and the means by which it is commonly used—that is, by smoking until the subjective sense of a satisfying degree of intoxication—it is difficult to determine precisely what doses of THC are required to produce specific effects. Therapeutic use of the FDA-approved form of THC, dronabinol, is commonly in doses of 2.5–40mg daily, with a maximum approved dose of 150mg daily.[59] Commercially available cannabidiol is often dispensed in doses of 10mg taken several times a day. I note, however that in a study of treatment of schizophrenia, patients were started on 40mg cannabidiol a day, and this was increased up to 1,280mg/day without adverse effects.[60]

6.5.4 TOXICITY

Cannabis appears to have very low acute toxicity. In rats, the intragastric LD50 of THC in oil vehicle was reported to be 800mg/kg, whereas the intravenous and inhaled LD50s were roughly the same at 36–40mg/kg.[61] In another study, the dried ethanolic extract of intact cannabis, which was 3% THC, was gavaged into the stomachs of male albino rats. The LD50 of that extract was 1,729.6mg/kg, or about 50mg THC/kg.[62] That finding compares well with the prior findings for intravenous and inhaled THC. Extrapolated to an adult human of 75kg, this would be a very large dose of about 3,600mg THC.

In experienced male cannabis smokers, daily oral THC doses of 10–30mg every 4 hours escalating to 210mg/day caused no obvious toxic effects but did begin to cause tolerance in subjective effects and physiological signs after several weeks.[63]

6.5.5 SAFETY IN PREGNANCY

Linn et al. found no statistical difference in likelihood of adverse pregnancy outcomes among women who continued to smoke cannabis. However, they advised against its use in pregnancy due to lack of definitive information.[64] A later study by Fergusson et al. drew a similar conclusion.[65] Many women have reported cannabis to be very effective in relieving the nausea of morning sickness during pregnancy.[66] Ironically, there have also been reports of cannabis causing the so-called cannabinoid hyperemesis syndrome during pregnancy.[67]

6.5.6 DRUG INTERACTIONS

CBD is metabolized primarily by the CYP3A4, CYP2C19, and CYP2C19 enzymes in the liver.[68] THC is metabolized primarily by CYP2C9 and CYP3A4.[69] Thus, cannabis can potentially alter blood levels of certain medications that are also metabolized by those enzymes.

Cannabis has also been reported to enhance the pain-relieving effects of opiates, which is of importance for treatment of both pain and substance abuse. This interaction is not due to competition for P450 enzymes in the liver but rather to synergistic interactions between respective G proteins within neurons.[70]

6.6   CENTELLA ASIATICA

Centella asiatica is commonly known as gotu kola. It is a perennial herbaceous creeper belonging to the family *Umbellifere*. It is found throughout India in moist places up to an altitude of 1,800m. It is found in swampy areas of other tropical and subtropical countries including Pakistan, Sri Lanka, Madagascar, South Africa, the South Pacific, and eastern Europe. Known as *mandukparni*, Indian pennywort, or *jalbrahmi*, it has been used as a medicine in the Ayurvedic tradition of India for thousands of years and was described in the ancient Indian medical text *Sushruta Samhita*. *Centella asiatica* was also known to the ancient Chinese herbalists and was referred to as a "miracle elixir of life." The herb has been used for the treatment of various skin conditions such as leprosy, lupus, varicose ulcers, eczema, psoriasis, diarrhea, fever, amenorrhea, diseases of the female genitourinary tract, and for relieving anxiety and improving cognition. In Ayurveda, it is one of the main herbs for revitalizing the nerves and brain cells, and it has been relied upon to treat emotional disorders such as depression.[71]

6.6.1 ANXIOLYTIC EFFECTS

Sudden loud noises cause people to lift their shoulders and duck their heads in what is called the startle response. People who are anxious and under stress are more easily startled by loud noises. A study found that a single dose of *Centella asiatica* significantly attenuates startle response in healthy human subjects. This suggests an anxiolytic effect of the herb.[72] A subsequent and more specific study found that 60 days of daily treatment with *Centella asiatica* significantly reduced symptoms of anxiety in individuals diagnosed with GAD per the Hamilton's Brief Psychiatric Rating Scale. The herb not only reduced anxiety but also significantly reduced symptoms of depression.[73] In yet another study, 500mg of *Centella asiatica* per day for 1 month significantly reduced subjective complaints of anxiety, muscle tension, fear, and insomnia.[74]

6.6.2 MECHANISM OF ACTION

The primary active constituents of *Centella asiatica* are thought to be triterpenoids. The total extract also contains tannins, sterols, flavonoids, and other components including brahmosides, brahminosides, madecassoside, β-caryophyllene, trans-β a-pharnesen, germachrene D, campesterol, sitosterol, stigmasterol, chercetin, kempferol, hydrochotine, and vallerine.[75] In vitro and in vivo research has found the triterpene asiaticoside to be the main active constituent responsible for the anxiolytic activity.[76]

Research in rats has linked triterpenes in *Centella asiatica* to increased brain levels of serotonin, noradrenaline, and dopamine together with reduced serum corticosterone levels.[77] Some of the anxiolytic effects of *Centella asiatica* were due to action at benzodiazepine receptors, as the anxiolytic effect of the extract in rats were diminished with flumazenil.[78] *Centella asiatica* also appears to enhance the effects of GABA in the brain by inhibiting GABA transaminase, the enzyme that breaks down GABA.[79]

6.6.3 DOSAGE

Easley and Horne recommend 500 to 1,000mg capsules of dried leaf powder three times a day. Alternatively, they suggest tincture of fresh plant (1:2 95% alcohol) or dried plant (1:5, 40% alcohol), 1 to 4ml, three times a day.[80]

6.6.4 TOXICITY

The LD50 of *Centella asiatica* in mice is reported be over 4,000mg/kg, which is far beyond the typical human dosage.[81]

6.6.5 SAFETY IN PREGNANCY

It has been reported that chronic treatment with *Centella asiatica* may prevent women from becoming pregnant by causing spontaneous abortion.[82] Because there is little or no information regarding the safety of *Centella asiatica* during breastfeeding, nursing mothers are advised to refrain from taking this herb.

6.6.6 DRUG INTERACTIONS

A 2010 review of the pharmacological effects of *Centella asiatica* noted "no reports documenting negative interactions between *Centella asiatica* and medications to date." The only caveat was that high doses can be sedating and that they could possibly enhance the effects of soporiphics and sedating anxiolytics.[83] However, at least one study has shown extracts of *Centella asiatica* to exert non-competitive inhibitory effects on CYP3A4 and CYP2D6 enzymes in human liver microsomes.[84]

6.7 CINNAMOMUM SPP

Cinnamon is a spice obtained from the inner bark of several tree species from the genus *Cinnamomum*. *Cinnamomum zeylanicum*, or "true cinnamon," is indigenous to Sri Lanka and southern parts of India. There is also *Cinnamomum cassia*, known as Chinese cinnamon. Cinnamon in its various forms was known by the ancients and highly prized. It has been used primarily as a food spice but also has a long history of use as a medicinal herb. In Ayurvedic medicine, cinnamon is considered a remedy for respiratory, digestive, and gynecological ailments. Modern research has established that *Cinnamomum* species can be used to lower blood sugar, kill bacteria, and reduce high blood pressure. A significant difference between "true" cinnamon and Chinese cinnamon is that Chinese cinnamon can contain much higher, even potentially dangerous, levels of coumarin.[85]

6.7.1 ANXIOLYTIC EFFECTS

Cinnamomum spp are some of the few herbs that have been shown to have antidepressant effects in humans. A study showed that patients who remained depressed during treatment with the antidepressant fluoxetine improved after the addition of cinnamon to their treatment regimen. In traditional Mexican folk medicine, cinnamon is one of a number of herbs used to treat *nervios*, which is the local term for anxiety. At least three published studies have demonstrated anxiolytic effects of cinnamon. However, each of those studies evaluated normal, healthy subjects, and none that had been diagnosed with an anxiety disorder.

In one study, the anxiolytic effect of cinnamon oil was compared with that of 5mg of diazepam in patients about to undergo surgery.[86] The Spielberger State-Trait Anxiety Inventory was administered before those treatments and 1 hour before surgery. Results shows that both treatments significantly reduced anxiety in those presurgical patients. There was no difference in the anxiety-reducing effects of the cinnamon versus the benzodiazepine diazepam. In a second study, the memories and levels of anxiety of high school students were tested before and after chewing gum infused with cinnamon. The cinnamon gum significantly improved memory and reduced anxiety as measured by the Hamilton Anxiety Rating Scale.[87]

6.7.2 MECHANISM OF ACTION

Among the phytochemicals in the various species of *Cinnamomum* are cinnamaldehyde—the predominant molecule—as well as cinnamic acid, cinnamyl alcohol, coumarin, eugenol, linalool, benzyl benzoate, and δ-cadinene.[88] Cinnamaldehyde extracted from cinnamon has been found on its own to have anxiolytic effects in animals.[89] Linalool, eugenol, cinnamic acid, and coumarin all enhance GABA activity in the brain, which offers an anxiolytic effect. Extracts of cinnamon have also been found to relive pain, and cinnamon is one of the few herbs that has been shown to significantly relieve symptoms of depression.[90] Both pain and depression can exacerbate anxiety.

6.7.3 DOSAGE

Easley and Horne suggest doses to be 0.5 to 2g cinnamon bark three times a day, 30 to 60 drops of tincture (1:5, 60% alcohol) up to three times daily, or 0.05 to 0.2g essential oil per day.[91]

6.7.4 TOXICITY

The LD50 in mice of essential oil is 2.65 to 3.5g/kg.[92] In tests of the toxicity of dried aqueous extracts of cinnamon in rats, it was found that kidney damage began to appear at doses as low as 0.1g/kg. There were no animal deaths at doses up to 2g/kg. However, there were signs of serious liver and kidney toxicity at that dose.[93] However, those doses are above typical doses of aqueous cinnamon in human studies, where 500mg of dried aqueous extract per day have been used. Moreover, it was noted, "In all the human studies involving cinnamon, or aqueous extracts of cinnamon, there have been no reported adverse events."[94]

6.7.5 SAFETY IN PREGNANCY

Traditional Chinese medical texts advise not to use cinnamon during pregnancy.[95] In animal studies, high doses of cinnamaldehyde isolated from cinnamon were found to increase rates of fetal malformations.[96]

6.7.6 DRUG INTERACTIONS

The *Botanical Safety Handbook* notes no known interactions with drugs.[97] However, one review has suggested caution when using with medications metabolized by P450 enzymes CY1A2 and CY2E1, as *Cinnamomum* species may interfere with their metabolism.[98]

6.8 CITRUS AURANTIUM

Citrus aurantium, known commonly as bitter orange, comes from China, where for centuries it was seen as a valuable medicinal herb. It later came to use by Arabian physicians and then on to Europe, where it was used most often as a perfume. Many parts of the orange tree are used as medicine. The volatile oils can be extracted from almost all parts, with subtle differences between those from the flower, leaves, or fruit. The oil extracted from the blossoms, called neroli oil after the princess that popularized it, contains large percentages of the fragrant terpenes linalool and limonene. Those two substances are also found in other fragrant herbs, most notably *Lavandula angustifolia*. The orange peel, while being a source of the essential oil bergamot, is also a rich source of flavonoids and alkaloids with medicinal properties. Caution must be exercised when the peel is used as medicine. Some of the sympathomimetic alkaloids in the peel can be used for weight loss but may cause significant heart problems, such as high blood pressure. Nonetheless, a preparation from the inner peel of the closely related bergamot orange is bergamot oil, the herbal fragrance and flavor in Earl Grey tea, and is recognized as safe for moderate consumption.[99]

6.8.1 ANXIOLYTIC EFFECTS

In the existing studies of human subjects, only the blossoms—not the fruit or rind—of *Citrus aurantium* were utilized. In one such study, patients about to undergo minor lower limb surgery drank a small glass of either salt water or distillate of petals and stamen of *Citrus aurantium*; 2 hours later, just before being taken to surgery, patients who had ingested the *Citrus aurantium* had significantly reduced levels of anxiety.[100]

6.8.2 MECHANISM OF ACTION

The flesh, peel, and essential oil of *Citrus aurantium* contain a wide variety of phytochemicals, including saponins, terpenes, flavonoids, and alkaloids.[101] Linalool from the oil is known to have anxiolytic properties. Some of linalool's effects are blocked by flumazenil, which indicates that it is acting as a weak benzodiazepine.[102] The oil also contains a variety of flavonoids and similar molecules called coumarins. Coumarin is the sweet smell of new-mowed hay. Many of these compounds are shared with other herbs and are known to act at GABA-A receptors. However, some of the most important biologically active constituents of the peel of bitter orange are substances like phenethylamine, octopamine, synephrine, tyramine, and N-methyltyramine that can mimic the fight-or-flight response.[103] Thus, care should be taken by those with major physical components to their anxiety response, such as heart racing, palpitations, sweating, and shaking.

6.8.3 DOSAGE

In the clinical study noted above,[100] flower petals and stamens of *Citrus aurantium* were steam distilled and standardized to 10ppm linalool, 3.3% phenolics, and 2.9% flavonoids. The dose each subject received was 1ml per kilogram of weight.

6.8.4 TOXICITY

Extract of *Citrus aurantium* appears to be very well tolerated. All female rats orally administered 5,000mg/kg of the extract survived. Administration at 2,000mg/kg per day to female rats over 4 days yielded no signs of toxicity.[104]

6.8.5 SAFETY IN PREGNANCY

The *Botanical Safety Handbook* notes that information of the safety of *Citrus aurantium* during pregnancy is limited. They do note that in traditional Chinese medicine, pregnant women are advised to avoid it.[105]

6.8.6 DRUG INTERACTION

Components of *Citrus aurantium* have been found to inhibit CYP3A4. However, the *Botanical Safety Handbook* found no indications of important drug interactions.

6.9 *CONVOLVULUS PLURICAULIS*

Convolvulus pluricaulis is one of several Ayurvedic herbs referred to as *shankha-pushpi*. (The herb sometimes appears in the literature as *shankhpushpi*.) It has been shown to have anxiolytic effects in humans and is a common ingredient in herbal combinations to treat a variety of mental illnesses. It is a species of morning glory. Another such herb, *Evolvulus alsinoides*—the dwarf morning glory—has also been found to have anxiolytic effects in human trials and is discussed later. *Convolvulus pluricaulis* is an ancient treatment and was recommended by Araya Charaka, the sage and developer of Ayurvedic medicine.[106]

6.9.1 ANXIOLYTIC EFFECTS

In a clinical study, subjects were diagnosed with GAD per *DSM* criteria. The symptoms were also consistent with the Ayurvedic diagnosis of *chittodvega*. Some subjects received 6 weeks of the active control treatment of *jaladhara*—that is, the pouring of warm water on the forehead. This treatment is similar to *shirodhara*, in which herb-infused oil is poured onto the forehead. The other group received 6 weeks of dried, powdered *Convolvulus pluricaulis* three times a day. Symptoms were measured using the Hamilton Anxiety Rating Scale, and each group showed significant improvement with treatment. The *jaladhara* treatment was somewhat more effective in relieving symptoms consistent with phobias and panic. However, *Convolvulus pluricaulis* was more effective in providing a full measure of relief from GAD. It must be noted that nearly half of the treatment group dropped out for reasons that were not given.[107]

6.9.2 MECHANISM OF ACTION

Among the bioactive components of *Convolvulus pluricaulis* are cinnamic acid and related phenylpropanoids, scopoletin and other coumarins, phthalic acid and other phenolics, β-sitosterol, tropane alkaloids, and kaempferol and various other flavonoids. Many of those substances have themselves been shown to exhibit anxiolytic effects. Extracts of the plant also have potent antioxidant and neuroprotective effects.[108]

6.9.3 DOSAGE

In the clinical study noted above,[107] 3gm of dried, powdered plant was given three times a day.

6.9.4 TOXICITY

Little is offered in the literature in regard to toxicity of *Convolvulus pluricaulis*. Indeed, various studies mention hepatoprotective, neuroprotective, and beneficial antioxidant effects. Nonetheless, the related species of morning glory, *Convolvulus arvensis*, is known to be toxic in grazing animals. The LD50 of the dried aqueous extraction in sheep was found to be about 410mg/kg, or about 30g for a 160-pound man. This is uncomfortably close to the 9g per day dosing in the study noted prior.[109] It is again worth noting that the use of *Convolvulus pluricaulis* is time honored in Ayurvedic medicine and the use of dried whole plant is likely to dilute toxic elements.

6.9.5 SAFETY IN PREGNANCY

Neither the *Botanical Safety Handbook* nor the *German Commission E Monographs* offer information about the safety of *Convolvulus pluricaulis* during pregnancy. Thus, its use is inadvisable.

6.9.6 DRUG INTERACTION

There is no readily accessible information in the literature about *Convolvulus pluricaulis* having possible drug interactions.

6.10 *CROCUS SATIVUS*

Saffron is the familiar spice made of the stigmas plucked from the flowers of the *Crocus sativus* plant. The plant is cultivated from the lands around the Mediterranean Sea and eastward across Iran, India, Tibet, and China. Nearly 80% of commercial saffron is grown in Iran, where much of the research into the herb's medicinal properties has been performed. *Crocus sativus* has traditionally been seen as an adaptogen, stimulant, aphrodisiac, and antidepressant.[110]

6.10.1 ANXIOLYTIC EFFECTS

Clinical studies have shown that *Crocus sativus* reduces anxiety in patients with GAD and other psychiatric conditions. Antidepressants are often prescribed to treat GAD, even in the absence of major depression. In one study of GAD, the addition of *Crocus sativus* to patients who had not benefitted from treatment with the antidepressant sertraline further and significantly reduced levels of anxiety over 6 weeks.[111]

 Crocus sativus is an herb that has been shown to be effective in relieving major depression in human patients. There are several studies showing that *Crocus sativus* relieves anxiety in the context of depression. A 50mg capsule of *Crocus sativus* extract twice daily for 12 weeks significantly reduced both anxiety and depression by standard tests—that is, by the Beck Anxiety and Depression scales.[112] In a similar study, 30mg of *Crocus sativus* extract per day over 6 weeks significantly reduced both anxiety and depression as shown by the Hamilton Anxiety and Depression scales. In fact, the herb was just as effective as treatment with the antidepressant citalopram.[113] Extract of *Crocus sativus* was also shown to reduce both anxiety and depression in depressed teenagers.[114]

6.10.2 MECHANISM OF ACTION

The principal phytochemical of *Crocus sativus* is safranal, which provides its characteristic flavor. Other active components are crocin and crocetin, which lend color to saffron, and the glucoside picrocrocin, which adds a slightly bitter flavor to the spice. Various antioxidant anthocyanins can be isolated from the blue flowers.[115] Safranal on its own exerts anxiolytic effects in animals, and this is likely by several mechanisms. It enhances GABA activity and likely acts like a benzodiazepine.[116] It also buffers glutamate activity,[117] which can produce a calming effect. Crocin, thought to be responsible for many of *Crocus sativus*'s effects, has both anxiolytic and antidepressant-like effects in animals. Some of the anxiolytic effects of crocin are prevented by the drug flumazenil, which suggests that these effects are partially due to action at benzodiazepine receptors in the brain.[118] Crocin also has anti-inflammatory effects that, over time, may contribute to its apparent antidepressant and anxiolytic effects.[119] Interestingly, crocetin isolated from *Crocus sativus* has been clinically shown to relieve insomnia in healthy adults with mild sleep complaints.[120]

6.10.3 DOSAGE

Easley and Horne state the dosage of *Crocus sativus* to be as tincture of dry herb (1:10, 40%), 5 to 20 drops, three times daily.[121] Available commercially are *Crocus sativus* extract capsules of 88.25mg, standardized to 0.3% safranal, to be taken twice a day.

6.10.4 TOXICITY

Crocus sativus is considered non-toxic, with an LD50 in mice of 27g/kg.[122]

6.10.5 SAFETY IN PREGNANCY

Crocus sativus has been used in folk medicine as an abortifacient and is thus not recommended during pregnancy.[123] The view in Chinese traditional medicine is also that *Crocus sativus* should be avoided in pregnancy.[124] Safety in lactation has not been established.

6.10.6 DRUG INTERACTIONS

The *Botanical Safety Handbook* notes no known interactions with commonly pre-scribed medications.[125] Nonetheless, crocin extracted from *Crocus sativus* signifi-cantly inhibited the activities of CYP3A, CYP2C11, CYP2B, and CYP2A enzymes in in rat liver microsomes, whereas safranal significantly enhanced the activities of CYP2B, CYP2C11, and CYP3A enzymes.[126]

6.11 *CURCUMA LONGA*

Curcuma longa is a rhizomatous herbaceous perennial plant of the ginger family that is cultured in tropical or subtropical regions worldwide. All parts of the plant are used for medical purposes, but greatest use comes from the dried rhizome. The deep yel-low-orange powder known as turmeric is produced by boiling and drying *Curcuma longa* rhizomes and is commonly used as a spice or traditional drug, especially in

Asia.[127] Similar species, including *Curcuma zedoria*, are used in traditional Chinese and Unani schools of medicine in the treatment of anxiety.[128]

6.11.1 ANXIOLYTIC EFFECTS

Although a mainstay in Chinese and Unani schools in treatment of anxiety, studies of the anxiolytic effects of *Curcuma longa* have been inconsistent. Two studies of *Curcuma longa* failed to show significant effects of the herb on symptoms of anxiety in otherwise healthy subjects.[129–130] In a randomized, double-blind, placebo-controlled study, individuals with major depressive disorder were treated with curcumin from *Curcuma longa* or placebo for 8 weeks. This treatment significantly reduced symptoms of major depression but showed only a trend in reducing symptoms of anxiety per the Spielberger State-Trait Anxiety Inventory.[131]

Other studies were more positive. In another clinical trial, a purified preparation of extract of *Curcuma longa*, which contained curcumin, demethoxycurcumin, and bisdemethoxycurcumin, was evaluated in obese individuals. Subjects did not necessarily suffer a formally diagnosed anxiety disorder. In this double-blind, cross-over trial, subjects received a month of treatment that was switched after a 14-day wash-out period. The mean scores on the Beck Anxiety Inventory test showed significant reductions in anxiety during treatment with the *Curcuma longa* preparation that was rich in cucurmin. Curiously, no such effects were seen in symptoms of depression.[132]

In a study of patients with anxiety and depression in the context of diabetic neuropathy, 8 weeks of daily treatment with curcumin significantly reduced both anxiety and depression.[133]

6.11.2 MECHANISM OF ACTION

A number of sesquiterpenes and other complex phytochemicals have been isolated from *Curcuma longa* rhizome, but it is richest in curcuminoids and furanodiene. Among the many phytochemical identified in *Curcuma longa* are ferulic acid, coumaric acid, pinene, sabinene, myrcene, phellandrene, careen, terpinene, cymene, limonene, cineole, zingiberene, sesquiphellandrene, nerolidol, santalenone, turmerol, germacrone, turmerone, bisabolone, trans-alpha-atlantone, stigmasterol, and sitosterol.[134–135] In a study of anxiolytic effects of extract of *Curcuma longa* in rats, the anxiolytic effects of the extract were blocked by flumazenil, suggesting mediation by benzodiazepine receptors.[136]

6.11.3 DOSAGE

The German Commission E gives the dosing of *Curcuma longa* root as 1.5 to 3g of root daily. The bioavailability of curcumin is quite low, but its absorption from the gut can be substantially increased by adding piperine, a phytochemical from black pepper.[137]

6.11.4 TOXICITY

In studies of the essential oil of *Curcuma longa* using rats and mice, no acute toxicity or mortality was seen in any animals up to the maximum dose of 5,000mg/kg body weight. Thus, the LD50 was deemed to be greater than 5,000mg/kg, which extrapolated to a 160-pound adult would be approximately 375g. Furthermore, repeated administration of the essential oil for 90 days in rats at a dose of 1,000mg/kg body weight did not induce any observable toxic effects, compared with corresponding control animals.[138]

6.11.5 SAFETY IN PREGNANCY

Reference texts from traditional Chinese medicine advise against use of either *Curcuma longa* or *Curcuma zedoaria* during pregnancy.[139–140]

6.11.6 DRUG INTERACTIONS

The *Botanical Safety Handbook* notes no known drug interactions with either *Curcuma longa* or *Curcuma zedoaria*.[141] Curcumin did inhibit recombinant human CYP1A2, CYP3A4, CYP2D6, CYP2C9, and CYP2B6 enzymes. However, this occurred at moderately high micromolar concentrations, and, due to relatively low exposure of the liver to ingested curcumin, effects on drug metabolism by the liver may be minimal.[142]

6.12 ECHINACEA ANGUSTIFOLIA

The well-known herb echinacea, with the scientific name *Echinacea angustifolia*, is a member of the sunflower family. It is native to the Great Plains of North America and was the most widely used medicinal plant of the Plains Indians. The root of *Echinacea angustifolia* was utilized for a variety of ailments, including toothache, coughs, colds, sore throats, snakebite, and as a painkiller. The fresh or dried flowering tops and the fresh pressed juice from the flowering tops of echinacea are also used for various purposes. An alterative herb is one that increases general health and vitality, much in the manner of the more modern term *adaptogen*. Indeed, in recent decades it has gained a reputation as an herb that can bolster resistance to illness. Scientific research on *Echinacea* species, mostly performed in Europe, has shown some ability of the herb to stimulate the immune system.[143]

6.12.1 ANXIOLYTIC EFFECTS

A study evaluated the effects of *Echinacea angustifolia* in healthy adults who had not been diagnosed with an actual anxiety disorder but had scored high on the State-Trait Anxiety Inventory, a standard test of anxiety. One week of daily treatment with 40mg of extract of *Echinacea angustifolia* significantly reduced levels of anxiety. This relief from anxiety began after 3 days of treatment and persisted for a week after treatment ended.[144]

6.12.2 MECHANISM OF ACTION

Echinacea angustifolia contains a variety of phytochemicals, and no single one is responsible for the medicinal effects of the herb. Flavonoids, including quercetin, kaempferol, and isorhamnetin, are present,[145] and these flavonoids have activity at GABA-A receptors in the brain. The volatile oils from the aerial parts of *Echinacea angustifolia* and closely related species also contain borneol, bornyl acetate, germacrene D, and β-caryophyllene. Interestingly, β-caryophyllene may have activity at cannabinoid receptors.[146] Also, the long-chained, nitrogen-containing alkylamides, caffeic acid derivatives, and alkenes may all contribute anxiolytic effects, perhaps in part due to action at cannabinoid receptors.[147]

6.12.3   DOSAGE

In the above noted study by Haller et al.,[144] 40mg per day of dried extract of *Echinacea angustifolia* had an anxiolytic effect.

6.12.4   TOXICITY

Studies have shown some toxicity of *Echinacea angustifolia* in mice at concentrations as low as 300mg/kg. However, the LD50 was found to be 3,800mg/kg.[148]

6.12.5   SAFETY IN PREGNANCY

The *Botanical Safety Handbook* states that the limited available data suggests no adverse effects of *Echinacea angustifolia* during pregnancy.[149] The German Commission E gives no warning about its use.

6.12.6   DRUG INTERACTION

The *Botanical Safety Handbook* notes no reports of drug interactions in the scientific literature.

6.13   *ECHIUM AMOENUM*

Echium amoenum is sometimes referred to as Iranian borage, but it is distinct from the *Borago officinalis* that is commonly referred to as European borage. Iranian borage is from the *Echium* genus, and it grows in the northern mountains of Iran in the Alborz hillsides. The herb has not yet been domesticated and cannot be cultivated with commercial success. Thus, it is still largely gathered from the wild. The flowers of this plant have long been used in folk medicine for their anti-inflammatory, analgesic, anxiolytic, and sedative effects.[150]

6.13.1   ANXIOLYTIC EFFECTS

In a somewhat unusual study, Iranian psychiatrists evaluated the ability of *Echium amoenum* to enhance the known anxiolytic effects of the prescription antidepressant fluoxetine.[151] In this study, patients formally diagnosed with GAD were randomly assigned to receive liquid extract of *Echium amoenum* plus fluoxetine or fluoxetine

(20mg/day) plus placebo. The patients were examined by psychiatrist before the trial and during the days 14, 28, 42, and 56. Effectiveness of the treatment was assessed using HAM-A14. By day 14, the combination of herb plus fluoxetine was more effective in relieving anxiety than the fluoxetine alone. In fact, the fluoxetine alone did not begin to relieve anxiety until the sixth week of treatment. The extra benefits of the herb continued throughout the study, and by the end of the study, on day 56, the combination remained significantly more effective than the antidepressant alone in relieving symptoms of anxiety.

There is also a report of modest efficacy of *Echium amoenum* in reducing symptoms of obsessive compulsive disorder as measured by the Yale-Brown Obsessive Compulsive Scale and Hamilton Anxiety Rating Scale.[152] Until quite recently, obsessive compulsive disorder was categorized as an anxiety disorder. However, that is no longer the case. It is now seen more as a disorder of thought and impulse control. Of final interest is a small but randomized controlled trial evaluating effects of *Echium amoenum* on major depression in human subjects. After 4 weeks of treatment, adults with mild to moderate major depressive disorder enjoyed significantly fewer symptoms of depression per the Hamilton Depression Rating Scale. This improvement was no longer significant at 6 weeks.[153] Nonetheless, it is possible that general improvements in mood may contribute to the apparent anxiolytic effects of the herb. As a cautionary note, the three studies here described were all performed by the same group. Though the results are promising, it would be more convincing if other researchers replicated those results.

6.13.2 MECHANISM OF ACTION

Among the phytochemicals that have been identified in *Echium amoenum* are cadinene and many similar terpenes, including amorphene, ledene, rythron, alloaromadendrene, viridiflorol, calacorene, and spathulenol. Cadinene terpenes are commonly found in the mint-like herbs, cinnamon, cannabis, and other fragrant herbs, many of which exert anxiolytic effects. *Echium amoenum* contains anthocyanidines, flavonoids, and trace amounts of alkaloids. It also contains the commonly found rosmarinic acid and β-caryophyllene.[154] Rosmarinic acid alone has anxiolytic and antidepressant effects. As previously noted, β-caryophyllene is a terpene active at cannabinoid receptors that is found in *Cannabis sativa* but also many other unrelated plants. B-caryophyllene also has pain- and anxiety-relieving effects.

In a laboratory study of the effects of restraint stress, pretreatment of rodents with the benzodiazepine-blocking drug flumazenil blocked the anxiolytic effects of the herb.[155] Thus, some of the effects of the herb are mediated by the benzodiazepine site on GABA-A receptors in the brain. However, in that same study, treatment with *Echium amoenum* prevented restraint-induced increases in plasma corticosterone levels and hippocampal levels of the inflammatory cytokines IL-1β and TNF-α. This suggests more wide-ranging effects of the herb. Extract of the herb has also been found to have some pain-relieving effects that are reversed by the opiate-blocking drug naloxone. Thus, some of the effects of *Echium amoenum* may be due to stimulation of opiate receptors.[156]

6.13.3   DOSAGE

In the study noted above of effects of *Echium amoenum* on depression, human subjects received 375mg of dried aqueous extract of *Echium amoenum* each day.[152]
There were no significant differences between placebo and drug-treated groups in
side effects observed.

6.13.4   TOXICITY

In the study of antioxidant effects in humans described prior, subjects received doses
of 7mg air-dried flowers/kg twice daily for 14 days without adverse effects. In rats,
the LD50 of intraperitoneally administered aqueous extract of *Echium amoenum*
was found to be 2.03g/kg, which extrapolates to approximately 140g in a 75kg human
adult.[157] Aside from those findings, the herb may contain trace amounts of pyrrolizidine alkaloids that can harm the liver. Thus, anyone with any form of liver disease
should avoid this herb.[158]

6.13.5   SAFETY IN PREGNANCY

Review of the literature reveals no studies of the safety of the use of *Echium amoenum*
in pregnancy. However, one study showed that the herb reduced the teratogenic effects
of high doses of lamotrigine in mice without adding additional adverse effects.[159]

6.13.6   DRUG INTERACTIONS

Review of the literature revealed no studies of the possible interactions of *Echium
amoenum* with commonly used medications.

6.14   *ELEUTHEROCOCCUS SENTICOSUS*

Eleutherococcus senticosus is a small shrub native to northeastern Asia. The herb is
commonly referred to as Siberian ginseng. However, the ginseng component of the
name is misleading. *Eleutherococcus senticosus*, or alternatively *Acanthopanax senticosus*, is not related to true ginseng, *Panax ginseng*. Nonetheless, *Eleutherococcus
senticosus* has long been used in traditional Chinese medicine, where it is known as
ciwujia. The roots, rhizomes, and stems of the plant are collected in the spring and
fall for use as a tonic to fight fatigue and enhance well-being. It is thought to stimulate *Qi*, strengthen the spleen, and nourish the kidney. Among the benefits attributed
to *Eleutherococcus senticosus* by modern herbalists are anti-inflammatory, antioxidative, anticarcinogenic, antifatigue, antidiabetic, hypolipidemic, immunoprotective,
and immunoregulatory effects.[160]

6.14.1   ANXIOLYTIC EFFECTS

For many years, in regions of what had been the Soviet Union, scientists pursued
substances that non-specifically enhance an organism's ability to withstand stress

and other adverse conditions. These substances, including various herbs, have been referred to as adaptogens. Whereas *Eleutherococcus senticosus* may offer some acute anxiolytic effects, the herb is seen as most helpful for building resiliency and the ability to cope with stress. For example, subjects described as suffering "neurosis" had significantly improved sleep, well-being, appetite, stamina, cognitive function, and mood after 4 weeks of treatment with *Eleutherococcus senticosus*.[161] In a randomized study of *Eleutherococcus senticosus* on quality of life in elderly patients, improvements in social functioning, mental health, and cognitive function were observed after 4 weeks of therapy, but these differences did not persist to the 8-week time point.[162] The herb has also been shown to enhance the ability to cope with specific forms of stress. In a double-blind study of healthy volunteers, 30 days of treatment with *Eleutherococcus senticosus* led to reduced heart rate and lower blood pressures during a stressful cognitive task, the Stroop Color and Word Test.[163] However, in one study participants suffering burnout and chronic stress were given *Eleutherococcus senticosus* root extract daily for 8 weeks. The herb gave those individuals no advantages over professional stress management training in the reduction of stress, restlessness, fatigue, insomnia, or other symptoms of chronic anxiety.[164]

6.14.2 MECHANISM OF ACTION

The many phytochemicals found in *Eleutherococcus senticosus* include sesamine, syringin, eleutherosides, eleutherans, isofraxidin, sinapaldehyde glucoside, coniferaldehyde glucoside, coniferin, caffeoylquinic acids, α-bergamotnen, δ-elemene, β-elemene, γ-cadinene, and α-pinene.[165] Some of the phytochemicals are unique to the herb, whereas others are common among plants.

Eleutherococcus senticosus is perhaps best known as an adaptogen, which over time builds resilience against stress and anxiety. The steroid-like triterpenes called eleutherosides in the herb have on their own been found to increase stamina and resiliency in animals.[166] There may also be more immediate anxiolytic effects of *Eleutherococcus senticosus*. For example, pinene, a monoterpene found in *Eleutherococcus senticosus*, has its own anxiolytic effects through rapid action at GABA receptors.[167] The herb also contains quantities of other flavonoids and coumarins that might contribute anxiolytic effects.[168] Indeed, in a study of mice, the acute hypnotic effects of *Eleutherococcus senticosus* were reversed by flumazenil, suggesting that components of the herb act immediately at GABA-A receptors as well as provide more persisting, anxiolytic effects by acting as an adaptogen.[169]

6.14.3 DOSAGE

Doses of *Eleutherococcus senticosus* extract standardized to contain 2.24mg eleutherosides improved fatigue in human subjects at doses of four 500mg capsules per day.[170] In a test for enhancement of athletic performance, subjects received 2ml (150mg of the dried material) of a 33% ethanol extract of *Eleutherococcus senticosus* twice daily for 8 days. This treatment improved performance and work capacity.[171]

6.14.4 TOXICITY

The oral LD50 of the 33% ethanolic extract is estimated to be 14.5g/kg, which, extrapolated to a 75kg human adult, would be approximately 1,000g. The extract is not considered to be teratogenic in mice at 10mg/kg.[172]

6.14.5 SAFETY IN PREGNANCY

The *Botanical Safety Handbook* notes no compelling evidence of adverse effects from using this herb during pregnancy. Animal studies are benign.[173]

6.14.6 DRUG INTERACTIONS

The *Botanical Safety Handbook* notes no known interactions with drugs. A study using normal human volunteers showed that standardized extracts of *Eleutheroccus senticosus* at generally recommended doses are unlikely to alter the metabolism of medications dependent on the CYP2D6 or CYP3A4 pathways for elimination.[174]

6.15 *ESCHSCHOLZIA CALIFORNICA*

Eschscholzia californica, with the common name of California poppy, is a delicate orange-to-yellow flowering plant in the family *Papaveraceae*. This makes it a cousin to the opium poppy. It is native to the United States and Mexico and has long been used by the Native Americans and rural populations of those areas for its analgesic and sedative properties. In the late 1800s, it was available in the Parke-Davis drug catalog and was described as "an excellent soporific and analgesic, above all harmless."[175]

6.15.1 ANXIOLYTIC EFFECTS

There are many references to the use of *Eschscholzia californica* for the treatment of anxiety and insomnia. It is one of the herbs most often recommended by members of the American Herbalists Guild for those purposes. It is also widely prescribed by herbalists in France for anxiety and insomnia. However, while numerous studies show it can relieve anxiety-like behaviors in animals, there are few clinical studies showing effectiveness in humans. One study showed that *Eschscholzia californica* in combination with *Crataegus oxyacantha* and supplemental magnesium was more effective than placebo in relieving anxiety in patients who had been diagnosed with GAD.[176] In reference to an unpublished study, another group of researchers reported that the combination of *Eschscholzia californica* and *Corydalis yanhusuo* relieved insomnia in human subjects. In fact, this combination has been marketed in Germany under the name Phytonoxon.[177]

6.15.2 MECHANISM OF ACTION

Eschscholzia californica contains a variety of phytochemicals, including flavonoids such as quercetin and isorhamnetin, that may contribute anxiolytic effects.[178]

However, it is perhaps most notable for containing alkaloids that are similar to those in other species of poppy. These include californidine, escholtzine, sanquinarine, chelerythrine, N-methylaurotetanine, glaucine, protopine, allocryptopine, and reticuline.[179] At one time it was suspected that it contained traces of morphine, but modern studies don't substantiate that. Some of its alkaloids can act at opiate receptors and likely provide some modest degree of pain relief. The anxiolytic effects of *Eschscholzia californica* have been traditionally attributed to the alkaloids protopine and allocryptopine, as they have been shown to affect GABA-A receptors. However, a recent study showed that the concentrations of those alkaloids in extracts of the herb are likely too low to be effective. The substance more likely to contribute anxiolytic effects is the alkaloid reticuline, which is known to enhance GABA-A activity.[180] In a study of rodents, the sedative and anxiolytic-like effects of *Eschscholzia californica* were dampened by flumazenil.[181]

6.15.3 DOSAGE

Standardized extracts of *Eschscholzia californica*, with approximately 200mg of herb per 1ml, are readily available in health stores and the internet. Hoffmann recommends dosing of 0.5 to 2ml of liquid extract up to three times a day.[182]

6.15.4 TOXICITY

In a rodent study noted above,[181] the aqueous alcohol extract (i.p. and p.o.) and the aqueous extract (i.p.) did not induce any acute toxic effects at doses suggesting the LD50 to be over 5,000mg/kg in mice.

6.15.5 SAFETY IN PREGNANCY

The German Commission E notes a scarcity of data about the safety of using *Eschscholzia californica* during pregnancy. Nonetheless, because of its similarity to opiate-containing herbs, they advise against its use by women who are pregnant.[183]

6.15.6 DRUG INTERACTION

The *Botanical Safety Handbook* notes no known drug interactions.[184]

6.16 EUPHYTOSE

This section has mostly discussed individual herbs that have been found in clinical trials to have anxiolytic effects. Euphytose is a combination of herbs including *Passiflora incarnata*, *Valeriana officinalis*, *Crataegus oxyacantha*, *Ballota nigra*, *Paullinia cupana*, and *Cola acuminata*. It is an herbal treatment for anxiety that has been available commercially in France since the 1920s. It is now produced by the Bayer company. Using combinations of herbs is the standard of practice in traditional Chinese and Ayurvedic medicine but is not uncommon in Western herbalism. Euphytose is somewhat unique in that it is not only born of the Western herbalism tradition but has also undergone a successful clinical trial and deserves discussion in this section.

6.16.1 ANXIOLYTIC EFFECTS

In a double-blind, placebo-controlled study, patients diagnosed with GAD received either Euphytose—2 tablets three times a day—or placebo over 4 weeks. Weekly evaluations, using the Hamilton Anxiety Rating Scale, determined that the treatment significantly reduced symptoms of anxiety, with relief appearing as early as the first week.[185]

6.16.2 MECHANISM OF ACTION

Some of the mechanism of action of Euphytose can be assumed to be due to effects of *Passiflora incarnata* and *Valeriana officinalis*, both of which have been shown to have anxiolytic activity. The likely mechanisms of action of those herbs are later discussed. *Crataegus oxyacantha* in this combination has also been used in combination with *Eschscholzia californica*, and the anxiolytic effect of that treatment is noted prior in discussion of the latter herb. Interestingly, *Paullinia cupana* and *Cola nitida* in Euphytose both have stimulant effects and ostensibly add benefits by countering the mildly sedating effects of the other herbs. Indeed, *Paullinia cupana* contains caffeine and related xanthines. It also contains catechin and epicatechin, as are found in *Camellia sinensis*.[186] In South America, *Paullinia cupana* is referred to as *guarana*, and it is commonly used in a coffee-like stimulating drink. *Cola nitida*, known commonly as the kola nut, also contains caffeine, as well as catechins, procyanidins, proanthocyanidins, and sterols.[187]

Of interest is a receptor-binding study that was performed using Euphytose. It was found that the phytochemicals in Euphytose interact with central benzodiazepine, alpha-2 adrenergic, and M1 muscarinic receptors with respective IC50 values of 37.1, 3.6, and 30.0µg/ml. Euphytose was found not to have significant binding at peripheral benzodiazepine, 5-HT1, 5 HT2, alpha-1 adrenergic, DA1 and DA2, or M2 muscarinic receptors.[188]

6.16.3 DOSAGE

The dose is standardized and appears on the container.

6.16.4 TOXICITY

This product has been used safely for many years. However, there is at least one report of fulminant hepatic failure occurring in a child who ingested Euphytose. It is not clear if the herbal product was being used as intended.[189]

6.16.5 SAFETY IN PREGNANCY

The manufacturer of Euphytose, Bayer, recommends against its use during pregnancy.

6.16.6 DRUG INTERACTIONS

There are no specific reports of interactions of Euphytose with drugs, except for what may be extrapolated from what is known about the individual herbs contained the product.

6.17 EVOLVULUS ALSINOIDES

Evolvulus alsinoides is a small, woody perennial herb belonging to the family *Convolvulaceae*. It is known to speakers of English as dwarf morning glory. The herb is native to subtropical areas of Asia, Indochina, Polynesia, sub-Saharan Africa, and the Americas. It has long been used in Ayurvedic medicine to improve brain power and memory and to treat various psychiatric disorders. There is some confusion about names in the Ayurvedic literature. There are several anxiolytic herbs that have each been called by the Punjabi-language name *shankpushpi*, and these include *Evolvulus alsinoides*, *Convolvulus pluricaulis* (another species of morning glory), *Clitorea ternatea*, and *Canscora decussata*. The local names also vary across India, with the names *shankhapushpi* and *sankhaholi* appearing to be interchangeable. It is possible that all these have been used with similar benefits by Ayurvedic herbalists.[190] In an animal study, *Evolvulous alsinoides* was found to have greater anxiolytic activity than *Convolvulus pluricaulis*.[191] Animal studies have also shown that *Clitorea ternatea*[192] and *Canscora decussatato*[193] have some anxiolytic effects.

6.17.1 ANXIOLYTIC EFFECTS

While several herbs referred to as *sankhaholi* or *shankpushpi* have been used for centuries in Ayurvedic medicine to treat anxiety and other nervous disorders, there is at least one formal study in which an herb clearly identified as *Evolvulus alsinoides* has been evaluated for anxiolytic effects. In individuals diagnosed as persistently suffering mild to moderate degrees of anxiety by the Hamilton Anxiety Rating Scale, 6 weeks of daily treatment with extract of *Evolvulus alsinoides* significantly reduced those symptoms of anxiety. Side effects were deemed to be negligible.[194]

6.17.2 MECHANISM OF ACTION

Evolvulus alsinoides contains phenolic compounds, flavonoids, and alkaloids thought to be active in the brain, including shankhapushpine, evolvine, scopoletin, umbelliferone, scopoline, 2-methyl-1,2,3,4-butanetetrol, caffeic acid, 6-methoxy-7-O-b-glucopyranoside coumarin, 2-C-methyl erythritol, kaempferol, and quercetin.[195] Scopoletin exerts anti-inflammatory effects and is able to reduce experimental inflammation-induced anxiety in mice. However, it also appears to act at GABA-A receptors.[196] Several other constituents of *Evolvulus alsinoides*, including kaempferol and quercetin, have long been known to enhance GABA activity in the brain. (See Chapter 5.) *Evolvulus alsinoides* may also buffer adrenergic activity that mediates the fight-or-flight response that underlies components of anxiety.[197] Evolvine may have some effects not unlike a very mild dose of nicotine.[198] Thus, *Evolvulus alsinoides* may act by multiple mechanisms, some rather unique among herbs, that would complement the effects of other herbs as well.

6.17.3 DOSAGE

In the study noted above, subjects received 3g of powdered dried *Evolvulus alsinoides* every night at bedtime.[194] Be aware that products sold on the internet labeled as *shankpushpi* are almost always identified as *Convolvulus pluricaulis*, which, while time honored, has not been evaluated in any clinical study. At least one product clearly identified as *Evolvulus alsinoides* is available online. Circumspection is advised.

6.17.4 TOXICITY

The LD50 of an alcoholic extract of *Evolvulus alsinoides* has been reported to be 7g/kg in mice. Thus, its toxicity appears to be quite low.[199]

6.17.5 SAFETY IN PREGNANCY

The *Botanical Safety Handbook* notes no information in the scientific literature about the safety of *Evolvulus alsinoides* during pregnancy. Thus, its use is inadvisable.[200]

6.17.6 DRUG INTERACTION

The *Botanical Safety Handbook* notes no information in the scientific literature about drug interactions.

6.18   *FOENICULUM VULGARE*

Foeniculum vulgare, commonly known as fennel, is a perennial plant in the carrot family. It is native to the shores of the Mediterranean, and it was a favorite of the ancient Romans. Over the centuries it has become widely cultivated in many parts of the world. Its leaves and seeds are used as spice, and its celery-like base is sometimes consumed as a vegetable. It has also been used as one of the main flavorings in the alcoholic drink absinthe. Pliny, the Roman naturalist and philosopher, wrote about the many medicinal effects of *Foeniculum vulgare*. The herb has been said to possess antifungal, antibacterial, antioxidant, blood-thinning, and liver-protective effects. It has been widely used as a carminative, digestive, lactogogue, and diuretic and in treating various respiratory and gastrointestinal disorders.[201] There is also modern data showing antidepressant effects of *Foeniculum vulgare* both in animals and in preliminary clinical studies.[202]

6.18.1 ANXIOLYTIC EFFECTS

There are no studies of effects of *Foeniculum vulgare* in human subjects diagnosed with any specific anxiety disorder. However, there are reports of effects of *Foeniculum vulgare* in women experiencing anxiety and other discomforts secondary to menopause and premenstrual syndrome. Menopausal women given 200mg of *Foeniculum vulgare* oil daily for 8 weeks experienced significant improvements in self-reported general quality of life, including psychological and sexual aspects.[203] In a similar study, menopausal women chronically treated with *Foeniculum vulgare* showed improvements in anxiety and depression scores, but these apparent improvements did not reach statistical significance.[204]

Reports on effects of *Foeniculum vulgare* on mood in premenstrual syndrome have been inconsistent. In one study, twice daily treatment with *Foeniculum vulgare* for a month provided significant improvement in mood.[205] In another study treatment with *Foeniculum vulgare* significantly improved symptoms of anxiety and depressed mood of premenstrual syndrome, particularly when paired with exercise.[206] In yet another study, modest improvements in mood and anxiety were noted, but they did not reach significance.[207]

6.18.2 MECHANISM OF ACTION

The highly aromatic plant is rich in phytochemicals, among which are fenchone, estragole, eugenol, p-anisaldehyde, α-phellandrene, and trans-anethole. Those estrogen-like compounds are responsible for the herb's ability to ease symptoms of menopause. *Foeniculum vulgare* also contains flavonoids and terpenes, including quercetin, kaempferol, caffeoylquinic acid, limonene, linalool, cineol, thujene, myrcene, pinene, rosmarinic acid, and luteolin.[208] Many of those phytochemicals have been found to exert anxiolytic effects on their own, and to do so by various mechanisms. Many act directly at GABA-A receptors and some at the benzodiazepine site on GABA-A receptors. Some affect serotonin and dopamine activity. Linalool may have weak effects at opiate receptors, whereas linalool and pinene are both somewhat active at cannabinoid receptors. Interestingly, both picrotoxin, a GABA antagonist, and tamoxifen, an estrogen blocker, were found to block the anxiolytic effects of extract of *Foeniculum vulgare* in rodents.[209] Notably, the natural estrogen in the human body, estradiol, is able to enhance activity at GABA-A receptors in the brain.[210]

6.18.3 DOSAGE

The German Commission E notes the daily dose of *Foeniculum vulgare* oil to be 0.1 to 0.6ml, which is equal to 0.1 to 0.6g of herb. Their suggested dose for *Foeniculum vulgare* seed is 5 to 7g.[211]

6.18.4 TOXICITY

The LD50 of essential oil of *Foeniculum vulgare* in mice is reported to be 1.038ml/kg.[212] This would be extrapolated to approximately 70ml for a 75kg adult human.

6.18.5 SAFETY IN PREGNANCY

The editors of the *Botanical Safety Handbook* stated their belief that *Foeniculum vulgare* is safe for use during pregnancy and lactation.[213]

6.18.6 Drug Interactions

The *Botanical Safety Handbook* notes no known interactions of *Foeniculum vulgare* with commonly used drugs in human subjects. However, extract of seed of *Foeniculum vulgare* has been found to inhibit the CY3A4 enzyme from human liver microsomes.[214]

6.19 GALPHIMIA GLAUCA

The medicinal plant *Galphimia glauca* is a small, evergreen shrub native to Mexico. In Mexico it is known as *calderona amarilla*, while in the United States it is referred to as thryallis. The most medicinally effective plants, which contain the highest concentrations of its main anxiolytic compound, galphimine B, are said to grow in only a few states in Mexico. It has been used for the treatment of anxiety and depression since pre-Hispanic times. However, it has also been used in the treatment of asthma, diarrhea, fever, hay fever, and seizures.[215]

6.19.1 Anxiolytic Effects

There are at least two clinical studies showing effectiveness of *Galphimia glauca* in anxiety disorders of human patients. In one clinical study of *Galphimia glauca*, it was found to relieve anxiety in young adults diagnosed with social anxiety disorder. Indeed, it was found to be as effective as the prescription antidepressant sertraline, which is commonly prescribed by doctors to treat that disorder.[216] In the other study, extract of the herb produced an anxiolytic effect in patients diagnosed with GAD. In fact, its anxiolytic effect was similar to that of the prescribed benzodiazepine lorazepam. The herb was also better tolerated, since many of the patients treated with lorazepam, but none who received the herb, withdrew from the study due to side effects.[217]

6.19.2 Mechanism of Action

Galphimia glauca contains the phenolic acids gallic acid, tetragalloylquinic acid, methyl gallate, and ellagic acid. Among the flavonoids in *Galphimia glauca* are quercetin, isoquercitrin, and hyperoside. The herb also contains various unique terpenes that as a class are referred to as the galphimine series, A through J. The related steroid-like triterpenoids, glaucacetalins A through D, have also been identified. The active component is thought to be galphimine-B. This substance, classified as a nor-seco-triterpenoid, acts in a unique way in the brain. It does not activate the GABAergic system, as do many other anxiolytic molecules. Its main effect is to modify the activity of the neurotransmitter dopamine. It may also block effects of glutamate at the NMDA receptor, which is a mechanism of ketamine, a medication recently found to exert powerful antidepressant effects.[218] *Galphimia glauca* also has antinociceptive effects that are mediated by opiate receptors.[219]

6.19.3 DOSAGE

In the clinical study above by Romero-Cerecero et al., subjects each day received extract of *Galphimia glauca* containing 0.374mg/dose of the active compound galphimine-B.[216] Similarly standardized preparations are available in specialty venues and on the internet.

6.19.4 TOXICITY

In rodents, the LD50 of the extract was found to be greater than 2,000mg/kg.[220]

6.19.5 SAFETY IN PREGNANCY

There are no references in the scientific literature about the safety of *Galphimia glauca* during pregnancy.

6.19.6 DRUG INTERACTION

There are no references in the scientific literature about drug interactions with *Galphimia glauca*.

6.20 GANODERMA LUCIDUM

Ganoderma lucidum, also known as *reishi* or *lingzhi*, is a large, dark mushroom with a glossy exterior and a woody texture. For over 2,000 years, the mushroom has been revered in China, Japan, and other Asian countries, where it has been thought to promote general health and longevity. Indeed, it has often been referred to as "the king of herbs."[221] (I note that several Chinese herbs possess that sobriquet.) According to the State Pharmacopoeia of the People's Republic of China (2000), it acts to replenish *Qi*, ease the mind, and relieve cough and asthma, and it is recommended for dizziness, insomnia, palpitation, and shortness of breath.

6.20.1 ANXIOLYTIC EFFECTS

Ganoderma lucidum is one of the herbs sometimes recommended for treatment of anxiety by members of the American Herbalists Guild. However, there are few studies in Western medical literature that show it is truly effective. In a study of breast cancer patients undergoing endocrine therapy, spore powder from *Ganoderma lucidum*—given in three daily doses over 4 weeks—significantly improved fatigue and physical well-being. These women also reported less anxiety and depression and better quality of life as revealed by the Hospital Anxiety and Depression Scale. None, however, had been diagnosed with an anxiety disorder. Moreover, the anti-inflammatory effects may have relieved some of the cancer-related symptoms these women suffered, and thus the mushroom may have only secondarily improved anxiety and sense of well-being.[222] However, two other studies showed little if any benefits on anxiety or overall mood. In a study on women with fibromyalgia, *reishi* offered no benefits on physical health and only tended to improve well-being and happiness.[223] In a study using *Ganoderma lucidum* to treat Alzheimer's disease, no benefits in quality of life were seen.[224]

6.20.2   MECHANISM OF ACTION

Ganoderma lucidum contains a variety of active phytochemicals, such as terpenoids, steroids, phenols, nucleotides and their derivatives, glycoproteins, and polysaccharides. Some are unique to the mushroom, such as the steroid-like terpenes ganoderic and lucidenic acids.[225] It also contains some common phenolic acids, such as chlorogenic, vanillic, caffeic, p-coumaric, and ferulic acids; as well as flavonoids, including rutin, quercetin, and kaempferol.[226] Rutin, quercetin, and kaempferol are known to act at GABA-A receptors with benzodiazepine-like effects. However, there is little basis to suggest that *Ganoderma lucidum* can offer any immediate relief from anxiety as a benzodiazepine would. It is possible that the mushroom might act primarily as an adaptogen and over time strengthen the system and improve resiliency that, in turn, reduces persisting anxiety.[227]

6.20.3   DOSAGE

In a study noted above, by Zhao et al., beneficial effects on mood and well-being were noted with a dose of 3g of dried *Ganoderma lucidum* given twice a day.[222] The carpophores of the mushroom—that is, the gill structures producing spores—were used. In the other case noted above (by Pazzi et al.), 1,000mg of spore powder was given three times a day.

6.20.4   TOXICITY

The aqueous extract of *Ganoderma lucidum* had an LD50 of 3.5g/kg body weight in Wistar rats. Thus, it has low toxicity and is apparently well tolerated.[228] One study showed a tendency of high doses—i.e., 3g per day of *Ganoderma lucidum*— to inhibit platelet aggregation, which could predispose the patient to bleeding.[229] Another study has shown that addition of high concentrations of extract to cells in culture can reduce cell viability.[230]

6.20.5   SAFETY IN PREGNANCY

The *Botanical Safety Handbook* noted that their review of existing scientific literature revealed no indications of adverse effects of *Ganoderma lucidum* during pregnancy. However, they added, "Although this review did not identify any concerns for use while pregnant or nursing, safety has not been conclusively established."[231]

6.20.6   DRUG INTERACTION

The *Botanical Safety Handbook* noted no clinical reports of drug interactions involving *Ganoderma lucidum*.

6.21 *GINKGO BILOBA*

Ginkgo biloba, also known as the maidenhair tree, is one of the oldest species of tree in the world. Indeed, the tree is the only living species in the division *Ginkgophyta*, all others being extinct. Native to China, the tree is widely cultivated and was cultivated early in human history. The trees can grow more than 130 feet tall and can live for over 1,000 years. Some trees in China are said to be over 2,500 years old. The seeds of *Ginkgo biloba* can be eaten, but it is the leaves that serve as a source of medicine.[232] A variety of health benefits have been attributed to *Ginkgo biloba*, and among the many uses are treating poor memory, dementia, dizziness, depression, cerebrovascular and cardiovascular insufficiency, oxidative damage, low cellular energy levels, inflammation, migraine, allergies, and asthma.

6.21.1 ANXIOLYTIC EFFECTS

In a study of patients diagnosed with GAD or adjustment disorder with anxious mood, 4 weeks of treatment with standardized extract of Ginkgo biloba L. (Egb 761) reduced scores in the Hamilton Anxiety Rating Scale and significantly relieved physical complaints associated with anxiety.[233] In a study of healthy young volunteers, a single dose of *Ginkgo biloba* reduced increases in blood pressure and release of stress hormone—i.e., cortisol—in response to physical and mental stresses. With consistent use, such effects could help provide resiliency against the development of anxiety and depression.[234]

6.21.2 MECHANISM OF ACTION

The leaves of *Ginkgo biloba* contain a variety of flavonol glycosides, biflavones, proanthocyanidins, alkylphenols, simple phenolic acids, and polyprenols. Some of these substances, such as quercetin, isorhamnetin, myricetin, rutin, luteolin, and kaempferol, are common in medicinal plants. Many of those molecules are known to enhance GABA activity. *Ginkgo biloba* also contains unique phytochemicals: e.g., the terpene trilactones ginkgolides A, B, C, and J.[235] The terpene bilobalide has been found to diminish GABA activity, and some ginkgolides have anxiolytic- and antidepressant-like effects in behavioral studies of laboratory animals.[236] In one such study, ginkgolide A produced anxiolytic effects that were not reversed by flumazenil.[237] Bilobalide and ginkgolides may have anti-inflammatory and neuroprotective effects, which in turn may mediate some of the herb's adaptogenic effects.[238]

6.21.3 DOSAGE

The German Commission E recommends 120 to 240mg of dried extract of *Ginkgo biloba* two to three times a day.[239] Authors have cautioned that the quality of various extracts of *Ginkgo biloba* can vary considerably. For this reason, standardized extracts such as the well-known Egb 761 have been developed and marketed. In such standardized extracts, high concentrations of ginkgolides A, B, C, and J and bilobalide are maintained while the mildly toxic ginkgolic acids are kept in concentrations less than 5mg/kg (5ppm).

6.21.4 TOXICITY

Ginkgo biloba appears to be quite non-toxic. In a study to determine LD50 of intra-peritoneal injection of *Ginkgo biloba* in rats, no animal deaths were seen until the dose of 8g/kg. This dose is well beyond typical human therapeutic doses.[240]

6.21.5 SAFETY IN PREGNANCY

The *Botanical Safety Handbook* notes no human studies of safety in using *Ginkgo biloba* during pregnancy and only limited animal studies. Caution is thus advised.

6.21.6 DRUG INTERACTIONS

Ginkgo biloba has been suspected of potentially dangerous interactions with medications that have included anticoagulants, monoamine oxidase (MAO) inhibitors, alprazolam, and haloperidol.[241] A study also revealed a significant inductive effect of ginkgo on CYP2C19 activity. In one case, this may have resulted in sub-therapeutic blood levels of erpinen and dilantin with a resulting fatal breakthrough seizure.[242]

6.22 *HUMULUS LUPULUS*

Humulus lupulus is a perennial plant in the hemp family. It is native to the temperate zones of Europe, Asia, and the Americas. Its flowers are commonly known as hops, and it is perhaps best known for its use in the brewing of beer. It lends a hearty, bitter flavor to the beverage and serves as a preservative owing to its antimicrobial properties. However, *Humulus lupulus* has also been used for centuries as a medicinal herb. Reports on the medicinal uses of *Humulus lupulus* date back to the Middle Ages. The oldest report may be an 11th-century book by the Arabic physician Mesue, who described anti-inflammatory properties of the herb. In the 13th century, the Arabic botanist Ibn Al-Baytar noted it as having soothing effects.[243]

6.22.1 ANXIOLYTIC EFFECTS

Many studies have shown *Humulus lupulus* to have anxiolytic-like effects in animals. The well-regarded German Commission E has approved *Humulus lupulus* for the treatment of restlessness, anxiety, mood disturbances, and sleep disturbances. Unfortunately, there are few studies of human subjects. In an open-labeled study, nightly consumption of non-alcoholic beer, a good source of hops, significantly improved sleep and eased anxiety in otherwise healthy students suffering the stresses of final exams.[244]

There is a report on the effects of *Humulus lupulus* on major depression in human subjects that also considered symptoms of anxiety. In a small but randomized, placebo-controlled, double-blind study, the effects of *Humulus lupulus* were tested in otherwise healthy young adults with evidence of mild depression or anxiety per the Depression Anxiety Stress Scale. After 4 weeks of treatment, *Humulus lupulus* produced significant improvements in both depression and anxiety scores.[245]

6.22.2 Mechanism of Action

Among the phytochemicals identified in *Humulus lupulus* are xanthohumol, humulone, cohumulone, adhumulone, lupulone, colupulone, adlupulone, catechin, quercetin, kaempferol, desmethylxanthohumol, 6-prenylnaringenin, 8-prenylnaringenin, ferulic acid, and resveratrol.[246] Several phytochemicals contained in *Humulus lupulus* have anxiolytic effects by different interactions with the GABA receptor. Humulone induces sleep by a mechanism that is blocked by flumazenil.[247] Xanthohumol interacts with midazolam, but not through the benzodiazepine receptor.[248] Radioligand binding and docking studies suggest that 6-prenylnaringenin extracted from *Humulus lupulus* acts at GABA-A receptors as a positive allosteric modulator as well as at a separate flumazenil-sensitive site on the GABA receptor complex.[249] Some of the other flavonoids and phenolics noted prior to be in *Humulus lupulus* also have anxiolytic effects mediated by GABA receptors. (See Chapter 5.) Thus, the various effects of *Humulus lupulus* on GABA activity are complex and likely synergistic.

6.22.3 Dosage

Marciano and Vizniak recommend a dosage of 1 cup three times a day of infusion from 1 teaspoon of *Humulus lupulus* per cup. Alternatively, they suggest tincture (1:5, 60% alcohol) of 2 to 3ml three times a day.[250]

6.22.4 Toxicity

Toxicological studies in animals stated that LD50 for orally administered *Humulus lupulus* extract in mice ranges from 500 to 3,500mg/kg.[251] Extrapolated to a 75kg human adult, these doses would be approximately 35 to 245g.

6.22.5 Safety in Pregnancy

The *Botanical Safety Handbook* notes there to be no definitive guidance from the literature concerning the safety of this herb during pregnancy.[252]

6.22.6 Drug Interactions

The *Botanical Safety Handbook* notes no known interactions with drugs. Extracts of *Humulus lupulus* do significantly inhibit a variety of cytochrome P450 enzymes, including CYP2C8, CYP2C9, CYP2C19, and CYP1A2.[253]

6.23 *HYPERICUM PERFORATUM*

Hypericum perforatum, commonly known as St. John's wort, is an herbaceous perennial plant native to Europe and Asia. It has been introduced into the United States, where it has naturalized. It has been used widely in both Chinese and Western herbal medicine.[254] In Chinese it is *guan ye lian qiao*, and, along with *Eleutherococcus senticosus*, it is an ingredient in the Chinese herbal treatment for depression called *shuganjieyu.* It was also known by Hippocrates and recommended by the great ancient Greek herbalist Dioscorides.

Hypericum perforatum has been used traditionally for the treatment of agitation, neuralgia, fibrositis, sciatica, menopausal neurosis, anxiety, and depression and as a nerve tonic. The herb has been very popular for the treatment of Major Depressive Disorder (MDD), both in the United States and Europe. In 1984, the German Commission E designated *Hypericum perforatum* as an approved herb, and its safety and effectiveness are reevaluated periodically. *Hypericum perforatum* is likely the best studied herbal antidepressant, with both preclinical and clinical studies lending support for its efficacy.

6.23.1 ANXIOLYTIC EFFECTS

Hypericum perforatum is widely known as an herbal treatment for major depression. Clinical studies have confirmed that to be the case. In at least one case, a study showed that while relieving symptoms of major depression, *Hypericum perforatum* also significantly reduced anxiety in those patients.[255]

In a study of patients suffering somatization disorder, a psychiatric condition in which people's anxieties lead to difficult-to-treat physical complaints, 6 weeks of treatment with *Hypericum perforatum* significantly reduced levels of both anxiety and physical symptoms as measured by the Hamilton Anxiety Rating Scale and the Clinical Global Impression questionnaire.[256]

There have been case reports of the herb being useful for the treatment of GAD.[257] However, in the only formal study to evaluate the effects of *Hypericum perforatum* on patients suffering social anxiety disorder, 12 weeks of treatment with *Hypericum perforatum* was found to be no better than placebo.[258]

6.23.2 MECHANISM OF ACTION

Hypericum perforatum contains a wide variety of phytochemicals, including anthraquinone derivatives, flavonoids, prenylated phloroglucinols, phenolic compounds, and tannins.[259] The primary and unique active components in *Hypericum perforatum* are thought to be hypericin (an anthraquinone) and hyperforin (a prenylated phloroglucinol). Both are likely to contribute to the well-known antidepressant effect of *Hypericum perforatum*. However, hyperforin may be most responsible for both the antidepressant and anxiolytic effects of *Hypericum perforatum*.[260] Hyperforin enhances release of four neurotransmitters in the brain: i.e., serotonin, norepinephrine, dopamine, and GABA.[261] The enhancement of mood may improve anxiety as a secondary effect. However, in a study of rats, a total extract of *Hypericum perforatum* produced anxiolytic effects that were blocked by flumazenil, suggesting that the herb has some rapidly acting anxiolytic effects mediated by benzodiazepine receptors.[262] Moreover, the plant also contains a variety of flavonoids, including kaempferol, quercetin, and luteolin, and phenolic compounds, including chlorogenic, p-coumaric, and ferulic, all of which may reduce anxiety by action at GABA-A receptors. (See Chapter 5.) Amentoflavone, a bioflavonoid in *Hypericum perforatum*, has high affinity binding at benzodiazepine receptors and has on its own exerted anxiolytic-like effects in animals.

6.23.3 DOSAGE

The German Commission E recommends 2 to 4g of herb per day, or 0.2 to 1.0mg of hypericin from standardized extract per day.[263]

6.23.4 TOXICITY

The LD50 of intraperitoneally administered dried methanolic extract of *Hypericum perforatum* is about 450mg/kg in mice.[264] Extrapolated to a 75kg human adult, this would be approximately 32g. Of note, consumption of *Hypericum perforatum* has been known to induce at times severe photosensitivity in susceptible individuals.[265]

6.23.5 SAFETY IN PREGNANCY

The *Botanical Safety Handbook* notes little basis for concern about the use of *Hypericum perforatum* during pregnancy. Animal studies have proven the herb to be benign, whereas a limited number of case reports noted no adverse effects on mother or newborn.[266]

6.23.6 DRUG INTERACTIONS

Clinically significant interactions with *Hypericum perforatum* have been identified with prescribed medicines including warfarin, phenprocoumon, cyclosporin, HIV protease inhibitors, theophylline, digoxin, and oral contraceptives, resulting in a decrease in concentration or effect of the medicines. These interactions are probably due to the induction of cytochrome P450 isoenzymes CYP2D6, CYP3A4, CYP2C9, and CYP1A2 and the transport protein P-glycoprotein.[267]

Hypericum perforatum is known to affect drug metabolism. Crude extracts of the herb demonstrated inhibition of the enzymes CYP2D6, CYP2C9, and CYP3A4 and to a lesser extent CYP1A2 and CYP2C19.[268] Many psychiatric medications are metabolized by these enzymes.[269] Thus, *Hypericum perforatum* might be expected to increase blood levels of such medications. This may explain some reports of serotonin syndrome in geriatric patients adding *Hypericum perforatum* to prescribed antidepressants.

6.24 *LAVANDULA ANGUSTIFOLIA*

There are 32 recognized species of the genus *Lavandula*. The species most commonly used in herbal medicines are *L. angustiflora*, *L. latifolia*, and *L. stoechas*. These plants grow naturally in a distribution that stretches from the Canary Islands and Cape Verde east across the Mediterranean, North Africa, Southwest Asia, and the Arabian Peninsula. Lavender has been used since ancient times, and the name is derived from the Latin word *lavare*, "to wash," as the Romans used the plant to perfume their bath water. For hundreds if not thousands of years, preparations of *Lavandula spp* have been used to treat anxiety, insomnia, arthritis, inflammation, indigestion, and headaches.[270]

6.24.1 ANXIOLYTIC EFFECTS

A variety of studies have found that *Lavandula spp* can reduce symptoms of anxiety. Orally administered lavender capsules relieved acute anxiety of emotionally disturbing films as measured by State-Trait Anxiety Inventory, galvanic skin response, and heart rate variation.[271] A more prolonged study found that in adults diagnosed with GAD, daily consumption of lavender oil in capsules over a 6-week period was as effective as the benzodiazepine lorazepam at reliving anxiety.[272] A similar study found that daily consumption of encapsulated lavender oil daily for 10 weeks was more effective than placebo, though somewhat less effective than the prescription antidepressant paroxetine, in relieving anxiety in adults who had been diagnosed with GAD.[273] I note that *Lavandula spp* also showed a pronounced antidepressant effect and improvement in general mental health and quality of life.

6.24.2 MECHANISM OF ACTION

Lavender oil is obtained from steam distillation of the stem, leaves, and flowers of the plant. The primary phytochemical components of the essential oil are linalool, linalyl acetate, ocimene, cineole, erpinene-4-ol, and camphor. Also found are pinene, borneol, myrcene, farnescene, β-caryophyllene, geraniol, and limonene.[274] Linalool is a major component of lavender oil, and, as discussed in Chapter 5, it has well-known anxiolytic-like effects. Its effects are wide ranging and appear to include action at benzodiazepine, muscarinic, opioid, dopamine, adenosine, NO2, and NMDA receptors. In an animal study, linalool, as well as borneol and camphene from lavender, produced significant anxiolytic-like effects.[275]

6.24.3 DOSAGE

Hoffman gives the dosing of preparations of *Lavandula angustifolia* as 1–2 teaspoons of flower per cup of water taken three times a day. It was advised that lavender oil not be taken internally, but rather inhaled or rubbed on the skin.[276] Easley and Horne note tincture of dried flower and leaf (1:5, 75% alcohol) 1 to 3ml, three times daily.[277]

6.24.4 TOXICITY

The LD50 of essential oil of lavender in rats is reported to be 3.55g/kg.[278] Extrapolated to a 75kg human adult, this dose would be approximately 250g.

6.24.5 SAFETY IN PREGNANCY

An expert review noted a lack of sufficient data about the use of *Lavandula angustifolia* by pregnant women. Yet it did advise against its use during pregnancy due to its purported properties as an emmenagogue.[279]

6.24.6 DRUG INTERACTIONS

Essential oil of lavender increases pentobarbital sleep time in rats, suggesting competition for P450 enzymes.[280] However, in healthy human volunteers, daily administrations of a proprietary formulation of lavender oil had no clinically relevant inhibitory or inducing effects on the CYP1A2, CYP2C9, CYP2C19, CYP2D6, or CYP3A4 enzymes in vivo.[281]

6.25 *LEONURUS CARDIACA*

Leonurus cardiaca, with the common name motherwort, is a member of the mint family. It is a perennial plant native to central Europe and Scandinavia but is also found in the temperate zones of Russia and central Asia. Because of its medicinal properties, it has been taken around the world for cultivation and now grows wild across North America. Traditionally, extracts of the herb have been used for digestive disorders and heart conditions. However, the herb is also known for its sedative and calming properties.[282] The renowned 17th-century herbalist Nicholas Culpeper said of the plant, "there is no better herb to take melancholy vapors from the heart and make a merry, cheerful soul."[283] Similarly, it has been known as a natural remedy for nervous disorders in women, including postpartum depression and premenstrual and menopausal anxieties.

6.25.1 ANXIOLYTIC EFFECTS

In at least one clinical study out of Russia, daily supplementation with oil extract of *Leonurus cardiaca* was found to relieve symptoms of anxiety and depression in at least half of patients given extract of the herb.[284] In another study, tincture of *Leonurus cardiaca* improved both anxiety and retinal light sensitivity in anxious young subjects.[285] This would suggest some utility in individuals suffering anxiety as a component of seasonal affective disorder.

6.25.2 MECHANISM OF ACTION

Leonurus cardiaca is rich in phytochemicals, including flavonoids and flavonoid glycosides, including apigenin, orientin, quercetin, hyperoside, rutoside, and isoquercitrin; phenolic acids such as ferulic acid, chlorogenic acid, caffeic acid, and cichoric acid; iridoid glycosides harpagide, ajugol, galiridoside, harpagide acetate, ajugoside, galiridoside, lavandulifolioside, and verbascoside; alkaloids, such as leonurinine and stachydrine; and terpenes, including β-caryophyllene, α-humulene, pinenes, linalool, and limonene.[286] Many of those flavonoid and phenolic compounds have an ability to dampen anxiety. (See Chapter 5.) Various preparations of *Leonurus cardiaca* have been found to have anxiolytic effects in both animals and human subjects. Several components of *Leonurus cardiaca*, including isoleosibirin, 7R-chloro-6-desoxy-harpagide, lavandulifolioside, and the alkaloids stachydrine and leonurine, bind with modest affinity to the GABA-A receptor. Since that binding is not blocked by the drug flumazenil, these substances do not act in the manner of benzodiazepines.[287]

6.25.3 DOSAGE

The German Commission E recommends 1.5g of dried *Leonurus cardiaca* three times per day.[288]

6.25.4 Toxicity

The toxicity of dried butyl alcohol extract from *Leonurus cardiaca* appeared low, with an LD50 of 2,000mg/kg in mice.[289]

6.25.5 Safety in Pregnancy

The *Botanical Safety Handbook* warns that *Leonurus cardiaca* be avoided during pregnancy due to its emmenagogue and uterine stimulation properties.[290]

6.25.6 Drug Interaction

The *Botanical Safety Handbook* notes no known clinical studies of drug interactions involving *Leonurus cardiaca*.

6.26 *LEPIDIUM MEYENII*

Maca is the root of the plant *Lepidium meyenii*, which grows at high altitude in the Andean region of Peru. It is a member of the mustard family, and the root resembles a parsnip. It may even be cooked and eaten, like other root vegetables, or dried and ground to use as flour. However, it is highly valued as medicine and has long had a reputation for fertility-enhancing and aphrodisiac effects. It is also thought to have adaptogenic properties and is sometimes referred to as Peruvian ginseng. One use of *Lepidium meyenii* that has been evaluated in studies is the ability to reduce symptoms of menopause, including the anxiety and depression that can sometimes occur.[291]

6.26.1 Anxiolytic Effects

In a randomized, double-blind, placebo-controlled, crossover study, postmenopausal women were given either 3.5g of powdered *Lepidium meyenii* or placebo for 6 weeks, then the treatment was switched, so that each woman was tried on *Lepidium meyenii* and had placebo to compare it against. Data were collected using the Greene Climacteric Scale, which included questions concerning anxiety, depression, and sexual function. During treatment with *Lepidium meyenii*, women reported a significant improvement in anxiety, depression, and sexual desire and pleasure.[292]

In another study, 2g of *Lepidium meyenii* per day gave similar results. The herb not only improved many of the physical discomforts of menopause, such as night sweats, flushing, and headache, but also significantly improved complaints of nervousness, heart palpitations, depression, and poor sleep.[293]

A study was also performed giving men *Lepidium meyenii* over 12 weeks.[294] As was seen in postmenopausal women, the herb appeared to enhance sexual in desire in those men. However, it had no beneficial effects on anxiety or depression. It must be noted that the participants were healthy men who did not begin with diagnoses of psychiatric disorders.

6.26.2 MECHANISM OF ACTION

The potentially bioactive ingredients in *Lepidium meyenii* include the alkaloids macaridine, lepidiline A, and lepidiline B. It also contains macamides, described as "benzylamides of long chain fatty acids," and such molecules are sometimes found to have effects at cannabinoid receptors. *Lepidium meyenii*, a member of the mustard family, contains nitrogen- and sulfur-containing molecules called glucosinolates, which is common among such plants. Some have attributed the effects of *Lepidium meyenii* on fertility to those compounds, though without compelling evidence.[295] It also contains anxiolytic flavonoids, perhaps most notably kaempferol and quercetin, and lignan derivatives.[296] However, while there are many phytochemicals in *Lepidium meyenii* that could have effects on brain chemistry, the main active component is unknown. Interestingly, tests performed in one of the studies described prior showed that *Lepidium meyenii* was not acting as a hormone to produce its beneficial effects on anxiety in postmenopausal women.

6.26.3 DOSAGE

In the aforementioned studies, participants received 2 to 4g of powdered *Lepidium meyenii* per day. *Lepidium meyenii* is available in bulk and in premeasured capsules in stores and on the internet at quite reasonable prices.[292–294] However, I suggest care be taken to choose a reputable brand.

6.26.4 TOXICITY

Lepidium meyenii has been reported to have low toxicity, with an LD50 for mice of over 16.3g/kg. Indeed, maca is consumed by natives of the Andean regions and may be considered safe.[297]

6.26.5 SAFETY IN PREGNANCY

The *Botanical Safety Handbook* notes that even large doses of *Lepidium meyenii* extract fed to pregnant rodents resulted in no birth abnormalities. There are no reports of adverse effects in human pregnancy.[298]

6.26.6 DRUG INTERACTION

The *Botanical Safety Handbook* notes no known drug interactions involving *Lepidium meyenii*.

6.27 *LILIUM BROWNII*

The Asian lily carries the scientific name *Lilium brownii*. In traditional Chinese medicine, the bulb of the lily, called *bai he*, has been used for hundreds of years to treat conditions as varied as heart palpitations, restlessness, insomnia, whooping cough, bronchitis, and pneumonia. In the Chinese tradition, the herb is thought to clear heat and restore lung *yin* deficiency. It is also said to clear heat from the heart and calm the spirit, or *Shen*. In most cases, traditional Chinese medicine uses herbs in combination. However, *bai he* is one of the few herbs that may at times be used on its own.[299]

6.27.1 ANXIOLYTIC EFFECTS

A study found that daily ingestion of tea made from dried *Lilium brownii* for 8 weeks significantly reduced symptoms of GAD as measured by the Hamilton Anxiety Rating Scale.[300] In fact, the herb was slightly but significantly more effective than 0.5mg (admittedly a modest dose) of the standard Western anxiolytic drug lorazepam.

6.27.2 MECHANISM OF ACTION

Lilium brownii contains a variety of phytochemicals, including steroidal saponins, polysaccharides, alkaloids, and flavonoids. It is not known which of them might be responsible for the anxiolytic effect.[301] However, in a study of *Lilium davidii*, a close cousin of *Lilium brownii*, extract of the bulb increased levels of serotonin and melatonin in rat brain, as well as increased the activity of GABA receptors.[302]

6.27.3 DOSAGE

There are no clear and consistent recommendations for dosage available in the Western literature. The excellent Me & Qi Chinese medicine website recommends 6 to 12g per day of boiled and then dried bulb.

6.27.4 TOXICITY

There are no searchable studies of toxicity of *Lilium brownii* to be found in the scientific literature. Of note, the bulb is widely eaten as food in China and can generally be considered as safe for consumption.

6.27.5 SAFETY IN PREGNANCY

The *Botanical Safety Handbook* notes no evidence from the scientific literature of any specific dangers of using *Lilium brownii* in pregnancy. At the same time, they note that the herb has not been proven safe.[303]

6.27.6 DRUG INTERACTION

The *Botanical Safety Handbook* notes no evidence from the scientific literature of any drug interactions involving *Lilium brownii*.

6.28 LIPPIA CITRIODORA

The common herb lemon verbena is known by several scientific names, including *Lippia citriodora*, *Lippia triphylla*, and *Aloysia citrodora*. It is a small flowering, perennial shrub native to South America but now cultivated around the world due to its pleasant lemony aroma and taste. Its leaves are used for the preparation of herbal tea or to extract essential oil. The plant has a long history of use in various folk medicines to treat asthma, spasms, colds, fever, flatulence, colic, diarrhea, indigestion, insomnia, and anxiety.[304]

6.28.1 ANXIOLYTIC EFFECTS

There have been no formal studies of the effects of *Lippia citriodora* in people diagnosed with an anxiety disorder. However, there is at least one study of the effects of the herb on mood including anxiety.[305] Healthy university students received 600mg of dried *Lippia citriodora* extract twice a day for 3 weeks. At the beginning and end of the treatment, data were collected using the Profile of Mood States questionnaire. In comparison to those who received placebo capsules, the students who received the herb extract had significantly lower scores for the tension-anxiety, anger-hostility, and fatigue-inertia sections of the questionnaire.

Another study evaluated the effects of essential oil of *Lippia citriodora* on sleep in elderly patients diagnosed as having sleep disorders.[306] Although insomnia is not considered an anxiety disorder, many of the same herbs and even prescription medications are used to treat both conditions. Elderly patients diagnosed with insomnia received a drop of oil of *Lippia citriodora* in a nostril twice a day for 4 weeks. By the end of that time, subjects who received the nasal drops of *Lippia citriodora* oil had significantly improved sleep.

6.28.2 MECHANISM OF ACTION

Among the main constituents of the essential oil of *Lippia citriodora* are sabinene, limonene, cineole, ocimene, terpineol, neral, geranial, β-caryophyllene, germacrene, curcumene, bicyclogermacrene, nerolidol, spathulenol, and cadinol.[307] One study showed that *Lippia citriodora* has several flavonoids that may be unique to the herb.[308] Iridoid glycosides from *Lippia citriodora*, including hastatoside, verbenalin, and verbascoside, all classified as iridoid glycosides, have each been found to induce sleep in laboratory mice.[309] Studies in mice have further shown that extract of *Lippia citriodora* has an anticonvulsant effect, and this effect can be reversed by flumazenil.[310] That finding indicates that at least some of the anxiolytic effects of *Lippia citriodora* are due to mimicking the anxiolytic benzodiazepines at GABA receptors in the brain. Other studies have shown that extract of *Lippia citriodora* has effects that can be blocked by drugs that reduce the activity of serotonin in the brain. *Lippia citriodora* also contains steroid-like triterpenes, particularly ursolic acid.[311] Ursolic acid is known to have anti-inflammatory effects and, like many plant triterpenes, may contribute adaptogenic effects.

6.28.3 DOSAGE

In the study of university students noted prior, each subject received 600mg of dried extract twice a day.[305] That dried extract was prepared specifically for that study.

However, liquid extract of *Lippia citriodora* is available in stores and on the internet to be used as directed. Essential oil is also readily available. Dried leaf may also be made into tea to suit the individual. It is worth noting that *Lippia citriodora* is a flavoring for many beverages and solid edibles, and the essential oil, perhaps the most concentrated form of the herb, is generally recognized as safe by the US Food and Drug Administration.

6.28.4 TOXICITY

A study found no deaths of mice at doses up to 800mg/kg.[312]

6.28.5 SAFETY IN PREGNANCY

The *Botanical Safety Handbook* notes no evidence from the scientific literature of any specific dangers of using *Lippia citriodora* in pregnancy. At the same time, they note that the herb has not been proven safe.[313]

6.28.6 DRUG INTERACTIONS

The *Botanical Safety Handbook* notes no evidence from the scientific literature of any significant drug interactions involving *Lippia citriodora*.

6.29 MAGNOLIA OFFICINALIS

Magnolia officinalis is a species of magnolia tree native to the mountains and valleys of China. It has long been used in traditional Chinese medicine and is an essential component of at least two classical herbal combinations, *ban xia hou pu* and *zhi zi hou po*, that are used to treat symptoms of major depression. Modern studies have shown aqueous and methanolic extracts of *Magnolia officinalis* to exhibit antioxidative, anti-inflammatory, antitumorigenic, antidiabetic, antimicrobial, antinociceptive, antineurodegenerative, and antidepressant properties.[314]

6.29.1 ANXIOLYTIC EFFECTS

There are no published studies of effects of *Magnolia officinalis* alone on mood in human subjects. However, there are two studies examining effects of the combination of *Magnolia officinallis* and *Phellodendron amurense* on general mood, cortisol, and stress. The earliest study showed that 6 weeks of administration of this herbal combination to overweight women who complained of "stress eating" had only minor effects. It reduced transitory episodes of anxiety but had no effect on long-standing feelings of anxiety or depression as measured using the Spielberger State-Trait Anxiety Inventory. It also had no effects on salivary cortisol, appetite, body morphology, or sleep. Part of these disappointing results may have been a very large dropout rate of nearly 50%.[315] In another study, 4 weeks of supplementation of the *Magnolia officinalis* and *Phellodendron amurense* extract reduced salivary cortisol as well as significantly reduced overall stress, tension, depression, anger, fatigue, and confusion.[316]

6.29.2 MECHANISM OF ACTION

The bark of the *Magnolia officinalis* tree is the major source of its medicinal phytochemicals. Among these chemicals, magnolol and its isomer, honokiol, are the most important. Other substances isolated from the bark are magnolianone, rythron-honokitriol, threo-honokitriol, magnaldehyde, magnatriol, randaiol, obovatol, magnolignan B, p-hydroxylbenzaldehyde, coniferaldehyde, coniferol, syringaldehyde, syringaresinol, and acteoside.[317–318]

A recent study has shown the combination of L-theanine extracted from green tea, lemon balm, and bark of *Magnolia officinalis* has potent anxiolytic-like effects in rats. These effects were not blocked by flumazenil, showing it was not mediated by benzodiazepine receptors. However, it was blocked by AM251, a cannabinoid receptor type 1 (CB1) antagonist, suggesting that the endocannabinoid system may be involved in the anxiolytic effects of that combination.[319] On the other hand, studies have shown that both honokiol and magnolol affect activity at GABA-A receptors, though perhaps at sites other than benzodiazepine receptors.[320]

6.29.3 DOSAGE

Powdered bark of *Magnolia officinalis* is commercially available under several brand names in 400mg capsules to be taken once daily.

6.29.4 TOXICITY

Toxicological studies of hydroethanolic extracts of the closely related plant *Magnolia grandiflora* were without deaths or obvious adverse effects in doses up to 5.7g/ kg.[321] Extrapolated to a 75kg human adult, that dose would be approximately 40g.

6.29.5 SAFETY IN PREGNANCY

Reference texts from traditional Chinese medicine advise against use of *Magnolia* species during pregnancy.[322–323]

6.29.6 DRUG INTERACTIONS

The *Botanical Safety Handbook* notes no known interactions of *Magnolia* species with drugs.[324] Honokiol and magnolol, the primary bioactive components of *Magnolia officinalis*, both potently inhibited the CYP1A2 isoenzyme but had little effect on the other cytochrome P450 enzymes.[325]

6.30 *MATRICARIA RECUTITA*

Chamomile is a member of the daisy family native to Europe and Western Asia. The use of chamomile as an herbal remedy dates at least as far back as ancient Greece and Rome. There are two herbs that go by this name, German and Roman chamomile. German chamomile, which scientists refer to as *Matricaria recutita*, is the most commonly used, best studied, and more potent of the two. The herb has long been used as a sedative, anxiolytic, antispasmodic, and treatment for mild skin inflammation. The renowned British herbalist Maud Grieve stated that chamomile is an "extremely efficacious remedy for hysterical and nervous affections in women." She further noted the herb to be "the sole certain remedy for nightmares."[326]

6.30.1 ANXIOLYTIC EFFECTS

Several controlled clinical studies have shown extract of *Matricaria recutita* to be effective in treating both acute and chronic symptoms of mild to moderate degrees of anxiety in adults diagnosed with GAD. In one such study, 8 weeks of daily 220mg doses of *Matricaria recutita* extract, standardized to a content of 1.2% apigenin, significantly reduced anxiety as measured by the Hamilton Anxiety Rating Scale.[327] In another study, 500mg capsules of standardized extract of *Matricaria recutita* three times a day over 12 weeks significantly reduced symptoms of anxiety in patients who had been diagnosed with moderate to severe GAD.[328] A similar study showed that 8 weeks of 1,500mg per day dosing of standardized *Matricaria recutita* extract significantly reduced anxiety in patients suffering moderate to severe GAD, as measured by the well-recognized Hamilton Anxiety Rating Scale and Beck Anxiety Inventory.[329] *Matricaria recutita* has also been shown to offer significant antidepressant effects in people suffering major depression. Thus, it is important to note that similar dosing of *Matricaria recutita* relieves depression as well as anxiety in patients diagnosed with both major depression and GAD.[330]

6.30.2 MECHANISM OF ACTION

There are a wide variety of phytochemicals contained in *Matricaria recutita*. Extracts of the herb contain the coumarins herniarin and umbelliferone; the phenylpropanoids chlorogenic acid and caffeic acid; and the flavonoids with derivatives apigenin, apigenin-7-O-glucoside, luteolin, luteolin-7-O-glucoside, quercetin, rutin, and naringenin. The essential oil is rich in terpenoids, including bisabolol.[331] The primary active phytochemicals in chamomile are likely to be the flavonoid apigenin and the monocyclic sesquiterpene alcohol bisabolol. The lesser amounts of luteolin, quercetin, rutin, and naringenin are all known to be bioactive. Bisabolol has an anxiolytic effect in mice that is reversed by flumazenil, suggesting action at benzodiazepine receptors.[332] However, the effects of chamomile on GABA-A receptor activity appear to be complex. As noted in Chapter 5, apigenin and (–)-epigallocatechin gallate enhance the effects of benzodiazepines. Some studies have found that apigenin itself can act like a benzodiazepine and thus provide anxiolytic effects. Borneol, a monoterpenoid present in the essential oil of *Matricaria recutita*, as well as other medicinal plants such as valerian and lavender, has also been found to enhance the effects of GABA. However, those effects of borneol are not blocked by flumazenil, meaning that its effects could be synergistic with the effects of those phytochemicals that mimic benzodiazepines.[333]

6.30.3 DOSAGE

Hoffman recommends infusion of 2–3 teaspoons of herb in 1 cup hot water, to be drunk up to four times a day. Alternatively, 3 to 10ml of tincture (1:5 in 50% ethanol) may be taken three times a day.[334]

6.30.4 Toxicity

In rats the LD50 of dried decoction of *Matricaria recutita* flowers was above 3,200mg/kg, as up to that dose, no toxic effects were observed.[335] In mice, the LD50 of the essential oil of *Matricaria recutita* was noted to be above 5,000mg/kg, as up to and including that dose, no animal deaths were noted.[336]

6.30.5 Safety in Pregnancy

In a study of Palestinian women, the use of *Matricaria recutita* during pregnancy was quite common. Nearly half of pregnant women used the herb. Although the sample was relatively small, i.e., 300 women, there was not a statistically significance in pregnancy outcomes between those who used *Matricaria recutita* and those who did not.[337] The *Botanical Safety Handbook* noted no concerns for use but also noted no firm evidence of safety.[338]

6.30.6 Drug Interaction

The crude essential oil of *Matricaria recutita* significantly inhibited the activity of the CYP1A2 isoenzyme and, to lesser extents, the CYP2C9, CYP2D6, and CYP3A4 isoforms.[339] However, the *Botanical Safety Handbook* notes no known interactions with drugs.

6.31 *MELISSA OFFICINALIS*

Lemon balm, with the scientific name *Melissa officinalis*, is a perennial plant of the mint family that is native to south-central Europe, the Mediterranean basin, Iran, and Central Asia. As noted by Maud Grieve in her famous book, *A Modern Herbal*, "It was highly esteemed by Paracelsus, who believed it would completely revivify a man. It was formerly esteemed of great use in all complaints supposed to proceed from a disordered state of the nervous system." She further noted, "The London Dispensary (1696) says: 'An essence of Balm, given in Canary wine, every morning will renew youth, strengthen the brain, relieve languishing nature and prevent baldness.'"[340] The herb has long been used for a wide range of human complaints, including depression, psychosis, hysteria, insomnia, epilepsy, headaches, vertigo, syncope, malaise, flatulence, indigestion, colic, nausea, anemia, asthma, bronchitis, amenorrhea, rheumatism, ulcers, and wounds.

6.31.1 Anxiolytic Effects

In an open-label study of volunteers with mild to moderate anxiety disorders and sleep disturbances, chronic administration extract of *Melissa officinalis* significantly reduced anxiety and improved insomnia. As many as 95% of subjects responded to treatment, and 70% achieved full remission from anxiety. About 85% of subjects reported better sleep.[341] Another study found *Melissa officinalis* to be effective in reducing anxiety and improving sleep in patients who had undergone coronary bypass surgery, a significant cause of anxiety and general distress.[342]

6.31.2 MECHANISM OF ACTION

Melissa officinalis is rich in polyphenolic phytochemicals, many of which have been identified as active components of extracts of various other herbs. Among the substances it contains are rosmarinic acid, caffeic acids, chlorogenic acid, metrilic acid, tannins, luteolin, apigenin, monoterpene glycosides, β-caryophyllene, germacrene, triterpenes, citronellal, citrals, ocimene, citronellol, geraniol, nerol, linalool, and ethric oil.[343] Many of those substances act directly at GABA receptors. However, there is also evidence that some component of *Melissa officinalis* may inhibit GABA transaminase, the enzyme that deactivates GABA, and thus enhance GABAergic activity.[344] Of note, neither methanolic nor aqueous extracts of *Melissa officinalis* displaced flumazenil from GABA receptors. There are reports that *Melissa officinalis* contains an inhibitor of monoamine oxidase, an enzyme that deactivates serotonin and norepinephrine.[345] Potent monoamine oxidase inhibitors have long been used as antidepressants but have also been known to reduce anxiety in depressed patients.

6.31.3 DOSAGE

Hoffman suggests dosing of tincture (1:5, 40%) to be 2 to 6ml three times a day. Alternatively, one may take as an infusion of 2 to 3 teaspoons of dried herb in a cup of water two to three times a day.[346]

6.31.4 TOXICITY

The LD50 of the dried alcoholic extract of *Melissa officinalis* in mice is reported to be 4.5g/kg.[347] This would extrapolate to be approximately 315g for a 75kg human adult.

6.31.5 SAFETY IN PREGNANCY

The *Botanical Safety Handbook* notes there to be no definitive guidance from the literature concerning the safety of this herb during pregnancy.[348]

6.31.6 DRUG INTERACTIONS

The *Botanical Safety Handbook* notes no known interactions with drugs.

6.32 *MENTHA PIPERITA*

Mentha piperita, commonly known as peppermint, is a hybrid plant. It is a cross between watermint and spearmint. The plant, indigenous to Europe and the Middle East, is now cultivated around the world. *Mentha piperita* has long been used medicinally. *Mentha haplocalyx*, an indigenous Chinese mint referred to as *bo he*, is associated with the lung and liver meridians. It has been used to expel wind and heat, clear the head and eyes, clear up rashes, and remove liver *Qi* stagnation. It is also taken as a means of stimulating the nervous system.[349] *Mentha piperita* has also long been used in Western herbalism. The German Commission E has approved the internal use of oil of *Mentha piperita* for a variety of conditions, including flatulence, gastro-intestinal and gallbladder disorders, and catarrhs of the upper respiratory tract, and external use for myalgia and neuralgia.[350] There is also evidence of anxiolytic effects of *Mentha piperita*, either through ingestion or aromatherapy. (See Chapter 10.)

6.32.1 ANXIOLYTIC EFFECTS

In a study on the anxiolytic effects of *Mentha piperita* decoction, participants were healthy college students experiencing the typical stresses of college life.[351] Indeed, any potential subjects who had been diagnosed with a psychiatric illness were elimi-nated from the study. The experimental group was asked to drink tea brewed from leaves of *Mentha piperita* once a day for 4 weeks, while the control group was asked not to consume any other forms of peppermint or any other herbs during the study. Anxiety, stress, memory performance, and sleep quality of the participating student were assessed by self-reported questionnaires before and after the *Mentha piper-ita* treatment. After 4 weeks scores obtained by the State-Trait Anxiety Inventory and the Pittsburgh Sleep Quality Index were both significantly better in the *Mentha piperita* group than in the control group.

6.32.2 MECHANISM OF ACTION

As is the case with many plants of the mint family, the concentrated oil of *Mentha piperita* has a high menthol content. The essential oil and extracts of the leaves also contain menthone, various menthyl esters, menthofuran, 1,8-cineol, limonene, pule-gone, β-caryophyllene, pinene, eriocitrin, hesperidin, luteolin, kaempferol, and other flavonoids.[352–353]

Menthol, the monoterpenoid in *Mentha piperita* oil, has interesting and complex actions in the body. It enhances activity of GABA-A receptors in the brain and also, to some degree, activity at glycine receptors.[354] Both are inhibitory and often act to calm the nervous system. In animal studies, menthol alone is effective in reducing anxiety-like behaviors.[355] Several of the flavonoids in the leaves of *Mentha piperita* are known to enhance GABA activity, and β-caryophyllene may have effects at can-nabinoid receptors.

6.32.3 DOSAGE

In the study described prior, participants once a day drank tea made from the infusion of 250mg of fresh leaves of *Mentha piperita* soaked for 10 minutes.[351] The German Commission E recommends a larger 3 to 6g dose per day or 5 to 15ml of tincture per day.[356] It is interesting to think that the slightly higher dose may have more of an anxiolytic effect.

6.32.4 TOXICITY

Mentha piperita is commonly consumed as a beverage and confectionary and is gen-erally regarded as safe. Use of the more concentrated oil may require circumspection.

6.32.5 SAFETY IN PREGNANCY

The German Commission E does not list pregnancy as a concern for use of either *Mentha piperita* oil or leaf. The *Botanical Safety Handbook* does recommend that caution be used with the more potent oil of *Mentha piperita* and that it be used only with expert guidance. It is likely that use of the oil as aromatherapy would be of less concern.[357]

6.32.6 DRUG INTERACTION

The *Botanical Safety Handbook* notes no reports of drug interactions involving *Mentha piperita*.

6.33 NARDOSTACHYS JATAMANSI

Nardostachys jatamansi, with the common English name spikenard, is native to the Himalayan foothills of India. There it is known as *jatamansi*, and it is one of the classical Ayurvedic herbs used in the treatment of anxiety and other psychiatric disorders. It has also been used in traditional Chinese medicine with the name *gansong*. *Nardostachys jatamansi* is a close cousin to the better-known herb valerian, and it has similar uses. It should be noted that there is considerable confusion in the literature about distinctions between *Nardostachys jatamansi* and *Valeriana jatamansi*, with some sources suggesting they are the same plant. However, this is not the case.[358] (See *Valeriana jatamansi* in this chapter.) There are also references to *Nardostachys chinensis* and *Nardostachys grandiflora*, as if they are synonyms of *Nardostachys jatamansi*. These may be varieties and do not appear to be distinct species.

6.33.1 ANXIOLYTIC EFFECTS

In a randomized, controlled study, the administration of capsules containing 530mg of *Nardostachys jatamansi* significantly relieved anxiety in otherwise normal patients on the night before and the morning of scheduled orthopedic surgery. Results were obtained using the Berger Anxiety Inventory.[359]

6.33.2 MECHANISM OF ACTION

Among the phytochemicals in *Nardostachys jatamansi* are jatamansic acid, nardostachone, nardol acaciin, ursolic acid, octacosanol, kanshone A, nardosinone-diol, nardosinone, aristolen-9 β-ol, oleanolic acid, and β-sitosterol.[360] A study found that nasal inhalation of a sesquiterpenoid isolated from *Nardostachys jatamansi*, aristolen-1(10)-en-9-ol, had a sedative effect in mice that was reversed by flumazenil.[361] Thus, those effects were due to mimicking the effects of benzodiazepines. The steroid-like triterpenoids known as oleanic and ursolic acid have anxiolytic effects that are not reversed by flumazenil, and they may act by mimicking natural, anxiolytic neurosteroids in the brain. Finally, there is evidence that some of the aristolane- and nardosinane- type sesquiterpenoids in *Nardostachys jatamansi* may act as inhibitors of serotonin reuptake sites.[362] That effect is the mechanism of action of the SSRI antidepressants, which can also help relieve anxiety as well as depression.

6.33.3 DOSAGE

In the study noted above, subjects were given single doses of 530mg dried root.[358] In the other study, *Nardostachys jatamansi* was administered by the unique Ayurvedic method of *shirodhara*—that is, dripping extract of the herb in oil upon the foreheads of the subjects. The latter method makes dosing difficult to estimate.

6.33.4 TOXICITY

In mice, the LD50 of methanolic extract of *Nardostachys jatamansi* was found to be very high at 2,000mg/kg of body weight.[363] Thus, it may be considered to have low toxicity.

6.33.5 SAFETY IN PREGNANCY

In traditional Ayurvedic medicine, *Nardostachys jatamansi* has been used to stimulate menstrual flow. Thus, it is generally seen as imprudent for use during pregnancy.

6.33.6 DRUG INTERACTION

The *Botanical Safety Handbook* notes no known or suspected cases of adverse drug interactions during use of *Nardostachys jatamansi*.[364]

6.34 OCIMUM SANCTUM

Ocimum sanctum, or, alternatively, *Ocimum tenuiflorum*, is a perennial plant native to the Indian subcontinent and widespread as a cultivated plant throughout the Southeast Asian tropics. Its common English name is holy basil. However, in Ayurvedic medicine, *Ocimum sanctum* is called *tulsi*, which in Sanskrit is "the incomparable one." The name reflects its special place in Hindu culture. *Ocimum sanctum* was also known in Western civilization and was used by the ancient Greeks and Romans

It has been used for the treatment of a variety of ailments, including bronchial asthma, chronic fever, colds, cough, malaria, dysentery, convulsions, diarrhea, arthritis, vomiting, and liver and heart conditions.[365] *Ocimum sanctum* is also sometimes used as a culinary spice. However, its close relative—sweet basil, or *Ocimum basilicum*—is more commonly used in cooking.

6.34.1 ANXIOLYTIC EFFECTS

There is at least one study in which the effects of *Ocimum sanctum* were evaluated in patients who had been diagnosed as suffering GAD. After 60 days of twice daily treatment, extract of *Ocimum sanctum* was shown to significantly reduce symptoms of GAD as well as to reduce feelings of depression and physical signs of stress.[366]

In a study of healthy adults, 15 days of once daily treatment with *Ocimum sanctum* reduced feelings of anxiety and stress during a challenging cognitive test. The herb also significantly improved performance and reduced levels of the stress hormone cortisol.[367]

6.34.2 MECHANISM OF ACTION

Leaves of *Ocimum sanctum* contain a variety of active phytochemicals, including apigenin, oleanolic acid, ursolic acid, rosmarinic acid, eugenol, carvacrol, linalool, luteolin, and β-caryophyllene. The essential oil consists mostly of eugenol, β-elemene, β-caryophyllene, and germacrene.[368] Some of its flavonoids and phenolic compounds, as discussed in Chapter 5, are known to act at the GABA-A receptor to produce anxiolytic effects. Indeed, studies have shown that some of the anxiolytic effects of its essential oil are reversed by the benzodiazepine antagonist flumazenil.[369] Linalool and β-caryophyllene contained in the herb have modest effects on cannabinoid receptors. *Ocimum sanctum* also contains steroid-like terpenes—i.e., ursolic acid and others—that are likely to give the herb adaptogenic effects that in turn would build resiliency to combat anxiety and stress.

6.34.3 DOSAGE

In the two successful human studies of *Ocimum sanctum* referred to above, one used 500mg capsules of dried alcohol extract twice a day,[366] whereas the other used 400mg capsules of standardized extract taken three times a day.[367]

6.34.4 TOXICITY

The LD50 in mice for essential oil of *Ocimum basilicum* was found to be 3.64mL per kilogram of weight.[370] Extrapolated to a 75kg human adult, this dose would be approximately 255ml.

6.34.5 SAFETY IN PREGNANCY

Traditional Chinese medicine doctrine warns against use of *Ocimum basilicum* during pregnancy.[371]

6.34.6 DRUG INTERACTIONS

The *Botanical Safety Handbook* notes no known interactions with drugs.[372]

6.35 *PANAX GINSENG*

The common name ginseng is used in reference to several plants of the genus *Panax*, including *Panax ginseng*, or Korean ginseng; *Panax notoginseng*, or

Chinese ginseng; and *Panax quinquefolius*, or American ginseng. The herb called Siberian ginseng is not in the Panax family but is rather another plant entirely, *Eleutherococcus senticosus*. *Panax spp* have been used for several thousand years in Asia as a tonic and, in traditional Chinese medicine, has been included as an ingredient in several classical herbal combinations for the treatment of depression. It is currently classified by many as an adaptogen, with alleged ability to enhance physical performance, promote vitality, increase resistance to stress and aging, and strengthen immune function.

Panax ginseng, *Panax notoginseng*, and *Panax quinquefolius* differ in several ways.[373] The most significant difference is the presence of ginsenoside R in *Panax ginseng* and *Panax notoginseng*, but not *Panax quinquefolius*. Moreover, pseudoginsenoside occurs in *Panax quinquefolius* but not in *Panax ginseng* or *Panax notoginseng*. Nonetheless, the Chinese saw American ginseng—that is, *Panax quinquefolius*—as sufficiently valuable such that large quantities of the North American species began being shipped to China as early as 1718. Hunters of wild American ginseng in Appalachia still profit from the demand. Although there are differences among the ginsengs, it has been suggested that the most important factor in determining the bioavailability and activity of the ginsengs may be differences in intestinal flora in individuals. Of note, the root of *Panax ginseng* is steamed and dried to prepare red ginseng, while the peeled roots dried without steaming are designated as white ginseng. The prepared ginseng can then be further treated through fermentation. In any case, most of the research has focused on the Korean species—that is, *Panax ginseng*.

6.35.1 ANXIOLYTIC EFFECTS

There have been several studies evaluating effects of *Panax ginseng* on mood and general sense of well-being. In some cases, evaluations included questions about anxiety. However, none of the studies focused on individuals with anxiety disorders.

In a study of healthy adults, 4 months of treatment with *Panax ginseng* improved mood and increased relaxation, which would suggest a decrease in anxiety.[374] In another 4-month study of health adults, the addition of powdered extract of *Panax ginseng* to vitamin and mineral supplements significantly improved reports on general quality of life.[375] In otherwise healthy postmenopausal women, 4 months of daily treatment with *Panax ginseng* extract also improved mood and general sense of well-being, though anxiety itself was not investigated.[376]

Unfortunately, the effects of *Panax ginseng* on anxiety or simply on one's sense of well-being have not been found to be uniformly beneficial. In a study of healthy adults, 4 weeks of treatment with *Panax ginseng* improved mood and social functioning, but the effect was no longer seen after 8 weeks.[377] In yet another, young healthy adults gained no benefits at all from 8 weeks of daily supplementation with *Panax ginseng*.[378] Though *Panax ginseng* may be useful to enhance general health and well-being, it does not seem to be a strong or reliable treatment for significant anxiety. It might best be added to more effective treatments to help build resiliency and restore health.

6.35.2 MECHANISM OF ACTION

Approximately 200 substances, such as steroid-like ginsenosides, polysaccharides, polyacetylenes, peptides, and amino acids, have been isolated from *Panax ginseng*, *Panax notoginseng*, and *Panax quinquefolius*.[379] Some ginsenosides are active at GABA-A receptors.[380] Accordingly, many ginsenosides on their own can relieve anxiety-like behaviors in animals or can enhance the effects of benzodiazepines. Ginsenosides also bind at GABA-B receptors.[381] Baclofen, a drug that stimulates GABA-B receptors, is generally used as a muscle relaxer, but it can also relieve anxiety to some degree.[382] Some of the steroid-like terpenes in *Panax spp* may also act as adaptogens and thereby enhance resiliency and the ability to endure stress.

6.35.3 DOSAGE

Hoffman recommends a dose of 200mg of 5:1 standardized *Panax ginseng* extract once a day, a 1 to 2ml tincture (1:5 in 60%) three times a day, or a standard decoction of 1/2 teaspoon powdered root in a cup of water three times a day.[383]

6.35.4 TOXICITY

The *Panax spp* appear quite non-toxic, with the LD50 in mice reported to be in a range between 10 and 30g/kg.[384] That is far beyond typical human dosage.

6.35.5 SAFETY IN PREGNANCY

At least two studies have described use of *Panax ginseng* in pregnant women with no adverse effects on mother or fetus.[385-386]

6.35.6 DRUG INTERACTIONS

There have been case reports of bleeding in patients after adding *Panax ginseng* to warfarin treatment.[387] However, more rigorous human studies of this possible interaction have shown no such effects.[388] In healthy human volunteers, 28 days of 500mg *Panax ginseng* twice daily significantly decreased serum levels of midazolam in comparison with controls. This was taken to be indicative of induction of the CYP3A family of cytochrome P450 enzymes.[389]

6.36 *PASSIFLORA INCARNATA*

The common name passionflower describes a variety of species of plants in the genus *Passiflora*. The German Commission E specifically considers the species *Passiflora incarnata*, but others of the genus contain similar phytochemicals and offer similar benefits. The majority of *Passiflora* species are found in Mexico and Central and South America, although there are additional representatives in the United States,

Southeast Asia, and Oceania. The herb has long been used in herbal medicine for the treatment of anxiety, dysmenorrhea, epilepsy, insomnia, neurosis, and neuralgia.[390] Maud Grieve, in her *A Modern Herbal*, noted that "its narcotic properties cause it to be used in diarrhea and dysentery, neuralgia, sleeplessness and dysmenorrhea."[391] There is more recent evidence of usefulness of *Passiflora* species in the treatment of mood disturbance.

6.36.1 ANXIOLYTIC EFFECTS

In a study out of Iran, *Passiflora incarnata* was found to be as effective as the benzodiazepine oxazepam in treating GAD. Those treated with the herb also reported less impairment of job performance than those who were given the benzodiazepine.[392] In two other Iranian studies, *Passiflora incarnata* was helpful in reducing acute anxiety prior to ambulatory surgery[393] and in anticipation of a dental procedure.[394]

6.36.2 MECHANISM OF ACTION

Among the phytochemicals that have been identified in *Passiflora incarnata* are homoorientin, orientin, vitexin, isovitexin, chrysin, schaftoside, isoschaftoside, chlorogenic acid, hyperoside, caffeic acid, quercetin, luteolin, rutin, scutelarein, vicenin, and their various glycoside products. The herb also contains small amounts of the harmala indole alkaloids, harman, harmin, armaline, harmol, and harmalol.[395] Some of those phytochemicals act at GABA-A receptors, and some of the effects of extract of *passiflora incarnata* can be reversed by the drug flumazenil, which blocks benzodiazepine receptors.[396]

6.36.3 DOSAGE

Hoffman recommends 1 to 4ml of tincture (1.5 in 40%) of *Passiflora incarnata* twice a day. Alternatively, he suggests up to 2g of dried herb four times a day.[397]

6.36.4 TOXICITY

The LD50 of intraperitoneally administered extract of *Passiflora incarnata* has been reported to be above 900mg/kg in mice.[398] Extrapolated to a 75kg human adult, this dose would above 70g. It was also reported that 3 weeks of oral administration of 5g/k per day of hydroalcoholic extract of *Passiflora incarnata* had no deleterious effects on rats.[399]

6.36.5 SAFETY IN PREGNANCY

The *Botanical Safety Handbook notes* there to be no definitive guidance from the literature concerning the safety of *Passiflora incarnata* during pregnancy.[400] No adverse developmental effects were observed in rats born to females administered 400mg/kg *Passiflora incarnata* extract daily on days 7 through 17 of pregnancy.[401]

6.36.6 DRUG INTERACTIONS

A benzoflavone moiety in *Passiflora incarnata* has been reported to inhibit aromatase, a member of the CYP3A4 isoenzyme family. This effect dampens the metabolic conversion of testosterone to its metabolites, thereby increasing serum levels of free testosterone and decreasing free estrogen. This may explain some reports of aphrodisiac effects of the herb.[402] However, the *Botanical Safety Handbook* notes no known interactions of *Passiflora incarnata* with commonly prescribed medications.

6.37 *PIPER METHYSTICUM*

Kava is the product of the pulverized roots of the *Piper methysticum* pepper plant that is native to the South Pacific islands. For centuries it has been used by Polynesian cultures as a ceremonial beverage for welcoming guests and honoring all degrees of social relationships. The effects of drinking kava have been described as inducing a "warm, pleasant and cheerful but lazy feeling making people sociable, though not hilarious or loquacious, and not interfering with reasoning."[403] Kava is described as having a wide range of pharmacological effects, including anxiolytic, anti-stress, sedative, analgesic, muscle relaxant, antithrombotic, neuroprotective, mild anesthetic, hypnotic, and anticonvulsant.

6.37.1 ANXIOLYTIC EFFECTS

Piper methysticum is one of the most studied herbs used for the treatment of anxiety. Most studies show that the herb is effective in relieving anxiety. Perhaps most notably, a Cochrane Review concluded that "kava extract is an effective symptomatic treatment for anxiety."[404] The effect was then seen as small. But subsequent studies have found more compelling effects. Jerome Sarris, a researcher and clinician in the Department of Psychiatry at the University of Melbourne, has published several reviews and clinical studies of the effects of *Piper methysticum* on anxiety.[405] *Piper methysticum* is native to the Polynesian islands in proximity to Australia, and thus Sarris has maintained a special interest in the herb. In one of Sarris's most recent studies, extract of *Piper methysticum* was found to significantly relieve anxiety in patients diagnosed with GAD.[406] In fact, at the end of the 6-week study, 26% of those receiving *Piper methysticum* no longer met criteria to diagnose that anxiety disorder. The extract was found to be safe and well tolerated, with no serious adverse effects.

6.37.2 MECHANISM OF ACTION

Among the many phytochemical constituents of *Piper methysticum* are those known collectively as kavalactones or kavapyrones. Six of these kavalactones, including kavain, dihydrokavain, methysticin, dihydromethysticin, yangonin, and desmethoxyyangonin, are thought responsible for nearly all the plant's pharmacological activity. The main mechanisms of action of *Piper methysticum* have been thought to be modulation of GABA activity via alteration of lipid membrane structure and sodium channel function,[407] monoamine oxidase B inhibition,[408] and noradrenaline and dopamine reuptake inhibition.[409-410] Recent research shows the constituent yangonin to be a novel cannabinoid.[411] Despite suggestions that *Piper methysticum* may enhance GABAergic activity, studies have found that the anxiolytic effects of extract of the root are resistant to flumazenil.[412]

6.37.3 DOSAGE

In the clinical study by Sarris et al. noted above, subjects received 2 tablets a day containing dried water extract of *Piper methysticum* standardized to contain 60mg of kavalactones per tablet for a total daily dose of 120mg of kavalactones.[406] After 3 weeks, this was increased to a dose of 240mg of kavalactones a day for those who did not respond to the lower dose. There are many preparations of *Piper methysticum* extract standardized by kavalactone content available in natural health stores and on the internet.

6.37.4 TOXICITY

Safety has been a major concern with the use of *Piper methysticum* after reports of liver damage emerged in the late 1990s. Indeed, at one time the herb was taken off the market in Europe. In the previous book, *Herbal Treatment of Major Depression*, it was advised to not use *Piper methysticum* to treat major depression because the availability of other more effective herbs and prescription medications made the risk unreasonable. Indeed, for full discussion of those concerns, see that text.[413] However, *Piper methysticum* is likely a better anxiolytic and sleep agent than it is an antidepressant, and the risk may be more worth taking to treat anxiety and insomnia. Moreover, steps can be taken to mitigate risk. Sarris, noted prior, has used *Piper methysticum* safely and effectively. He has concluded that the use of only the peeled roots from *Piper methysticum* plants grown specifically for therapeutic use, with subsequent water extraction of the medicinal phytochemicals, produced an herbal medicine that was both safe and effective. Certainly, no one with established liver disease should use *Piper methysticum*. Anyone starting *Piper methysticum* should occasionally be monitored by a doctor, including assays of transaminases if deemed necessary. It would also be prudent to augment any treatment using *Piper methysticum* with the liver-protecting herb milk thistle or supplement with the live-protecting agent N-acetylcysteine, which is available over the counter in many pharmacies.[414–415]

6.37.5 SAFETY IN PREGNANCY

The *Botanical Safety Handbook* notes that treatment of pregnant rodents with significant doses of various components of *Piper methysticum* caused no birth defects. Yet they prudently advise against its use except under expert supervision.[416] However, the German Commission E advises against its use in pregnant women.

6.37.6 DRUG INTERACTIONS

The *Botanical Safety Handbook* further states that *Piper methysticum* can interfere with activity of CYP2E1. Among the drugs metabolized in part by CYP2E1 are ethanol, nicotine, acetaminophen, acetone, aspartame, chloroform, chlorzoxazone, and some antiepileptic drugs like phenobarbital.[417]

6.38 *PORIA COCOS*

The *Poria cocos* mushroom, also known alternatively as *Wolfiporia extensa*, is a time-honored ingredient in many traditional Chinese medicine formulas. In China it is known as *wuling*, but it may also be seen as *fu ling* or *hoelen*. In the English language it is sometime referred to as China root. In traditional medicine, *Poria cocos* filaments have been used to treat loss of memory, anxiety, restlessness, fatigue, tension, nervousness, dizziness, urination problems, fluid retention, insomnia, stomach problems, diarrhea, and tumors and to control coughing.[418]

6.38.1 ANXIOLYTIC EFFECTS

There are at least two studies of the effects of *Poria cocos* on anxiety. In one case, the patients in the study were diagnosed with GAD. Patients with anxiety were given either capsules of poria mushroom three times a day or the Western drug Deanxit once a day for 2 months. Deanxit is a potent combination of two psychoactive agents—the antipsychotic drug flupentixol and the antidepressant drug melitracen. This drug is not approved by the FDA for use in the United States. The mushroom produced relief from anxiety similar to that of Deanxit, but without side effects or undue sedation.[419] In another study, women experiencing symptoms of menopause, including complaints of anxiety and depression, were given either *Poria cocos* or the traditional Chinese medicine herbal combination, *geng ni an chun*. *Geng ni an chun* consists of *Rehmannia glutinosa*, *Alisma orientale*, *Ophiopogon japonicus*, *Scrophularia ningpoensis*, *Paeonia suffruticosa*, *Poria cocos*, pearl shell, *Curculigo orchioides*, *Schisandra chinensis*, ground magnetite, *Polygonum multiflorum*, *Uncaria rhynchophylla*, immature wheat grain, and cured *Polygonum multiflorum*. After 6 weeks of treatments three times a day, both groups showed significant improvement in anxiety and other symptoms. However, *Poria cocos* alone, with improvement in 90% of patients, was significantly better than the herbal combination, in which 77% of patients improved. The effects of treatment were evaluated with the Kupperman Index concerned with menopause, the Self-Rating Depression Scale, and the Self-Rating Anxiety Scale before treatment and after 6 weeks of treatment.[420]

6.38.2 MECHANISM OF ACTION

The *Poria cocos* mushroom is rich in steroid-like triterpenes, which are likely responsible for much of its pharmacological activity.[421] Pachymic acid, the triterpene in *Poria cocos*, is known to enhance GABA activity.[422] Some of the triterpenes may also reduce glutamate activity in the brain, which may contribute a calming effect.[423] Other triterpenes in *Poria cocos* may reduce activity at a specific serotonin receptor in the brain called the 5-HT3 receptor.[424] This is a major mechanism of action of a prescribed antidepressant called mirtazapine. Several studies have found that mirtazapine is an effective treatment for GAD. Finally, many triterpenes in *Poria cocos* are known to have potent anti-inflammatory effects.[425] It is becoming clearer that inflammation plays a significant role in chronic psychiatric conditions such as depression and persistent anxiety disorders. Thus, the anti-inflammatory, adaptogenic effects of *Poria cocos* triterpenes may be partially responsible for its anxiolytic effects. Perhaps most important about *Poria cocos* is that it appears to act by rather unique mechanisms that can be additive to the mechanisms of action of other herbs.

6.38.3 DOSAGE

There are no reports of doses of *Poria cocos* alone for treatment of GAD, as it is traditionally used in combination for this application. I note that informal references in the literature for conditions such as edema show human subjects taking 3g of dried mushroom three times daily with good results.

6.38.4 TOXICITY

The oral LD50 of dried warm water extract in mice is 10g/kg.[426] In a human adult weighing 75kg, this would extrapolate to approximately 700g.

6.38.5 SAFETY IN PREGNANCY

Review of the literature revealed no studies of the safety of *Poria cocos* during human or animal pregnancy.

6.38.6 DRUG INTERACTIONS

Poria cocos has been found to inhibit the CYP3A4 enzyme.[427] A variety of neuroleptics, including aripiprazole, haloperidol, pimozide, and risperidone, are metabolized by this enzyme.[428] The enzyme is also involved in the metabolism of SSRIs and tricyclic antidepressants.[429] Thus, chronic use of *Poria cocos* could affect blood levels of a variety of important psychiatric medications.

6.39 *PSILOCYBE SPP*

Psilocybe is a genus of mushrooms that contains the psychoactive substance psilocybin. There are many species of *Psilocybe* that contain effective amounts of psilocybin, including *Psilocybe cubensis*, *Psilocybe cyanescens*, *Psilocybe semilanceata*, and *Psilocybe azurescens*. Psilocybin is considered a prodrug, as it must be converted to psilocin in the body. It is psilocin that has the dramatic psychoactive effects. Psilocin stimulates a specific type of serotonin receptor in the brain, the 5-HT2A receptor, that mediates the so-called psychedelic effects. The effects are similar to those produced by the synthetic molecule Lysergic acid diethylamide, or LSD; mescaline, from *Lophophora williamsii*, or peyote cactus; and dimethyltryptamine from *Banisteriopsis caapi*, also known as *ayahuasca*, from South America.[430]

Psilocybin-containing mushrooms can be used in two very different ways. One way is to ingest the mushroom in a large dose to produce the so-called psychedelic effect.

There are reports of quite remarkable results of scientific studies using psychedelic doses of *Psilocybe* mushrooms to treat several psychiatric disorders. Another purported way to use these mushrooms is through so-called microdoses of the mushroom.

Caution must be taken in presenting information about *Psilocybe* mushrooms. This is for two reasons. First, in most states these mushrooms are illegal to possess and use. Laws must not be broken. The second reason for caution is that *Psilocybe* mushrooms can have very powerful effects that must be respected and treated with due diligence. The use of these mushrooms for purposes of psychedelic-mediated personal growth should take place only under supervision of an expert knowledgeable about the effects of the mushroom. Careless or mere recreational use of this sacred plant is ill advised.

6.39.1 ANXIOLYTIC EFFECTS

There are several well-designed and controlled clinical studies of the effects of single large, "psychedelic" doses of psilocybin on anxiety and depression. In one such study, two oral doses of psilocybin (10 and 25mg, 7 days apart) provided significant relief from anxiety and depression in patients suffering severe, unipolar, treatment-resistant major depression. Data was collected using the State-Trait Anxiety Index and Beck Depression Inventory. This relief persisted for at least 6 months.[431] In another study, two treatments of 22 or 30mg/70 kg of psilocybin separated by 5 weeks provided significant and sustained relief from anxiety in patients diagnosed with life-threatening cancer. All patients in this controlled study also had a *DSM-IV* diagnosis of chronic adjustment disorder with anxiety, chronic adjustment disorder with mixed anxiety and depressed mood, GAD, major depressive disorder, or a dual diagnosis of GAD and depression. Results were obtained through a battery of tests that included the Hamilton Anxiety Rating Scale and Hamilton Depression Rating Scale, the State-Trait Anxiety Inventory, the Life Attitude Profile Death Acceptance survey, and other standard tests.[432] Psilocybin has also shown promise in the treatment of obsessive compulsive disorder[433] and PTSD.[434]

To date, there have been no controlled, clinical studies of the effects of psilocybin microdosing on anxiety or any other specific psychiatric condition. There have been several investigations in which individuals who have microdosed psilocybin on their own have been sought out and interviewed by researchers wanting to learn of their experiences.[435–436] But there are weaknesses in their methods. First, none of these subjects were formally diagnosed with any anxiety disorder. Second, methods of microdosing could not be monitored and controlled as would be the case in standard clinical trials. Some of those interviewed in various survey studies reported microdosing daily, every other day, or on a three-day cycle of one day on and two days off. There is no scientifically established basis for any of those regimens. It has also been noted that many microdosers simply estimate the dose of mushroom they are taking. Finally, those individuals who took steps to start microdosing on their own were likely to have had biases about the value of microdosing psilocybin, and their reports may need to be viewed with a certain degree of skepticism.

There is one fully controlled study of psilocybin microdosing.[437] Unfortunately, the study did not focus on anxiety or mood but rather "feelings of awe and aesthetic emotions." Participants engaged in a 3-week microdosing schedule in which they took 5–7 microdoses of psilocybin or placebo. Doses were approximately 0.7g of dried psilocybin-containing truffles that contained 1.5mg of psilocybin. This was considered to be in the high range for microdosing. After 3 weeks, the treatment each participant received was switched. They did not observe a consistent effect of microdosing on perception of art. In an interesting but not fully controlled study of microdosing of psychedelics—i.e., LSD or psilocybin—an attempt was made to introduce randomized control into what was otherwise a survey study. Participants were given instructions on how to blindly supply themselves with active microdosed psychedelic versus placebo. That study found no overall significant differences between active treatment and placebo throughout the trial. Some significant effects on anxiety (per the Spielberger State-Trait Anxiety Inventory) and mood (per the Warwick-Edinburgh Mental Wellbeing Scale and the Quick Inventory of Depressive Symptomatology) were noted on days when active drug was taken. However, those effects did not persist beyond the few hours of having taken the drug, which ostensibly is the intention of such treatment. There were also several problems in this study. First, only 23% of participants used psilocybin, with the rest using LSD. Data were then collapsed into "LSD equivalents," which eliminated any possibility of identifying effects specific to psilocybin. Second, the purity and dosing could not be guaranteed, and finally, it was noted that many—beyond chance—were able to guess whether they had taken active treatment versus placebo. The authors of the study concluded that any benefits of microdosing of psychedelics were likely due to placebo effect.[438] Of some relevance is a study of intermittent psilocybin microdosing in rats, who are arguably incapable of a placebo response. Standard rodent models of anxiolytic and antidepressant effects—the light/dark conflict and open field tests and the forced swim test respectively—revealed no significant effects.[439] All in all, it may be concluded that while psychedelic doses of psilocybin may produce powerful and long-lasting effects on anxiety and mood, there is yet to be compelling evidence of microdosed psilocybin offering similar benefits.*

6.39.2 Mechanism of Action

The fundamental mechanism of action for the so-called psychedelic effect of *Psilocybe spp* is well known.[440] This is due to stimulation of 5-HT2A receptors in the brain. However, explaining the pharmacological mechanism does not capture the nature of the psychedelic experience. It is likely that psilocybin, like other serotonergic psychedelic substances, alters consciousness by causing changes in what areas of the brain are active and connected to each other. Of particular interest is the so-called default mode network. It has been found that the functional connectivity of the default mode network is altered in patients suffering anxiety and depression.[441] It is thought that serotonergic psychedelics, like psilocybin, make connectivity in the brain more global and allow a persisting "re-set" of the default mode network.[442] The acute produces an "altered state of consciousness" that, with proper guidance, can be very conducive to insight and change. The "re-setting" of the default mode network allows persisting changes in interactions among the prefrontal cortex, cingulate, and amygdala that dampen anxiety and depression.

What remains mysterious is the possible mechanism of action of microdoses of *Psilocybe spp* or any of the other psychedelic substances. The effect is likely due to low-level stimulation of 5-HT2A receptors, but not to the extent of causing the psychedelic effect. Thus, the high dose and microdose are almost certainly effective through different mechanisms. The microdosing effect is not likely due to being "a little high." Indeed, to elaborate upon an old saying, having a subthreshold psychedelic experience is like having a subthreshold pregnancy.

One possibility is that daily, low-level stimulation of 5-HT2A receptors with small doses of *Psilocybe spp* may begin to make the 5-HT2A receptors less sensitive. That is, they down-regulate. Thus, the anxiolytic and antidepressant effects reported using microdoses may in fact be due to the very opposite of what high doses do, despite the fact that remarkable antidepressant and anxiolytic effects are reported for those high doses. This seems paradoxical. However, I note that antidepressant treatment tends to down-regulate 5-HT2A receptors. The tricyclic antidepressants, such as amitriptyline and nortriptyline, have components that block 5-HT2A receptors; and the atypical antipsychotics used to strengthen the effects of antidepressants that are not working well also act, in part, by blocking 5-HT2A receptors.[443] Nonetheless, it must be concluded that we do not know exactly how microdosing psychedelic drugs might actually work, if it does at all.

6.39.3 DOSAGE

In the clinical studies noted prior, doses of pure psilocybin of 10 to 25mg, or 22 to 30mg per 70kg, were utilized with significant effects. The translation of such doses to the *Psilocybe spp* mushroom itself is problematic. The dose necessary to produce a full, psychedelic effect is commonly said to be about 15 to 30g of fresh mushroom, or about one tenth that weight of dried mushroom.[444] Another authoritative reference states that the psychedelic dose of dried *Psilocybe* mushroom is between 3 and 5g.[445] However, a paper by Bigwood and Beug notes that psilocybin content in both wild and cultivated *Psilocybe* mushrooms can vary considerably—as much as sevenfold. Drying and storage methods may also affect psilocybin content.[446] Thus, considerable caution must be exercised in using whole mushroom, fresh or dried, and graduating doses in a series of trials using a single batch of mushroom is advisable. Microdosing is defined as a dose one tenth that required to produce a full, psychedelic effect. For psilocybin, this microdose is about 250mg of dried mushroom. In one report, a dose of 650mg dried mushroom produced mild psychedelic effects. Thus, it would be wise to avoid doses above 400mg of dried *Psilocybe spp* mushroom for microdosing. In any case, trials of graduated doses from a single batch are advisable.

6.39.4 TOXICITY

There is one reference in the literature to an intravenous injection of extract of *Psilocybe* mushroom having an LD50 of 280mg/kg in mice.[447]

With little physiological risk, it must be stated that the greatest danger of *Psilocybe spp* is potential psychological injury from too high a dose of mushroom or, at least, a dose higher than one is prepared for. Indeed, it is well established that increasingly high doses of psilocybin make the phenomenon of ego dissolution more likely. This in itself may be therapeutic.[448] However, it must be something an individual is willing and prepared to experience.

6.39.5 SAFETY IN PREGNANCY

There appear to be no formal studies of the effects of *Psilocybe spp* mushroom, either in psychedelic dosing or in microdosing, on mothers or fetuses during human pregnancy. One group of researchers stated, "Because psilocin was eliminated slowly from the fetal tissues of rats, human consumption of magic mushrooms should be avoided during pregnancy." The latter is in reference to large doses of psilocybin, not microdosing. Nonetheless, it is prudent to advise against use during pregnancy.[449]

6.39.6 DRUG INTERACTION

A review of the literature reveals no information about drug interactions involving *Psilocybe spp.*

6.40 RHODIOLA ROSEA

Rhodiola rosea is a perennial flowering plant in the family *Crassulaceae*. It grows naturally in wild Arctic and mountainous regions of Europe, Asia, and North America. It has been popular in traditional medical systems in eastern Europe and Asia, with a reputation for stimulating the nervous system, decreasing depression, enhancing work performance, and eliminating fatigue. It has thus been categorized by some as an adaptogen due to its ability to increase resistance to a variety of stressors. Its benefits have been said to include antidepressant, anticancer, cardioprotective, and central nervous system enhancement effects. It has particularly been recommended for asthenic conditions—decline in work performance, sleep difficulties, poor appetite, irritability, hypertension, headaches, and fatigue—as consequences of intense physical or intellectual strain.[450]

6.40.1 ANXIOLYTIC EFFECTS

Rhodiola rosea has a reputation of being an adaptogen and thus reducing anxiety by increasing the body's resiliency. There is only one small study of benefits of *Rhodiola rosea* in patients actually diagnosed with GAD.[451] These patients were given powdered extracted of *Rhodiola rosea* daily for 10 weeks, and at the end of the study, these patients showed significant reductions in anxiety per the Hamilton Anxiety Rating Scale, the Four-Dimensional Anxiety and Depression Scale, and the Clinical Global Impression Scale. The weakness of the study is that results were not compared against a control group. Indeed, it was possible that simply being in a study where they were attended to and given a treatment they thought might help was enough to improve symptoms.

Nonetheless, there are other studies suggestive of anxiolytic effects of *Rhodiola rosea*. In one such study, subjects were described as "mildly anxious," as measured by the Spielberger State-Trait Anxiety Inventory. *Rhodiola rosea* significantly reduced their symptoms of anxiety.[452] Another study showed that *Rhodiola rosea* significantly improved and increased sense of general well-being in healthy young students during a stressful examination period.[453] Several clinical studies have shown *Rhodiola rosea* to have significant, albeit modest, antidepressant effects in people suffering major depression.[454-455] Because anxiety sometimes arises from states of depression, *Rhodiola rosea* might help alleviate anxiety indirectly by improving overall mood.

6.40.2 MECHANISM OF ACTION

Rhodiola rosea contains a variety of phytochemicals, some of which are somewhat unique to the herb. It contains flavonoids, including rhodiosin and herbacetin; monoterpenes, such as geraniol; triterpenes; phenylethanol derivatives, such as salidroside and tyrosol; and phenylpropanoid glycosides including rosin, rosavin, rosdirin, and rosarin that are specific to this plant.[456] Interestingly, whereas many herbs contain flavonoids and terpenes that are active at benzodiazepine receptors, this may not be the case with *Rhodiola rosea*. In a study of rats, the anxiolytic effects of *Rhodiola rosea* were not reversed by flumazenil, suggesting a non-benzodiazepine mediation.[457] Salidroside alone may produce many of the beneficial effects of *Rhodiola rosea*. In animals, it offers both anxiolytic- and antidepressant-like effects.[458] It also has neuroprotective effects against a variety of brain insults, such as inflammation and oxidation.[459] That ability to protect the brain may be responsible for some of *Rhodiola rosea*'s well-known adaptogenic effects. Curiously, salidroside is not a steroid-like compound as many adaptogenic phytochemicals appear to be. Various constituents of *Rhodiola rosea* may act as monoamine oxidase inhibitors, which may further mediate some of the herb's antidepressant and anxiolytic effects.[460] Indeed, several clinical studies have shown *Rhodiola rosea* to be an herb that can significantly improve symptoms of major depression in human subjects.[461] That effect may help alleviate persistent symptoms of anxiety.

6.40.3 DOSAGE

Marciano and Vizniak recommend tincture (1:5, 40%) 1 to 3 ml three times a day or standard extract (3% rosavin 1% saluidroside) 300 to 600mg a day.[462]

6.40.4 TOXICITY

The oral LD50 of *Rhodiola rosea* extract in mice is reported to be 3,360mg/kg.[463] Extrapolated to the weight of a human adult of 75kg, this would be approximately 230g.

6.40.5 SAFETY IN PREGNANCY

Evidence on the safety and appropriateness of *Rhodiola rosea* supplementation during pregnancy and lactation is currently unavailable.[464]

6.40.6 DRUG INTERACTIONS

In vitro studies have shown *Rhodiola rosea* to inhibit CYP3A4 and P-glycoprotein.[465] Nonetheless, a recent review notes that human studies have given no indications that such interactions have clinical significance.[466]

6.41 *ROSMARINUS OFFICINALIS*

Rosmarinus officinalis, synonymous with *Salvia osmarinus* and more commonly known as rosemary, is a member of the mint family *Lamiaceae* that is native to the Mediterranean region. It is perennial herb with fragrant, evergreen, needle-like leaves and white, pink, purple, or blue flowers. Its medicinal properties were known to the ancients. The Greeks and Romans believed it strengthened the memory. Hippocrates, Galen, and Dioscorides prescribed the herb for various ailments, and it was an essential part of the apothecary's repertoire during the Renaissance. *Rosmarinus officinalis* has found wide use in traditional herbal medicine and has been used to treat depression, anxiety, tiredness, defective memory, rheumatic complaints, circulatory disorders, headache, menstrual disorders, nervous menstrual complaints, sprains, and bruises.[467] Maud Grieve noted a 1607 description of rosemary: "It helpeth the brain, strengtheneth the memorie, and is very medicinal for the head."[468]

6.41.1 ANXIOLYTIC EFFECTS

No studies have been performed to evaluate anxiolytic effects of *Rosmarinus officinalis* in patients diagnosed with an anxiety disorder. However, several have evaluated anxiolytic effects in healthy adults. In a double-blind, randomized controlled trial, extract of *Rosmarinus officinalis* given twice daily for a month significantly reduced anxiety and depression and improved memory in healthy university students. Results were obtained with use of the Hospital Anxiety and Depression Scale and the Prospective and Retrospective Memory Questionnaire.[469] In another study of young and healthy volunteers, daily intake of strong rosemary tea for 10 days brought reductions in blood levels of cortisol and other chemical markers of stress.[470] For completeness, it must be noted that not all studies show anxiolytic effects of *Rosmarinus officinalis*. A Japanese study of the effects of daily treatment with extract of the herb found some improvement in mood but no specific effects on anxiety.[471]

6.41.2 MECHANISM OF ACTION

Phytochemicals found in *Rosmarinus officinalis* include rosmarinic acid, camphor, linalool, cineol, caffeic acid, chlorogenic acid, ursolic acid, apigenin, luteolin, pinene, borneol, betulinic acid, carnosic acid, carnosol, and myrcene.[472] A number of the constituent phytochemicals in *Rosmarinus officinalis* have anxiolytic effects. Rosmarinic acid on its own has been found to have such effects in laboratory animals.[473] Those effects are likely mediated in part by enhancing activity at GABA-A receptors.[474] Rosmanol, cirsimaritin, and salvigenin have all been found on their own to have anxiolytic effects in rodents. However, those effects were not reversed by flumazenil.[475] Linalool, also on its own, has been found to have anxiolytic effects in animals and, along with action at GABA-A receptors, may also have effects on opiate and cannabinoid receptors in the brain. Indeed, among the other molecules in *Rosmarinus officinalis* with their own anxiolytic effects are apigenin, luteolin, pinene, and borneol. (See Chapter 5.) Collectively, those phytochemicals enhance GABA and dopamine activities, reduce inflammatory processes in the brain, and have antidepressant-like effects. Thus, *Rosmarinus officinalis* has many components contributing to its anxiolytic effects, likely through actions at various neurotransmitter systems in the brain.

6.41.3 DOSAGE

Hoffman states the standard dosing of *Rosmarinus officinalis* to be 1 to 2ml three times a day of tincture (1:5, 40%) or infusion of 1 to 2 teaspoons per cup of water, taken three times a day.[476]

6.41.4 TOXICITY

Neither methanolic or aqueous extracts of *Rosmarinus officinalis* were found to be toxic in mice in oral doses of up to 5,000mg of dried extract per kg of weight. Thus, the LD50 was deemed to be above 5,000mg/kg.[477] Extrapolated for a human adult of 75kg, this would be approximately 350g. Oral administration of essential oil up to 2,000mg/kg also resulted in no animal deaths.[478]

6.41.5 SAFETY IN PREGNANCY

The *Botanical Safety Handbook* notes conflicting evidence concerning the safety of *Rosmarinus officinalis* during pregnancy. Their conclusion is that while the dried herb and decoction are likely safe, the use of essential oil should be avoided during pregnancy.[479]

6.41.6 DRUG INTERACTIONS

The essential oil of *Rosmarinus officinalis*, its dried leaves, and various extracts have been found to induce several P450 enzymes, particularly the CYP2B family.[480] Among the major drug substrates of the CYP2B family are bupropion, cyclophosphamide, ifosfamide, pethidine, ketamine, and propofol.[481] The *Botanical Safety Handbook* notes no known interactions of *Rosmarinus officinalis* with commonly used medications.

6.42   *SALVIA OFFICINALIS*

Salvia officinalis is often referred to as garden sage, common sage, or culinary sage. It is a perennial, evergreen subshrub in the mint family and native to Mediterranean lands. It has a pleasant, spicy odor and flowers of various shades of blue. It has been used for likely thousands of years, both as a spice for food and a time-honored source of healing. In ancient Greece and Rome, and later in medieval Europe, *Salvia officinalis* was used to treat conditions as various as pain, rheumatism, convulsions, arthritis, dizziness, diarrhea, breathing problems, poor memory, and mental disorders. In India, it is known as *karpooravalli* and has been used for the treatment of asthma, bronchitis, migraine, and the common cold. It is used for similar purposes in traditional Chinese medicine, where it is known as *dan shen*. The leaves of *Salvia officinalis* can be used for tea or for extraction of essential oil.[482]

6.42.1 ANXIOLYTIC EFFECTS

There are no studies of the effects of *Salvia officinalis* on people who have been diagnosed with anxiety disorders. However, there have been several studies on the ability of the herb to reduce anxiety in otherwise healthy people under stressful circumstances. In one such study, normal subjects given dried *Salvia officinalis* leaf exhibited reductions in feelings of anxiety, though this was not dose dependent and tended to diminish when the subjects engaged in a challenging mental exercise.[483] Another study revealed a similar mild calming effect of *Salvia lavandulaefolia*, or Spanish sage, a species closely related to *Salvia officinalis*. Healthy volunteers who received essential oil of *Salvia lavandulaefolia* reported increased sense of calmness and positive mood, as well as exhibited improvement in cognitive performance.[484] In a study of postmenopausal women, daily treatment with dried extract of *Salvia officinalis* in tablet form over 3 months significantly improved anxiety, depression, and insomnia as well as other menopausal symptoms such as flushing, night sweats, heart palpitations, and muscle and joint pain. It also enhanced sexual desire, though this may have simply been due to feeling better in general.[485]

6.42.2 MECHANISM OF ACTION

Among the many phytochemicals contained in *Salvia officinalis* are, in descending order of concentration, camphor, α-thujone, sclareol, α- and β-thujone, 1,8-cineole, γ-selinene, α-humulene, β-caryophyllene, borneol, limonene, humulene epoxide, and lesser amounts of ursolic acid, carnosol, carnosic acid, fumaric acid, chlorogenic acid, and caffeic acid.[486]

As previously noted, β-caryophyllene has mild activity at cannabinoid receptors, whereas borneol, limonene, fumaric acid, chlorogenic acid, and caffeic acid are known to enhance GABA activity. Two diterpenes found in *Salvia officinalis*, 7-methoxyrosmanol and galdosol, were found to have significant affinity for human benzodiazepine receptors, with IC50 values of 7.2µM and 0.8µM, respectively.[487]

Two of the predominant phytochemicals in *Salvia officinalis*, camphor and α- and β-thujones, can be toxic. Camphor can cause seizure at high doses.[488] α-Thujone, a major component of the notoriously famous absinthe drink, is neurotoxic. It also appears to reduce activity at GABA-A receptors and in high doses can cause convulsions in animals.[489] It is unlikely, however, that common use would be dangerous.

6.42.3 Dosage

In the prior studies, *Salvia officinalis* was administered in several different forms and doses. In the study above by Kennedy et al., *Salvia officinalis* was taken as single daily doses of 300 or 600mg of dried leaf.[483] In the study by Zeidabadi et al., it was administered as a tablet of 100mg dried extract given three times a day.[484] The study by Tildesley et al.[485] evaluated oral doses of 25 or 50μl of essential oil, whereas the other studies evaluated essential oil on cloth inhaled to effect.

6.42.4 Toxicity

Salvia officinalis is a culinary herb and generally regarded as safe. The oral median LD50 of the plant extract was determined to be 4,361mg/kg in mice.[490]

6.42.5 Safety in Pregnancy

The German Commission E advises against use of alcohol extracts or essential oil of *Salvia officinalis* during pregnancy.[491]

6.42.6 Drug Interaction

The *Botanical Safety Handbook* notes no clinical reports of drug interactions involving *Salvia officinalis*.[492]

6.43   SCHISANDRA CHINENSIS

Schisandra chinensis, known as magnolia vine or schizandra, and in China as *wu wei zi*, is a deciduous woody vine native to forests of northern China and the Russian Far East. The fruit of the plant, known as magnolia berry and by the Chinese as five-flavor-fruit, is used in the manufacture of juices, wines, and sweets and for medicinal purposes. It is a common component in traditional Chinese and Ayurvedic herbal combinations used to treat anxiety. (See Chapters 7 and 8.) It is also one of many plants evaluated by Russian scientists for having characteristics of an adaptogen—that is, for an apparent ability to give non-specific stress resistance and resiliency to cells and organ systems. Many such plants have been used in folk medicine for treatment of weakness, depression, and the ravages of age. *Schisandra chinensis* is alleged to increase work capacity and protect against a broad spectrum of harmful factors including heat shock, skin burn, cooling, frostbite, immobilization, aseptic inflammation, irradiation, and heavy metal intoxication.[493]

6.43.1 Anxiolytic Effects

Schisandra chinensis has long been used in traditional Chinese medicine to calm and quiet the spirit. It is also among the herbs commonly recommended by members of the American Herbalists Guild to treat anxiety. However, there are few clinical studies of the effects of *Schisandra chinensis* on anxiety disorders. In one study,

3 months of treatment with a combination of extract of *Schisandra chinensis*, polyunsaturated fatty acids, and vitamin D3 significantly improved confidence and reduced measurements of anxiety and stress in athletes during training.[494]

6.43.2 MECHANISM OF ACTION

A multitude of polyphenolic phytochemicals have been isolated from *Schisandra chinensis*. The principle components of the essential oil are ylangene, β-himachalene, and α-bergamotene.[495] The plant also contains flavonoids and flavonoid derivatives, including hyperoside, isoquercitrin, rutin, quercetin, and kaempferol; and organic acids, such as chlorogenic, caffeic, and other such acids.[496] Some of those phytochemicals in the herb themselves have anxiolytic-like effects in animals due in part to action at GABA-receptors. (See Chapter 5.) Lignans—some of which are so-called phytoestrogens—are the major and characteristic constituents of the genus *Schisandraceae*. Schisandrins are lignans unique to this herb.[497] Schisandrins have been found to reduce anxiety- and depression-like behaviors in rodents. Schisandrin B is thought to have anxiolytic effects through increasing the GABA/glutamate ratio and upregulating the expression of GABA-A receptors.[498] Some anxiolytic effects of *Schisandra chinensis* may be due in part to antioxidant and anti-inflammatory effects in the brain.[499] Finally, extracts of the herb have been reported to exert adaptogenic effects.[500] Thus, *Schisandra chinensis* may offer relief from anxiety by several complimentary mechanisms that may both act rapidly and increase over time.

6.43.3 DOSAGE

Therapeutic dosages are 400–450mg powdered herb in capsules three times daily or 1–2 ml of 1:3 EtOH tincture of *Schisandra chinensis* three times daily.[501]

6.43.4 TOXICITY

LD50 value of dried ethanolic extract of *Schisandra chinensis* was estimated to be 35.63 ± 6.46g/kg.[502] In addition, it was observed that chronic feeding of *Schisandra chinensis* fruit to mice in doses as high as 4g/kg had no adverse effects.[503]

6.43.5 SAFETY IN PREGNANCY

The *Botanical Safety Handbook* noted the report that women who took *Schisandra chinensis* during pregnancy experienced less postpartum hemorrhaging, without adverse effects to themselves or their newborns.[504] *Schisandra chinensis* was also noted to be safe for mothers and infants when used to successfully induce labor.[505]

6.43.6 DRUG INTERACTIONS

Schisandra chinensis is metabolized primarily by the P450 enzyme CYP3A.[506] A variety of neuroleptics, including aripiprazole, haloperidol, pimozide, and risperidone, are metabolized by this enzyme.[507] The enzyme is also involved in the metabolism of SSRIs and tricyclic antidepressants.[508] Thus, chronic use of *Schisandra chinensis* could affect blood levels of a variety of important psychiatric medications.

6.44 *SCUTELLARIA BAICALENSIS*

Skullcap refers to two medicinal plants, western skullcap, *Scutellaria lateriflora*, and Chinese skullcap, *Scutellaria baicalensis*. *Scutellaria baicalensis* has long been a mainstay in Chinese medicine and has been used for anxiety, depression, neurological conditions, and gastric distress. *Scutellaria lateriflora* has been used in traditional Native American medicine for nervous tension and various psychiatric and neurological problems. There are differences between the two species in the percentages of certain phytochemicals they contain.[509] Maud Grieve discusses several species of *Scutellaria* available in England and other areas of Europe. She noted, "It is considered a specific for the convulsive twitches of St. Vitus's dance, soothing the nervous excitement and inducing sleep when necessary, without any unpleasant symptoms following."[510]

6.44.1 ANXIOLYTIC EFFECTS

Scutellaria spp are favored remedies for anxiety among British and Irish herbalists, but generally in combination with other herbs. Similarly, *Scutellaria baicalensis* is used as one of several herbal ingredients in two of the most commonly used traditional Chinese medicine herbal combinations for the treatment of major depression—i.e., *tiao qi* and *chai hu jia long gu mu li*. Unfortunately, there is a lack of strong clinical data showing that it is effective as treatment for anxiety and depression. Two studies have shown anxiolytic effects of the herbs, but in people who had not been formally diagnosed with anxiety disorder.[511–512] The relief from symptoms of anxiety appeared to be modest.

6.44.2 MECHANISM OF ACTION

The main phytochemicals in *Scutellaria spp* are the flavonoids and glycosides scutellarin, scutellarein, baicalin, baicalein, wogonin, wogonoside, apigenin, chrysin, and oroxylin A.[513] The plants also contain serotonin, melatonin, and various alkaloids. Animal studies have shown that wogonin has an anxiolytic effect in rodents.[514] Wogonin is known to act at benzodiazepine receptors, and its anticonvulsant effects are blocked by the benzodiazepine antagonist flumazenil.[515] Interestingly, the anxiolytic effects of baicalein in mice are not reversed by flumazenil but are reversed by the neurosteroid, DHEAS.[516] Thus, the anxiolytic effects of those two flavonoids in *Scutellaria baicalensis* may have additive or even synergistic effects.

6.44.3 DOSAGE

Easley and Horne state the dose of *Scutellaria baicalensis* to be 10 drops to 5ml of tincture of dried leaf and flower (1:2 60% alcohol) two to four times daily. Alternatively, they suggest a standard infusion of 4 to 8 ounces three times daily.[517]

6.44.4 TOXICITY

In tests of acute LD50 of aqueous extract of *Scutellaria baicalensis* root in mice, no deaths or adverse effects were seen in doses up to 2,000mg/kg.[518] That would extrapolate to a dose of 140g for a 75kg human adult. I note a report from a traditional Chinese medical hospital in Beijing in which a very small percentage (0.12%) of patients suffered elevations in transaminases after treatment with *Scutellaria baicalensis radix*. In most cases, these elevations were mild, but there was at least one case in which fivefold increases were noted.[519]

6.44.5 SAFETY IN PREGNANCY

Reference texts from traditional Chinese medicine advise against use of *Scutellaria baicalensis* during pregnancy.[520]

6.44.6 DRUG INTERACTIONS

Some phytochemicals isolated from *Scutellaria baicalensis* have been found to inhibit the cytochrome enzyme CYP2D6.[521] The CYP2D6 enzyme catalyzes the metabolism of a large number of clinically important drugs, including antidepressants, neuroleptics, and opioids.[522]

6.45 SILYBUM MARIANUM

Milk thistle, with the scientific name *Silybum marianum*, is a biennial plant of the *Asteraceae* family. The plant is native to the low mountains of Mediterranean Europe but is now cultivated throughout the world. The herb has been used as a healing substance for the last 2,000 years. It is mentioned in the writings of the famous physicians and herbalists of the past, Dioscorides, Pliny the Elder, Hieronymus Bock, Jacobus Theodorus, and Nicholas Culpepper. It has been used primarily for treatment of liver diseases, including alcoholic liver disease, cirrhosis, steatohepatitis, and non-alcoholic toxic and drug-induced hepatitis.[523] The German Commission E recommends its use primarily for dyspeptic complaints and liver conditions, including toxin-induced liver damage and hepatic cirrhosis, and as a supportive therapy for chronic inflammatory liver conditions.[524]

6.45.1 ANXIOLYTIC EFFECTS

Curiously, there are at least two reports on the use of *Silybum marianum* in the treatment of obsessive compulsive disorder, or OCD, in human subjects. OCD can be very difficult to treat and has at times been categorized among the anxiety disorders. In a double-blind, randomized trial, adults diagnosed with OCD through the Yale-Brown Obsessive Compulsive Scale received either extract of silymarin or an active fluoxetine control. At the end of 8 weeks, both treatments significantly reduced the Yale-Brown Obsessive Compulsive Scale scores.[525] In a published description of three cases, the authors described success in treating resistant OCD with 150mg of

Silybum marianum twice a day.[526] In one of the cases, *Silybum marianum* was used for the remission of symptoms after failure of treatment with antidepressants.

6.45.2 MECHANISM OF ACTION

The extract of *Silybum marianum* contains the flavonolignans silybin, isosilybin, silydianin, and silychristine.[527] The herb also contains small quantities of kaempferol, apigenin, and quercetin, all of which are known to have anxiolytic effects likely mediated by enhancing GABA activity (See Chapter 5.) However, the amount of those flavonoids may not be sufficient to be meaningful. At least one laboratory study suggests that some of the effects of *Silybum marianum* may be due to increased activity at a certain serotonin receptor in the brain known as the 5-HT1A receptor.[528] This is thought to be the mechanism by which the prescribed medication buspirone acts to reduce anxiety. A British study showed that silybin alone reduces anxiety in patients undergoing treatment for hepatitis C.[529] Nonetheless, the exact mechanism by which *Silybum marianum* might relieve OCD or forms of anxiety remains unknown.

6.45.3 DOSAGE

The German Commission E notes the daily dosage of silymarin to be 200 to 400mg a day, standardized to silybin content.[530]

6.45.4 TOXICITY

Silymarin appears to have quite low acute toxicity. In rats, the LD50 of orally administered silymarin was 10g/kg.[531] This would extrapolate to an approximate dose of 700g for a 75kg human adult.

6.45.5 SAFETY IN PREGNANCY

The *Botanical Safety Handbook* cites evidence of relative safety of the use of *Silybum marianum* during pregnancy. Limited human and animal studies of the use of silymarin during pregnancy reveal no adverse effects.[532-533]

6.45.6 DRUG INTERACTIONS

The *Botanical Safety Handbook* notes no known interactions with drugs.[534] Indeed, at moderate doses, extract of *Silybum marianum* has little if any ability to either inhibit or induce P450 enzymes from human liver microsomes.[535]

6.46 *TINOSPORA CORDIFOLIA*

Guduchi is a time-honored herb in Ayurvedic medicine. It carries the scientific name of *Tinospora cordifolia* and is commonly known to the English-speaking world as heart-leaved moonseed. The herb is native to India and is an ancient remedy for anxiety and other nervous disorders. It is considered a *rasayana*, with the ability to rejuvenate and build resiliency.[536]

6.46.1 ANXIOLYTIC EFFECTS

Although *Tinospora cordifolia* has been used for thousands of years in Ayurvedic medicine, there are few clinical studies of its ability to relieve chronic anxiety. In one such study, daily ingestion of the herb for 1 month significantly reduced subjective complaints of insomnia, fear, tension, and heart palpitations in patients diagnosed with GAD.[537] In another study, subjects had all been diagnosed as suffering depression and persistent "mental stress" as measured by the Symptom Distress Scale, the State-Trait Anxiety Inventory Scale for assessment of anxiety, and the Beck Depression Inventory for assessment of depression. Powdered dried herb twice daily over 2 months significantly reduced anxiety and depression scores. In fact, relief from anxiety with the herb was similar to that of 10mg a day of the anxiolytic drug valium. When combined with yoga practice, *Tinospora cordifolia* was even more effective.[538]

6.46.2 MECHANISM OF ACTION

The leaves and stems of *Tinospora cordifolia* contain a variety of phytochemicals, including flavonoids, terpenes, steroids, diterpenoid lactones, lignans, and alkaloids, some of which are unique to the herb. Among its phytochemicals are giloinsterol, β-sitosterol, tinosporicide, atrorrhizine, palmatine, berberine, tembeterine, tinocordifolioside, tinosporic acid, tinosporal, tinosporon, and tinosporide.[539] Tinosporicide has been found to dampen the effects of glutamate, one of the excitatory neurotransmitters in the brain, which may mediate some of the herb's calming effects.[540] The alkaloid berberine, found in a number of other herbs, has anxiolytic effects in animal models.[541] Palmatine produces an antidepressant-like effect in rodents, and such an effect may over time contribute to an anxiolytic effect.[542] *Tinospora cordifolia* has long been seen as an adaptogen, which is likely due in part to the steroid-like triterpenes it contains.[543] That quality may allow building of resistance to anxiety-provoking stress over time. It would likely blend well with herbs that produce effects by direct action at GABA receptors in the brain, such as *Matricaria recutita* or *Passiflora incarnata*.

6.46.3 DOSAGE

In one study prior, patients received 500mg of dried *Tinospora cordifolia* three times each day.[537] In the other study, patients received 3g of dried and powdered stems of the herb twice daily.

6.46.4 TOXICITY

The LD50 of *Tinospora cordifolia* has been determined to be more than 1,000mg/kg.[544]

6.46.5 SAFETY IN PREGNANCY

The *Botanical Safety Handbook* notes no information on safety of *Tinospora cordifolia* during pregnancy. In modern Ayurvedic practice, *guduchi* is being touted as a valuable treatment to prevent gestational diabetes in pregnant women. However, there are no studies specifically addressing the safety of the herb during pregnancy. Other opinions state that any herb containing significant concentrations of berberine, as *Tinospora cordifolia* does, should be avoided during pregnancy. If the herb is used pregnancy, it must be under the guidance of an expert.[545]

6.46.6 DRUG INTERACTION

The *Botanical Safety Handbook* notes no information on drug interactions of *Tinospora cordifolia*.

6.47 *TRIFOLIUM PRATENSE*

Trifolium pratense, with the common name red clover, is a perennial plant native to Europe, Western Asia, and Northwest Africa. Extracts of *Trifolium pratense* have been found to have antioxidant and anti-inflammatory effects. The herb may also have anticancer properties. Chinese and Russian folk healers have used the herb to treat respiratory problems such as asthma and bronchitis. In the Ayurvedic tradition of India, *Trifolium pratense* has been used as a calming herb, as well as to treat asthma and skin conditions.[546]

Perhaps most important is the use of *Trifolium pratense* for the discomforts of menopause. It is not uncommon for women to begin to experience emotional symptoms, such as anxiety and depression, when they reach menopause. These symptoms are often associated with troubling physical symptoms, such as hot flashes, sweating, and sleep disturbances, that exacerbate those emotional symptoms. These symptoms are generally attributed to changes in hormones, and estrogen replacement therapy is often started to relieve those problems. However, this treatment has been controversial due to concerns about increased risk for cancers of the breast and uterus. Thus, many women have sought herbal treatments to reduce their discomfort. Such herbal treatments are used to replace lost estrogen with so-called phytoestrogens. *Trifolium pratense* contains compounds known as isoflavones that act as phytoestrogens. It has been found to be helpful in relieving the anxiety of menopause.[547]

6.47.1 ANXIOLYTIC EFFECTS

One group found that for menopausal women suffering anxiety and depression, 12 weeks of twice daily treatment with extract of *Trifolium pratense* significantly reduced anxiety per the Hospital Anxiety and Depression Scale.[548] Indeed, symptoms of anxiety were reduced by 76%. The extract also significantly reduced symptoms of depression per the Zung Self-Rating Depression Scale. In a similar study, 90 days of twice daily treatment with *Trifolium pratense* extract significantly reduced scores on the Kupperman Index, a test designed to evaluate a variety of symptoms menopausal women suffer.[549] The subscales of nervousness and depression symptoms in the Kupperman scale showed significant improvements compared to women in the placebo group. There is experimental evidence that *Trifolium pratense* can reduce some of the physical symptoms of menopause, such as hot flashes, and that, in turn, would be expected to reduce the general discomfort that only makes anxiety worse.[550] However, at least two studies have found no benefits of *Trifolium pratense* in reducing anxiety in women suffering anxiety related to postmenopausal changes.[551-552]

6.47.2 MECHANISM OF ACTION

Trifolium pratense has been found to reduce anxiety in the context of menopausal symptoms. It is thought to relieve emotional and physical symptoms of menopause because it contains isoflavones that acts as phytoestrogens. Phytoestrogens are plant-derived molecules that mimic the estrogen that is diminished in menopause. Daidzein, genistein, formononetin, and biochanin A are among the isoflavones in *Trifolium pratense* known to exert estrogen-like effects.[553] However, there is evidence that some isoflavones could have anxiolytic effects apart from action as phytoestrogens. For example, studies have shown that GABA mediates some effects of such isoflavones. In any case, some of the flavonoids contained in *Trifolium pratense*, such as quercetin, kaempferol, and myricetin, themselves have anxiolytic effects, likely through GABA receptors.[554] There is also evidence that some component of *Trifolium pratense* may stimulate opiate receptors, which may add a component of relief from both pain and anxiety.[555] Although *Trifolium pratense* may act by a variety of mechanisms to reduce anxiety, whether it might offer anxiolytic benefits in men or women not suffering from issues of menopause is not known.

6.47.3 DOSAGE

In the studies prior in which *Trifolium pratense* extract was found to reduce anxiety, the subjects received 80mg a day of red clover isoflavones.[548,549] Most commercial preparations of *Trifolium pratense* are not pure isoflavone but rather dried intact blossoms.

6.47.4 TOXICITY

Trifolium pratense appears to be very well tolerated and has been found to have an oral LD50 on 4,327mg/kg in mice.[556] In the clinical trials noted prior, no adverse effects were noted.

6.47.5 SAFETY IN PREGNANCY

The *Botanical Safety Handbook* notes no indications of adverse effects of *Trifolium pratense* during pregnancy but adds that information is quite limited. Prudence is advised.[557]

6.47.6 Drug Interaction

The *Botanical Safety Handbook* notes no reports of adverse drug interactions involving *Trifolium pratense*.

6.48 *VALERIANA JATAMANSI*

Valeriana jatamansi Jones, also known as *Valeriana wallichii*, is a small perennial herb native to Himalaya and distributed from Afghanistan to southwest China, India, Nepal, Bhutan, and Myanmar. It carries the common names Indian valerian or *tagar*. It is of the same genus as the better-known herb *Valeriana officinalis*. Each has found a similar niche in herbal medicine with use as a restorative, antispasmodic, carminative, sedative, stimulant, stomachic, and nervine.[558] *Valeriana jatamansi* has long been used in both Ayurvedic and traditional Chinese schools of herbal medicine.

6.48.1 Anxiolytic Effects

There is at least one clinical study of anxiolytic effects of *Valeriana jatamansi* in human subjects. This study involved induction of presurgical anxiolysis in patients not otherwise diagnosed with any formal anxiety disorder. Moreover, the rating scales used were rather simple and not standard evaluations of state or trait anxiety. Nonetheless, the study is compelling in that the results were strong and those who administered the herbal treatment, anesthesiologists, were experienced in gauging preparedness for surgery. Patients were given hydroalcoholic extract of *Valeriana jatamansi* on the evening before surgery and on the morning of surgery. Control subjects received 10mg of diazepam on the evening prior to surgery and 5mg the following morning. Both treatments gave significant relief from pretreatment levels of anxiety and did not significantly differ from each other in that respect.[559]

6.48.2 Mechanism of Action

The plant is rich in complex phytochemicals, including flavonoids, iridoid glycosides, sesquiterpenes, steroids, and lignins.[560] Among the anxiolytic phytochemicals that have been identified in *Valeriana jatamansi* are hesperidin, isochlorogenic acid isoforms, and chlorogenic acid.[561] Valeric acid contained in *Valeriana jatamansi* itself exhibits GABAergic activity, as well as antagonistic effects of the NMDA receptor.[562] A study in mice showed that anxiolytic effects of the herb were blocked by flumazenil.[563]

6.48.3 Dosage

In the clinical study noted above, adult patients received 500mg of dried hydroalcoholic extract of *Valeriana jatamansi* in each dose, with children receiving 250mg.[559]

6.48.4 TOXICITY

Acute administration of up to 2,000mg per kg of hydroethanolic extract of *Valeriana jatamansi* rhizome was found to have no adverse effects in mice. Sub-chronic dosing up to 1,800mg/kg/body did not exhibit any toxicity in healthy animals.[564]

6.48.5 SAFETY IN PREGNANCY

The *Botanical Safety Handbook* combines the various subspecies of *Valeriana* into a single group. It noted human and animal studies that found no adverse effects of even high doses of *Valeriana officinalis* root during pregnancy.[565]

6.48.6 DRUG INTERACTION

Review of the literature revealed no studies of the possible interactions of *Valeriana officinalis* with commonly used medications. Extract of *Valeriana officinalis* has no significant effect on the activities of the human CYP1A2, CYP2D6, CYP2E1, or CYP3A4 isoenzymes.[566]

6.49 *VALERIANA OFFICINALIS*

Valeriana officinalis is a perennial flowering plant native to Europe and Asia. The ancients knew the plant. The Greek physician and herbalist Dioscorides recommended the root to treat myriad disorders, including heart palpitations, digestive problems, epilepsy, and urinary tract infections. During the second century, Galen recommended *Valeriana officinalis* as a treatment for insomnia. The major modern uses for the herb continue to be those of a sedative and anxiolytic, generally in the form of valerian root tea. Indeed, during World War I, valerian tea was used to prevent and treat shell shock in frontline troops. During World War II, it was used to help calm civilians subjected to air raids.[567]

6.49.1 ANXIOLYTIC EFFECTS

Despite its reputation as an effective herbal treatment of anxiety, reports on the effects of the root of *Valeriana officinalis* on anxiety have been surprisingly inconsistent if not outright disappointing. In one study of the herb, some benefits were observed, but it was not significantly better than placebo in relieving symptoms of anxiety.[568] Interestingly, there is at least one report of *Valeriana officinalis* being helpful for the treatment of OCD, an illness that overlaps to some degree with symptoms of GAD. After 8 weeks of treatment, subjects given daily doses of 765mg of extract of *Valeriana officinalis* were significantly relieved of symptoms as measured by the standard Yale-Brown Obsessive Compulsive Scale.[569] Uncertainty also exists in regard to the use of *Valeriana officinalis* as a treatment for insomnia. Nonetheless, there are some studies that have found it to be helpful for getting to sleep.[570–572]

6.49.2 MECHANISM OF ACTION

The chemistry of *Valeriana officinalis* is complex, and there are likely over 150 different phytochemicals, many of which are pharmacologically active.[573] It contains a wide range of phytochemicals, including the predominant iridoid valepotriates: valtrates, isovaltrate, didrovaltrate, valerosidate, and others. The volatile essential oil contains bornyl isovalerenate and bornyl acetate; valerenic, valeric, isovaleric, and acetoxyvalerenic acids; valerenal, valeranone, and cryptofaurinol; and other monoterpenes and sesquiterpenes. The plant also contains alkaloids, such as valeranine, chatinine, alpha-methyl pyrrylketone, actinidine, skyanthine, and naphthyridylmethylketone, and lignans, such as hydroxypinoresinol.

Hydroalcoholic and aqueous extracts of the root have shown affinity for the GABA-A receptor in the brains of rats.[574] Valerenic acid has complex effects at GABA-A receptors, as it can both enhance or dampen activity and may act selectively at subtypes of GABA-A receptors.[575] The anxiolytic effects of valerenic acid and the similar compound valerenol are resistant to flumazenil.[576]

6.49.3 DOSAGE

The German Commission E recommends the dose of *Valeriana officinalis* to be 2 to 3g of dried root per cup in infusion, one to several times day; 1 to 3ml of tincture, one or more times daily; or extract equivalent to 1 to 3g of drug daily.[577]

6.49.4 TOXICITY

In a test of acute toxicity of *Valerian officinalis*, doses of extract up to 2,000mg/kg caused no deaths in mice.[578] This dose would extrapolate to 140g in a 75kg human adult.

6.49.5 SAFETY IN PREGNANCY

See *Valeriana jatamansi* prior.

6.49.6 DRUG INTERACTIONS

See *Valeriana jatamansi* prior.

6.50 *VITEX AGNUS-CASTUS*

The Chaste tree, or *Vitex agnus-castus*, is a shrub native to Mediterranean Europe and Central Asia. The berries have been used since ancient times for treatment of many women's health problems. Hippocrates recommended the herb for disorders of the uterus, as did the great Renaissance herbalist Gerard. In recent times, extract of *Vitex agnus-castus* berries have been used to treat menstrual disorders, premenstrual syndrome, infertility, acne, discomforts of menopause, and disrupted lactation.[579]

6.50.1 ANXIOLYTIC EFFECTS

There are no formal studies of the effects of *Vitex agnus-castus* berries on any specific anxiety disorder. However, there is a large literature concerning its use in premenstrual and menopausal mood disorders, both of which are characterized as causing anxiety, irritability, and agitation.

Many of the complaints of menopause are physical in nature, such as hot flashes, night sweats, breast changes, and vaginal dryness. However, mood disorders are common. Despite the herb's reputation for relieving the discomforts of menopause, there is only one study that has evaluated the effects of essential oil of the berries on menopausal symptoms. It was found to reduce both physical and emotional symptoms, including anxiety.[580]

Far more work has been done in evaluating the use of *Vitex agnus-castus* in the treatment of premenstrual dysphoric disorder (PMDD). Symptoms of PMDD include unstable mood, persistent irritability or anger, and anxiety, nervous tension, and depressed mood. There have been at least seven formal evaluations of chronic, 3-month courses of administration of extract of the fruit of *Vitex agnus-castus* on the symptoms of PMDD. Uniformly, these studies found that such extracts offered significant improvement of emotional and physical symptoms of PMDD.[581–587]

6.50.2 MECHANISM OF ACTION

The fruit and leaves of *Vitex agnus-castus* contain a complicated mix of phytochemicals, including flavonoids, iridoid glycosides, alkaloids, diterpenoids, and steroids. Among those phytochemicals are vitexin, casticin, agnuside, aucubin, apigenin, thujene, pinene, sabinene, myrcene, terpinene, limonene, cineole, linalool, cryptone, citronellol, cumin aldehyde, carvacrol, β-caryophyllene, farnesene, myristicin, and scores of others.[588] Some of those substances, including apigenin, casticin, quercetagetin, and isovitexin, are known to be active at GABA-A receptors and exert anxiolytic effects. The anticonvulsant effect of vitexin from *Vitex agnus-castus* was reversed with flumazenil.[589] Some are also thought to act as phytoestrogens. However, those phytochemicals only weakly mimic estrogen and are present in relatively low levels.[590] Thus, it has been suggested that other mechanisms, such as stimulation of dopamine receptors,[591] stimulation of opioid receptors,[592] or enhancement of melatonin release,[593] may be at least partially responsible for the benefits the herb has long been found to offer women suffering premenstrual emotional distress.

6.50.3 DOSAGE

Hoffman recommends 2.5ml of tincture (1:5 in 60% ethanol) three times a day. He also notes the German Commission E recommendation of 175mg per day of 20:1 fruit extract standardized to 0.5% aguniside. He goes on to say that benefits may be seen within 2 to 3 weeks but more often require 3 to 6 months of treatment.[594]

6.50.4 TOXICITY

The oral LD50 value of the essential oil of *Vitex agnus-castus* in mice was estimated to be more than 5g/kg.[595] In humans, the most frequent adverse events associated with the use of *Vitex agnus-castus* are nausea, headache, gastrointestinal disturbances, menstrual disorders, acne, pruritus, and erythematous rash. The adverse events following *Vitex agnus-castus* treatment are mild and reversible.[596] The German Commission E has approved its use for treatment of mastalgia.[597]

6.50.5 SAFETY IN PREGNANCY

The *Botanical Safety Handbook* notes that *Vitex agnus-castus* has traditionally been used to prevent miscarriage in pregnant women. Thus, one might suspect that it is safe in pregnancy. They also note, however, that no follow-up studies have been performed to assess rates of adverse outcomes.[598]

6.50.6 DRUG INTERACTIONS

The *Botanical Safety Handbook* notes no known interactions with drugs.

6.51 *WITHANIA SOMNIFERA*

Withania somnifera, often referred to as *ashwagandha*, is a medicinal herb from the nightshade family. The Sanskrit word *ashwagandha* means the smell of horses, as the strong odor is said to resemble that of horse urine. The plant is native to India, China, and Nepal and is commonly used in Ayurvedic medicine to calm the mind, relieve weakness and nervous exhaustion, build sexual energy, and promote healthy sleep. It has been used for over 3,000 years and was described in the ancient texts from which Ayurvedic medicine was first formulated. It has long been considered to be a *rasayana*, meaning an herb that bestows longevity and vitality. In more modern terms, it is considered to act as an adaptogen.[599]

6.51.1 ANXIOLYTIC EFFECTS

Clinical studies have shown *Withania somnifera* to be effective in treating both anxiety and depression in humans. It has been shown to significantly reduce levels of anxiety in patients diagnosed with anxiety disorders including GAD, mixed anxiety and depression, adjustment disorder with anxiety, and panic disorder.[600]

Similar results were seen in a subsequent study in which anxiety scores were substantially reduced after 30 days of treatment with extract of *Withania somnifera*. Interestingly, blood levels of C-reactive protein, a marker of inflammation, were also reduced.[601] It must be noted that the author of the study was an employee of the company that made the extract. Thus, the results may need to be interpreted cautiously.

Other studies have shown anxiolytic effects in people not necessarily diagnosed as having an anxiety disorder. In one study, daily ingestion of *Withania somnifera* reduced subjective sense of stress. However, as a far more objective measurement, the treatment also significantly reduced blood levels of the stress hormone cortisol.[602]

In a similar study, daily treatment with *Withania somnifera* in combination with B-complex vitamins reduced subjective stress as well as lowered blood levels of stress hormones.[603]

Withania somnifera has often been used to treat insomnia. The herb improved sleep in a group of patients who had long had difficulty getting to sleep and staying asleep. It also reduced scores on a standard test of anxiety, the Hamilton Anxiety Rating Scale, though none of the subjects had been diagnosed as suffering an anxiety disorder.[604]

6.51.2 MECHANISM OF ACTION

Withania somnifera is rich in various phytochemicals, including withanolides, steroidal lactones, phenolics, and flavonoids.[605] Extract of *Withania somnifera* is known to displace GABA from its own receptor. The sedating effects of extract of *Withania somnifera* are enhanced by valium and reversed by the GABA antagonist picrotoxin but not blocked by the benzodiazepine blocker flumazenil.[606] Thus, components of the herb mimic the effects of GABA, but not by stimulating benzodiazepine receptors. This suggests it may be additive to herbs that act more directly at benzodiazepine receptors, such as *Matricaria recutita*, *Passiflora incarnata*, and others.

However, most likely responsible for any unique effects of *Withania somnifera* are the 138 steroid-like withanolides that have been isolated from its aerial parts, roots, and berries. Withaferin-A, one of the primary withanolides, on its own produces anxiolytic effects in rodents.[607] Withanolides, as well as ferulic acid esters found in the herb, activate GABA-A receptors.[608–609]

Withania somnifera may also lessen anxiety over time through acting as an adaptogen. The ability of *Withania somnifera* to rejuvenate and enhance resiliency has been recognized for centuries, particularly by practitioners of Ayurvedic medicine.[610] Studies of laboratory animals have shown that daily administration of *Withania somnifera* extract protects animals from the ravages of chronic stress that include hyperglycemia, glucose intolerance, increase in plasma corticosterone levels, gastric ulcerations, sexual dysfunction, cognitive deficits, immunosuppression, and signs of mental depression.[611] The steroid-like withanolide molecules may buffer against exhaustion of the adrenal glands and perhaps modifies the brain's response to high levels of steroids the body itself can release during periods of high stress. On the other hand, a withanolide-free extract of *Withania somnifera* has also been found to exhibit adaptogenic effects in rodents.[612] Thus, *Withania somnifera* may act in complex ways to reduce anxiety quickly but also build resistance to anxiety and stress over time.

6.51.3 DOSAGE

The recommended dosage, per Easley and Horne, is 1 to 10ml of tincture of dried root or 1 to 3g dried root powder three times daily.

6.51.4 TOXICITY

Withania somnifera appears to have quite low toxicity. The LD50 intraperitoneal injection of alcohol extract of the herb is reported to be 1,260mg/kg.[613] Extrapolated to a 75kg human adult, this dose would be approximately 88g.

6.51.5   SAFETY IN PREGNANCY

Easley and Horne suggest caution when using during pregnancy.[614] The *Botanical Safety Handbook* advises that information of the safety of using *Withania somnifera* during pregnancy is conflicting. Some traditional sources have described the herb as an abortifacient, while others have noted its use in preventing miscarriage. It does appear safe in lactation, with traditional use in stimulating lactation.[615]

6.51.6   DRUG INTERACTIONS

The *Botanical Safety Handbook* notes no known interactions with drugs. At least one study showed no interactions of extracts of *Withania somnifera* with CYP3A4 or CYP2D6 enzyme activity in human liver microsomes.[616]

6.52   *ZIZYPHUS JUJUBA*

Jujuba is the fruit of *Zizyphus jujuba* Mill. It is also known as Chinese date or red date, and it has been widely used as food and in Chinese herbal medicine for over 3,000 years. *Zizyphus jujuba* was first described in the ancient Chinese text *Classic of Poetry* from 1000 BCE. In the book *Shennong Bencao Jing*, from 300 BCE, it was considered as one of the superior herbal medicines that prolonged human life span by nourishing blood, improving quality of sleep, and regulating the digestive system. It is thought to calm the mind and relieve mental tension.[617] *Zizyphus jujuba* is commonly prescribed in traditional Chinese medicine, either as single herb or, more commonly, in tranquilizing formulas combined with other herbal medicines, for the treatment of insomnia and forgetfulness.

6.52.1   ANXIOLYTIC EFFECTS

Zizyphus jujuba is most often used in combination with other herbs, and there are studies showing the significant benefits of those herbal formulas. (See Chapter 7.) Because of this traditional method of use, there are few reports of the effects of *Zizyphus jujuba* on its own. The literature contains only one reference to a controlled clinical study of *Zizyphus jujuba* in patients diagnosed with GAD. This is a poorly documented study from China that describes comparing the effects of boiled fruit of *Zizyphus jujuba* with the effects of an active control treatment, the drug doxepin. The researchers reported that both groups significantly reduced anxiety as revealed by use of the Hamilton Anxiety Rating Scale, a standard method of assessment of anxiety.[618] I note that doxepin is an old antidepressant medication that currently is most often used in low doses to treat insomnia. It is rarely used to treat anxiety.

6.52.2   MECHANISM OF ACTION

Zizyphus jujuba contains a number of common medicinally significant flavonoids, including kaempferol, quercetin, catechin, epicatechin, and apigenin, as well as some unusual ones, such as swertisin, spinosin, and puerarin.[619] Many of those flavonoids and derivatives have been shown to have anxiolytic effects (See Chapter 5.) It also contains many alkaloids, phenolics, and a family of saponins called jujubosides that are known for their sedating effects. In a study of mice, the anxiolytic effects of a methanolic extract of *Zizyphus jujuba* were reversed by flumazenil.[620] Jujuboside A is known to enhance GABAergic activity[621] and increase GABA receptor density in the hippocampus with repeated treatment.[622] Jujuboside A also dampens activity of glutamate.[623] Jujubosides A and B are thought to be major contributors to the sedating and anxiolytic effects of the traditional Chinese herbal combination *suanzaoren*.[624] (See Chapter 7.) In fact, the word *suanzaoren* itself means the seed of *Zizyphus jujuba*. The seed is sometimes used on its own, but in combination it lends its name to the formula. It has been suggested that jujubosides do not readily cross the blood-brain barrier. Thus, some hydrolyzed derivatives may be most responsible for such effects.[625]

6.52.3 DOSAGE

The *Zizyphus jujuba* fruit and its seeds boiled in water to produce a strong tea is the most commonly prepared form to be drunk several times daily. Standardized liquid extracts are also available in various venues, including the internet. The usual dose is about 30ml two or three times daily.

6.52.4 TOXICITY

Zizyphus jujuba appears to have a high margin of safety, with the dry ethanolic extract of *Zizyphus jujuba* being determined to have LD50 above 5,000mg/kg in rats.[626]

6.52.5 SAFETY IN PREGNANCY

Based in part on opinions derived from the long experience of traditional Chinese medicine, the *Botanical Safety Handbook* advises against the use of *Zizyphus jujuba* during pregnancy.[627]

6.52.6 DRUG INTERACTIONS

The *Botanical Safety Handbook* notes no reports of significant drug interactions involving *Zizyphus jujuba*.

6.53 ANXIOLYTIC HERBS RECOMMENDED BY EXPERTS THAT REMAIN UNTESTED

In evidence-based medicine, expert opinion is recognized as valid but is seen as the least reliable basis upon which to plan treatment. There are many herbs that have long had reputations as being useful for treatment of anxiety but have never been scrutinized in clinical studies. In his excellent doctoral dissertation, Luke Einerson, Ph.D., gathered the names of many anxiolytic herbs favored by master herbalists of the American Herbalists Guild.[628] Many of those herbs have been studied and are among those discussed prior. However, many have not been proved in clinical trials.

Among the most favored anxiolytic herbs that lack solid scientific basis for recommendation—and thus were not included earlier in this chapter—are *Borago officinalis*, *Lactuca virosa*, *Mimosa pudica*, *Nepeta cataria*, *Paeonia lactiflora* (discussed in Chapter 7 as a mainstay of Chinese herbal treatment), *Piscidia piscipula*, *Taraxacum officinale*, and *Tilia spp*. Although expert opinion alone is considered weak, if bolstered by compelling preclinical evidence of anxiolytic effects or strong indications of a specific mechanism of action, then such evidence is more reasonable to consider as basis for treatment. Thus, these herbs will be briefly considered.

6.53.1 *BORAGO OFFICINALIS*

Borago officinalis is native to the Mediterranean region but has naturalized in many other locales. The leaves are edible, and the plant is grown in gardens for that purpose in some parts of Europe. The plant is also commercially cultivated for borage seed oil extracted from its seeds.[629] The plant contains a variety of flavonoids, including myricetin, rutin, and daidzein, as well as phenolic acids, including gallic, pyrogallol, salicylic, rosmarinic, syringic, sinapic, ferulic, cinnamic, and caffeic. It is also one of the few rich sources of the essential fatty acid γ-linolenic acid.[630]

Studies have shown extract of *Borago officinalis* to have anxiolytic-like effects in rats. In one typical study, rats showed increased activity in the elevated plus maze 30 minutes after an intraperitoneal injection of extract.[631] In a quite different paradigm, 9 days of treatment with extract of *Borago officinalis* dampened the severity of naloxone-induced withdrawal from morphine.[632] Together those studies suggest a complex set of actions. Many of the phytochemicals found in *Borago officinalis* have on their own been found to have anxiolytic effects. Of note, γ-linolenic acid extracted from the seeds of *Borago officinalis* is known to have anti-inflammatory effects. Plant oils rich in γ-linolenic acid have been used to treat some of the symptoms of PMDD.[633]

6.53.2 *LACTUCA VIROSA*

Lactuca virosa, or wild lettuce, is a species recognized by many herbal traditions as a sedative and pain reliever. In Unani medicine, the plant is prescribed for loss of appetite and insomnia. The 16th-century Western herbalist John Gerard wrote: "Lettuce cooleth the heat of stomacke, called the heart-burning; and helpth it when troubled with choler; it quencheth thirst, and causeth sleepe."[634] The latex released from damaged leaves or stems of the flowering plants dries into a brown gummy product known as lactucarium or lettuce opium. This "lettuce opium" has been prized for its analgesic, antitussive, and sedative properties. It contains the sesquiterpene lactones lactucin, lactucopicrin, and 11β,13-dihydrolactucin, which are thought to be the most important active constituents of *Lactuca virosa*. Extracts of *Lactuca virosa* produced both analgesic and anxiolytic-like effects in mice.[635] Acute administration of dried extract of the closely related plant *Lactuca sativa* similarly produced significant anxiolytic effects in mice in the elevated plus maze. Indeed, its effects were comparable to those of diazepam.[636] The sleep-enhancing effects of extract of *Lactuca sativa* were reversed by flumazenil, suggesting that plants of this genus may act through benzodiazepine receptors.[637] The exact mechanisms of action of *Lactuca virosa*, and the degree to which it may affect opiate receptors, are unknown. However, it can have toxic effects, which are suspected to be due to the anticholinergic effects of hyoscyamine.[638]

6.53.3 MIMOSA PUDICA

Mimosa pudica, sometimes called touch-me-not or sensitivity plant, is a creeping perennial herb of many tropical areas of the world. It has been valued in various folk medicines around the world, including Ayurvedic medicine. It has been used for its sedative as well as anti-asthmatic, aphrodisiac, analgesic, and antidepressant properties.[639] Among its constituent flavonoids are isorientin, orientin, isovitexin, and vitexin,[640] all of which have been found to exert anxiolytic-like effects in rodents. Several studies have found that extracts of the herb have anxiolytic-like effects in rodents, demonstrated primarily in the elevated plus maze.[641] The mechanism by which *Mimosa pudica* might exert anxiolytic effects is unclear. However, the effect may be mediated in part by a benzodiazepine-like effect. In an electrophysiological study, extract of *Mimosa pudica* enhanced the ability of the GABA agonist, 4,5,6,7-tetrahydroisoxazolopyridin-3-ol, to reduce firing of serotonergic neurons in the dorsal raphe. This effect was similar to that of diazepam.[642]

6.53.4 NEPETA CATARIA

Nepeta cataria, more commonly known as catnip, is a species in the family *Lamiaceae*, which includes many medicinal herbs. The plant is native to southern and eastern Europe, the Middle East, Central Asia, and parts of China. However, it has become widely cultivated in northern Europe and North America. Among the phytochemicals found in *Nepeta cataria*, many of which themselves exert anxiolytic effects, are apigenin, luteolin, quercetin, chlorogenic acid, rosmarinic acid, β-sitoserol, caffeic acid, β-caryophyllene, and humulene. However, it is the various nepetalactones in *Nepeta cataria* that are so attractive to cats.[643] 4aα,7α,7aα-nepetalactone extracted from *Nepeta cataria* also has sedative and analgesic effects in rodents that are reversed by naloxone. However, this was apparently mediated by a non-μ opioid receptor.[644]

Nepeta cataria, and several other herbs in that genus, produce anxiolytic effects in rodents. Acute and long-term dosing of *Nepeta cataria* increased both rearing and locomotion frequencies of mice in an open field.[645] Intraperitoneal administration of an hydroalcoholic extract of the closely related herb *Nepeta persica* also showed anxiolytic-like effects on mice in the elevated plus maze.[646] In one study, *Nepeta cataria* did not exhibit anxiolytic effects in rodents in the open field but did show indications of antidepressant-like effects.[647] Finally, an extract of *Nepeta glomerulosa* increased pentobarbital-induced sleep in mice, and this effect was blocked by flumazenil, suggesting some mediation by benzodiazepine receptors.[648]

6.53.5 *Piscidia piscipula*

Piscidia piscipula, formerly called *Piscidia erythrina*, is commonly referred to as Jamaican dogwood. However, the genus *Piscidia* itself is Latin for "fish killer" due to its occasional use for narcotizing and disabling fish that can then be scooped up by hand. Indeed, another name for this plant is Florida fishpoison tree.[649] The bark and wood of the root and stem of this tree have long been used by the natives of the Antilles as an analgesic.[650] Extracts, primarily of bark, contain a variety of complex and rather unique isoflavonoids, including rotenone, ichthynone, jamaicin, piscidone, piscerythrone, 2′-deoxypiscerythrone, 6′-prenylpiscerythrone, and 3′,5′-diprenylgenistein.[651] The component thought to produce the narcotizing effect on fish, as well as insects and various pests, is rotenone and possibly some derivatives.[652]

The effects of *Piscidia piscipula* in humans have been known for centuries. In his 1832 description of an episode of self-experimentation with the herb, William Hamilton noted,

> I became sensible of a burning in the epigastric region spreading rapidly to the surface, and terminating in a copious diaphoresis in the midst of which I was surprised by a sleep so profound that I was utterly unconscious of existence from about eight o'clock at night till eight the following morning, when I awoke free from pain of every description, and found myself still grasping the uncorked phial in one hand from which not a drop had been spilled.[653]

In modern times, the herb has commonly been recommended for relief of pain and insomnia, as well as for anxiety.[654] Unfortunately, rotenone in the herb has been shown to produce a Parkinson's-like syndrome in rodents and is used experimentally for such.[655] Thus, with so many other herbs as effective options, I discourage any use or experimentation unless under care of experts highly familiar with the use of this herb.

6.53.6 *Taraxacum officinale*

Taraxacum officinale, or the common dandelion, is an herb widely distributed in the warmer temperate zones of the Northern Hemisphere. It is a plant in the *Asteraceae* family, which includes a wide variety of medicinal plants including *Lactuca vurosa*—a plant that has some similarities with *Taraxacum officinale*. Both the leaves and root of the plant are used medicinally, and among the herb's active constituents are isovitexin, apigenin, hesperidin, naringenin, kaempferol, sinapinic, gallic acid, and various triterpenoids and phytosterols.[656] The perennial weed has been known since ancient times for its curative properties and has been utilized for the treatment of various ailments such as dyspepsia, heartburn, spleen and liver complaints, hepatitis, and anorexia. Many of the phytochemicals found in *Taraxacum officinale* might be expected to offer anxiolytic or mildly sedative effects. Unfortunately, there is virtually no experimental evidence, either clinical or preclinical, to support this possibility.

6.53.7 *Tilia spp*

Tilia is a genus of about 30 species of trees or bushes native throughout most of the temperate Northern Hemisphere.[657] The tree is known as linden for the European species and basswood for North American species. Tea made from linden flower is commonly recommended for anxiety and sleep. However, the leaves and bark also have medicinal properties. Among the phytochemicals in *Tilia spp*—in this case the representative species, *Tilia tomentosa*—are flavonoids, mainly quercetin, rutin, isoquercitrin, and kaempferol; the flavonoid derivative tiliroside; phenolic acids, including caffeic, p-coumaric, and chlorogenic acids; and various terpenoids.[658]

In one study, extract of one of the more commonly used varieties of *Tilia, T. tomentosa*, was found not only to produce anxiolytic effects in mice in both the elevated plus maze and hole board tests but also to displace ligand from benzodiazepine receptors in a binding experiment.[659] In another study evaluating extract of *Tilia americana*, treatment produced anxiolytic-like effects in mice in the elevated plus maze and open field tests. In addition, it was found that the anxiolytic-like effects were blocked by antagonists of either the 5-HT1A or 5-HT2A receptor.[660] Thus, there is evidence that the apparent anxiolytic effects of *Tilia spp* may be mediated by both benzodiazepine and serotonergic activation. Indeed, an electrophysiological study found that effects of extract of *Tilia tomentosa* buds were blocked by flumazenil.[661]

NOTE

* As this book was in press, a double-blinded, placebo-controlled study (Marschall J, Fejer G, Lempe P, et al. Psilocybin microdosing does not affect emotion-related symptoms and processing: A preregistered field and lab-based study. *J Psychopharmacol.* 2021;36(1):97–113) found psilocybin microdosing ineffective in treating anxiety.

REFERENCES

1. Rajput SB, Tonge MB, Karuppayil SM. An overview on traditional uses and pharmacological profile of *Acorus calamus* Linn. (Sweet flag) and other *Acorus* species. *Phytomedicine.* 2014;21:268-276.
2. Bhattacharyya D, Sur TK, Lyle NA, et al. clinical study on the management of generalized anxiety disorder with *Vaca* (*Acorus calamus*). *Indian J Tradit Know.* 2011;10:668–671.
3. Chellian R, Pandy V, Mohamed Z. Pharmacology and toxicology of alpha- and beta-Asarone: A review of preclinical evidence. *Phytomedicine.* 2017;32:41–58.
4. Balakumbahan R, Rajamani K, Kumanan K. *Acorus calamus*: An overview. *J Med Plants Res.* 2010;4(25):2740–2745.
5. Sharma V, Sharma R, Gautam D, et al. Role of *Vacha* (*Acorus calamus Linn.*) in neurological and metabolic disorders: Evidence from ethnopharmacology, phytochemistry, pharmacology and clinical study. *JCM.* 2020;9(4):1176.
6. JECFA. *WHO Food Additive Series No. 16.* Monograph on β-Asarone, Toxicological Evaluation of Certain Food Additives; 1981.
7. Kumar R, Sharma S, Sharma S. A review in *vacha*: An effective medicinal plant. *World J Pharm Res.* 2020;9(6):842–849.
8. Katyal J, Sarangal V, Gupta YK. Interaction of hydroalcoholic extract of *Acorus calamus* Linn with sodium valproate and carbamazepine. *Indian J Exp Biol.* 2012;50(1):51–55.
9. Raguindin PF, Itodo OA, Stoyanov J, et al. A systematic review of phytochemicals in oat and buckwheat. *Food Chem.* 2021;338:127982.
10. Kennedy DO, Jackson PA, Forster J, et al. Acute effects of a wild green-oat (*Avena sativa*) extract on cognitive function in middle-aged adults: A double-blind, placebo-controlled, within-subjects trial. *Nutr Neurosci.* 2017;20:135–151.

11. Xochitl AF, Rosalía RC, Minerva RG, et al. Polyphenols and avenanthramides extracted from oat (*Avena sativa* L.) grains and sprouts modulate genes involved in glucose and lipid metabolisms in 3T3 L1 adipocytes. *J Food Biochem.* 2021;26:e13738.

12. Peterson DM, Emmons CL, Hibbs AH. Phenolic antioxidants and antioxidant activity in pealing fractions of oat groats. *J Cereal Sci.* 2001;33:97–103.

13. Singh R, De S, Belkheir A. *Avena sativa* (Oat), A potential neutraceutical and therapeutic agent: An overview. *Crit Rev Food Sci Nutr.* 2013;53:2, 126–144.

14. Pursell JJ. *The Herbal Apothecary.* Portland, OR: Timber Press; 2016. p. 139.

15. Ramaiah M, Nagaphani K, Preeth V, et al. Screening for antidepressant-like effect of methanolic seed extract of *Avena Sativa* using animal models. *Phcog J.* 2014;6(3):86–92.

16. Gardner Z, McGuffin M, editors. *Botanical Safety Handbook*, 3rd edition. Boca Raton, FL: CRC Press; 2013. p. 115.

17. Aguiar S, Borowski T. Neuropharmacological review of the nootropic herb *Bacopa monnieri. Rejuvenation Res.* 2013;16(4):313–326.

18. Calabrese C, Gregory WL, Leo M, et al. Effects of a standardized *Bacopa monnieri* extract on cognitive performance, anxiety, and depression in the elderly: A randomized, double-blind, placebo-controlled trial. *J Altern Complement Med.* 2008;14(6):707–713.

19. Stough C, Lloyd J, Clarke J, et al. The chronic effects of an extract of *Bacopa monniera (Brahmi)* on cognitive function in healthy human subjects. *Psychopharmacology* (Berl). 2001;156(4):481–484.

20. Sathyanarayanan V, Thomas T, Einöther SJL, et al. *Brahmi* for the better? New findings challenging cognition and anti-anxiety effects of *Brahmi (Bacopa monniera)* in healthy adults. *Psychopharmacol.* 2013;227:299–306.

21. Roodenrys S, Booth D, Bulzomi S, et al. Chronic effects of *Brahmi (Bacopa monnieri)* on human memory. *Neuropsychopharmacol.* 2002;27:279–281.

22. Al-Snafi AE. The pharmacology of *Bacopa monniera.* A review. *IJPSR.* 2013;4(12):154–159.

23. Mathew J, Balakrishnan S, Antony S, et al. Decreased GABA receptor in the cerebral cortex of epileptic rats: Effect of *Bacopa monnieri* and bacoside-A. *J Biomed Sci.* 2012;19(1):1–3.

24. Panayotis N, Freund PA, Marvaldi L, et al. β-sitosterol reduces anxiety and synergizes with established anxiolytic drugs in mice. *Cell Rep Med.* 2021;2(5):100281.

25. Girish C, Oommen S, Vishnu R. Evidence for the involvement of the monoaminergic system in the antidepressant-like activity of methanolic extract of *Bacopa monnieri* in albino mice. *Int J Basic Clin Pharmacol.* 2016;5(3):914–922.

26. Easley T, Horne S. *The Modern Herbal Dispensary.* Berkeley, CA: North Atlantic Books; 2016. p. 180.

27. Dar A, Channa S. Relaxant effect of ethanol extract of *Bacopa monniera* on trachea, pulmonary artery and aorta from rabbit and guinea-pig. *Phytother Res.* 1997;11(4):323–325.

28. Gardner Z, McGuffin M, editors. *Botanical Safety Handbook*, 3rd edition. Boca Raton, FL: CRC Press; 2013. p. 123.

29. Ramasamy S, Kiew LK, Chung LY. Inhibition of human cytochrome P450 enzymes by *Bacopa monnieri* standardized extract and constituents. *Molecules.* 2014;19(2):2588–2601.

30. Namita P, Mukesh R, Vijay KJ. *Camellia Sinensis* (green tea): A review. *Glob J Pharmacol.* 2012;6:52–59.

31. Mancini E, Beglinger C, Drewe J, et al. Green tea effects on cognition, mood and human brain function: A systematic review. *Phytomedicine.* 2017;34:26–33.

32. Williams JL, Everett JM, D'Cunha NM, et al. The effects of green tea amino acid l-theanine consumption on the ability to manage stress and anxiety levels: A systematic review. *Plant Foods Hum Nutr.* 2020;75:12–23.

33. Chan SP, Yong PZ, Sun Y, et al. Associations of long-term tea consumption with depressive and anxiety symptoms in community-living elderly: Findings from the diet and healthy aging study. *J Prev Alzheimers Dis.* 2018;5:21–25.
34. Unno K, Hara A, Nakagawa A, et al. Anti-stress effects of drinking green tea with lowered caffeine and enriched theanine, epigallocatechin and arginine on psychosocial stress induced adrenal hypertrophy in mice. *Phytomedicine.* 2016;23:1365–1374.
35. Nobre AC, Rao A, Owen GN. L-theanine, a natural constituent in tea, and its effect on mental state. *Asia Pac J Clin Nutr.* 2008;17 (S1):167–168.
36. Sarris J, Byrne GJ, Cribb L, et al. L-theanine in the adjunctive treatment of generalized anxiety disorder: A double-blind, randomized, placebo-controlled trial. *J Psychiat Res.*2018;110:31–37.
37. Yadav KC, Parajuli A, Khatri BB, et al. Phytochemicals and quality of green and black teas from different clones of tea plant. *J Food Qual.* 2020;2020:1–13.
38. Williams JL, Everett JM, D'Cunha NM, et al. The effects of green tea amino acid l-theanine consumption on the ability to manage stress and anxiety levels: A systematic review. *Plant Foods Hum Nutr.* 2020;75:12–23.
39. Dietz C, Dekker M. Effect of green tea phytochemicals on mood and cognition. *Curr Pharm Design.* 2017;23(19):2876–2905.
40. Lucas M, O'Reilly EJ, Pan A, et al. Coffee, caffeine, and risk of completed suicide: Results from 3 prospective cohorts of American adults. *World J Biol Psychiat.* 2014;15(5):377–386.
41. Nie SP, Xie MY. A review on the isolation and structure of tea polysaccharides and their bioactivities. *Food Hydrocolloid.* 2011;25(2):144–149.
42. PDR. *The Physicians Desk Reference for Non-Prescription Drugs and Dietary Supplements*, 27th edition. Montvale, NJ: Medical Economics Co; 2006.
43. Jeppesen U, Loft S, Poulsen HE, et al. A fluvoxamine-caffeine interaction study. *Pharmacogenetics.* 1996;6(3):213–222.
44. Carrillo JA, Benitez J. Clinically significant pharmacokinetic interactions between dietary caffeine and medications. *Clin Pharmacokinet.* 2000;39(2):127–153.
45. Butrica J. The medicinal use of cannabis among the Greeks and Romans. In: E Russo, F Grotenherman (Eds.), *The Handbook of Cannabis Therapeutics: From Bench to Bedside.* New York: Haworth; 2006. pp. 23–42.
46. Warf B. High points: An historical geography of cannabis. *Geograph Rev.* 2014;104(4):414–438.
47. Acharya R. Vijaya (*Cannabis sativa* Linn.) and its therapeutic importance in Ayurveda; a review. *JDRAS.* 2015;1:1–2.
48. Hall W, Solowij N, Lemon J. *The Health and Psychological Consequences of Cannabis Use.* National Drug Strategy Monograph Series no 25, Australian Government Publishing Service, Canberra; 1994.
49. Piper BJ, DeKeuster RM, Beals ML, et al. Substitution of medical cannabis for pharmaceutical agents for pain, anxiety, and sleep. *J Psychopharmacol.* 2017;31:569–575.
50. Karniol IG, Shirakawa I, Kasinski N, et al. Cannabidiol interferes with the effects of delta 9—tetrahydrocannabinol in man. *Eur J Pharmacol.* 1974;28:172–177.
51. Martin-Santos R, Crippa JA, Batalla A, et al. Acute effects of a single, oral dose of d9-tetrahydrocannabinol (THC) and cannabidiol (CBD) administration in healthy volunteers. *Curr Pharm Design.* 2012;18:4966–4979.
52. Bergamaschi MM, Queiroz RHC, Chagas MHN, et al. Cannabidiol reduces the anxiety induced by simulated public speaking in treatment-naive social phobia patients. *Neuropsychopharmacology.* 2011;36:1219–1226.
53. Crippa JA, Derenusson GN, Ferrari TB, et al. Neural basis of anxiolytic effects of cannabidiol (CBD) in generalized social anxiety disorder: A preliminary report. *J Psychopharmacol.* 2011;25:121–130.

54. Niesink RJ, van Laar MW. Does cannabidiol protect against adverse psychological effects of THC? *Front Psychiat.* 2013;4:130.
55. El Sohly MA, Radwan MM, Gul W, et al. Phytochemistry of *Cannabis sativa* L. *Prog Chem Org Nat Prod.* 2017;103:1–36.
56. Szkudlarek HJ, Rodríguez-Ruiz M, Hudson R, et al. THC and CBD produce divergent effects on perception and panic behaviours via distinct cortical molecular pathways. *Prog Neuro-Psychopharmacol Biol Psychiat.* 2021;104:110029.
57. de Mello Schier AR, de Oliveira Ribeiro NP, de Oliveira e Silva AC, et al. Cannabidiol, a *Cannabis sativa* constituent, as an anxiolytic drug. *Rev Bras Psiquiatr.* 2012;34(Suppl 1):S104–S117.
58. Ofir R. Cannabis-derived terpenes and flavonoids as potential pharmaceuticals. *Israel J Plant Sci.* 2021;68(1–2):29–37.
59. PDR staff. *Physicians Desk Reference*, 60th edition. Montvale, NJ: Thomson; 2006. pp. 3334–3336.
60. Zuardi AW, Hallak JEC, Dursun SM, et al. Cannabidiol monotherapy for treatment-resistant schizophrenia. *J Psychopharmacol.* 2006;20:683–686.
61. Rosenkrantz H, Heyman IA, Braude MC. Inhalation, parenteral and oral LD50 values of Δ9-tetrahydrocannabinol in Fischer rats. *Toxicol Appl Pharm.* 1974;28(1):18–27.
62. Yassa HA, Dawood AEA, Shehata MM, et al. Subchronic toxicity of cannabis leaves on male albino rats. *Hum Exp Toxicol.* 2010;29(1):37–47.
63. Jones RT, Benowitz N, Bachman J. Clinical studies of cannabis tolerance and dependence. *Ann N Y Acad Sci.* 1976;282:221–239.
64. Linn S, Schoenbaum SC, Monson RR, et al. The association of cannabis use with outcome of pregnancy. *Am J Public Health.* 1983;73(10):1161–1164.
65. Fergusson DM, Horwood LJ, Northstone K. Maternal use of cannabis and pregnancy outcome. *BJOG.* 2002;109(1):21–27.
66. Westfall RE, Janssen PA, Lucas P, et al. Survey of medicinal cannabis use among childbearing women: Patterns of its use in pregnancy and retroactive self-assessment of its efficacy against 'morning sickness.' *Complement Ther Clin.* 2006;12(1):27–33.
67. Andrews KH, Bracero LA. Cannabinoid hyperemesis syndrome during pregnancy: A case report. *J Reprod Med.* 2015;60(9–10):430–432.
68. Jiang R, Yamaori S, Takeda S, et al. Identification of cytochrome P450 enzymes responsible for metabolism of cannabidiol by human liver microsomes. *Life Sci.* 2011;89(5–6):165–170.
69. Watanabe K, Yamaori S, Funahashi T, et al. Cytochrome P450 enzymes involved in the metabolism of tetrahydrocannabinols and cannabinol by human hepatic microsomes. *Life Sci.* 2007;80(15):1415–1419.
70. Cichewicz DL. Synergistic interactions between cannabinoid and opioid analgesics. *Life Sci.* 2004;74(11):1317–1324.
71. Gohil KJ, Patel JA, Gajjar AK. Pharmacological review on *Centella asiatica*: A potential herbal cure-all. *Indian J Pharm Sci.* 2010;72(5):546–556.
72. Bradwejn J, Zhou Y, Koszycki D, et al. A double-blind, placebo-controlled study on the effects of gotu kola (*Centella asiatica*) on acoustic startle response in healthy subjects. *J Clin Psychopharmacol.* 2000;20(6):680–684.
73. Jana U, Sur TK, Maity LN, et al. A clinical study on the management of generalized anxiety disorder with *Centella asiatica*. *NMCJ.* 2010;12(1):8–11.
74. Vishal G, Shetty SK. A comparative study on *guduchi vati* and *mandookaparni vati* in the management of *chittodvega* (generalized anxiety disorder). *IAMJ.* 2015;3(7):2030–2040.
75. Brinkhaus B, Lindner M, Schuppan D, et al. Chemical, pharmacological and clinical profile of the East Asian medical plant *Centella aslatica*. *Phytomedicine.* 2000;7(5):427–448.

76. Wijeweera P, Arnason JT, Koszycki D, et al. Evaluation of anxiolytic properties of Gotu kola—(*Centella asiatica*) extracts and asiaticoside in rat behavioral models. *Phytomedicine*. 2006;13(9):668–676.
77. Chen Y, Han T, Rui Y, et al. Effects of total triterpenes of *Centella asiatica* on the corticosterone levels in serum and contents of monoamine in depression rat brain. *J Chinese Med Materials*. 2005;28(6):492–496.
78. Ceremuga TE, Valdivieso D, Kenner C, et al. Evaluation of the anxiolytic and antidepressant effects of asiatic acid, a compound from Gotu Kola or *Centella asiatica*, in the male Sprague Dawley rat. *AANA J*. 2015;83(2):91–98.
79. Umamageswari M, Latha K, Sathiya Vinotha AT, et al. Evaluation of anti-convulsant activity of aqueous leaf extract of *Centella asiatica* in Wistar Albino rats. *Int J Pharmacog Phytochem Res*. 2015;7(4):690–695.
80. Easley T, Horne S. *The Modern Herbal Dispensary*. Berkeley, CA: North Atlantic Books; 2016. p. 242.
81. Chauhan PK, Singh V. Acute and subacute toxicity study of the acetone leaf extract of *Centella asiatica* in experimental animal models. *Asian Pac J Trop Biomed*. 2012;2(2):S511–S513.
82. Dutta T, Basu UP. Crude extract of *Centella asiatica* and products derived from its glycosides as oral antiferility agents. *Indian J Exp Biol*. 1968;6:181–182.
83. Gohil KJ, Patel JA, Gajjar AK. Pharmacological review on *Centella asiatica*: A potential herbal cure-all. *Indian J Pharm Sci*. 2010;72(5):546–556.
84. Savai J, Varghese A, Pandita N, et al. Investigation of CYP3A4 and CYP2D6 interactions of *Withania somnifera* and *Centella asiatica* in human liver microsomes. *Phytother Res*. 2015;29(5):785–790.
85. Mishra N, Srivastava R. Therapeutic and pharmaceutical potential of cinnamon. Therapeutic and pharmaceutical potential of cinnamon. In: *Ethnopharmacological Investigation of Indian Spices*; Hershey, PA: IGI Global; 2020. pp. 124–136.
86. Shahinfar J, Zeraati H, Zahrab M, et al. The efficiency of Cinnamomum versus diazepam on pre-operative anxiety in orthopedic surgery. *JIITM*. 2016;7(2):207–214.
87. Rajan UK. *Effectiveness of Cinnamon Chewing Gum on Memory and Anxiety Among Adolescents at Selected Seventh Day Adventist High Schools, Andhra Pradesh*. Masters Thesis, Dhanvantri College of Nursing, Namakkal; 2012.
88. Singh G, Maurya S, deLampasona MP, et al. A comparison of chemical, antioxidant and antimicrobial studies of cinnamon leaf and bark volatile oils, oleoresins and their constituents. *Food Chem Toxicol*. 2007;45(9):1650–1661.
89. Etaee F, Komaki A, Faraji N, et al. The effects of cinnamaldehyde on acute or chronic stress-induced anxiety-related behavior and locomotion in male mice. *Stress*. 2019;22(3):358–365.
90. Shen Y, Jia L-N, Honma N, et al. Beneficial effects of cinnamon on the metabolic syndrome, inflammation, and pain, and mechanisms underlying these effects—a review. *J Tradit Comp Med*. 2012;2(1):27–32.
91. Easley T, Horne S. *The Modern Herbal Dispensary*. Berkeley, CA: North Atlantic Books; 2016. p. 212.
92. Price L, Price S. *Aromatherapy for Health Professionals E-Book*. London: Churchill, Livingstone; 2012.
93. Ahmad RA. Assessment of potential toxicological effects of cinnamon bark aqueous extract in rats. *Int J Biosci Biochem Bioinform*. 2015;5(1):36–44.
94. Anderson RA. Chromium and polyphenols from cinnamon improve insulin sensitivity. *P Nutr Soc*. 2008;67:48–53.
95. Bensky D, Clavey S, Stoger E. *Chinese Herbal Medicine: Materia Medica*, 3rd edition. Seattle, WA: Eastland Press; 2004.

96. Mantovani A, Stazi AV, Macri C, et al. Prenatal (segment II) toxicity study of cinnamic aldehyde in the Sprague-Dawley rat. *Food Chem Toxicol.* 1989;27:781–786.

97. Gardner Z, McGuffin M, editors. *Botanical Safety Handbook*, 3rd edition. Boca Raton, FL: CRC Press; 2013. p. 216.

98. Ulbricht C, Seamon E, Windsor RC, et al. An evidence-based systematic review of cinnamon (Cinnamomum spp.) by the natural standard research collaboration. *J Diet Suppl.* 2011;8(4):378–454.

99. Suntar I, Khan H, Patel S, et al. An overview on *Citrus aurantium* L.: Its functions as food ingredient and therapeutic agent. *Oxi Med Cell Longev.* 2018;78:642–669.

100. Akhlaghi M, Shabanian G, Rafieian-Kopaei M, et al. *Citrus aurantium* blossom and preoperative anxiety. *Rev Bras Anestesiol.* 2011;61(6):702–712.

101. Suryawanshi JAS. An overview of *Citrus aurantium* used in treatment of various diseases. *African J Plant Sci.* 2011;5(7):390–395.

102. Cline M, Taylor JE, Flores J, et al. Investigation of the anxiolytic effects of linalool, a lavender extract, in the male sprague-dawley rat. *AANA J* 2008;76:47–52.

103. Mercader J, Wanecq E, Chen J, et al. Isopropylnorsynephrine is a stronger lipolytic agent in human adipocytes than synephrine and other amines present in *Citrus aurantium. J Physiol Biochem.* 2011;67(3):443–452.

104. Deshmukh NS, Stohs SJ, Magar CC, et al. *Citrus aurantium* (bitter orange) extract: Safety assessment by acute and 14-day oral toxicity studies in rats and the Ames test for mutagenicity. *Reg Toxicol Pharmacol.* 2017;90:318–327.

105. Gardner Z, McGuffin M, editors. *Botanical Safety Handbook*, 3rd edition. Boca Raton, FL: CRC Press; 2013. p. 224.

106. Agarwa P, Sharma B, Fatima A, et al. An update on Ayurvedic herb *Convolvulus pluricaulis* choisy. *Asian Pac J Trop Biomed.* 2014;4(3):245–252.

107. Dass RK. A clinical study to compare the role of *Jaladhara* and *Shankhpushpi Rasayana* in the management of *Chittodvega* (Anxiety disorder.) *Int J Res Ayurveda Pharm.* 2012;3:872–875.

108. Rachitha P, Krupashree K, Jayashree GV, et al. Chemical composition, antioxidant potential, macromolecule damage and neuroprotective activity of *Convolvulus pluricaulis. J Trad Comp Med.* 2018;8(4):483–496.

109. Al-Snafi AE. The chemical constituents and pharmacological effects of *Convolvulus arvensis* and *Convolvulus scammonia*- A review. *IOSR J Pharm.* 2016;6(6):64–75.

110. Schmidt M, Betti G, Hensel A. Saffron in phytotherapy: Pharmacology and clinical uses. *Wein Med Wochenschr.* 2007;157(13–14):315–319.

111. Jafarnia N, Ghorbani Z, Nokhostin M, et al. Effect of saffron (*Crocus sativus* L.) as an add-on therapy to sertraline in mild to moderate generalized anxiety disorder: A double blind randomized controlled trial. *Arch Neurosci.* 2017;4(4):e14332.

112. Mazidi M, Shemshian M, Mousavi SH, et al. A double-blind, randomized and placebo-controlled trial of saffron (*Crocus sativus* L.) in the treatment of anxiety and depression. *J Complement Integr Med.* 2016;13:195–199.

113. Ghajar A. *Crocus sativus* L. versus citalopram in the treatment of major depressive disorder with anxious distress: A double-blind, controlled clinical trial. *Pharmacopsych.* 2017;50(04):152–160.

114. Lopresti AL, Drummond PD, Inarejos-García AM, et al. Affron®, a standardised extract from saffron (*Crocus sativus* L.) for the treatment of youth anxiety and depressive symptoms: A randomised, double-blind, placebo-controlled study. *J Affect Disorders.* 2018;232:349–357.

115. Srivastava R, Ahmed H, Dixit RK, et al. *Crocus sativus* L.: A comprehensive review. *Pharmacogn Rev.* 2010;4(8):200–208.

116. Hosseinzadeh H, Noraei NB. Anxiolytic and hypnotic effect of *Crocus sativus* aqueous extract and its constituents, crocin and safranal, in mice. *Phytother Res.* 2009;23(6):768–774.

117. Pitsikas N. Constituents of Saffron (*Crocus sativus* L.) as potential candidates for the treatment of anxiety disorders and schizophrenia. *Molecules*. 2016;21(3):303.
118. Pitsikas N, Tarantilis PA. The GABAA-benzodiazepine receptor antagonist flumazenil. Abolishes the anxiolytic effects of the active constituents of *Crocus sativus* L. Crocins in Rats. *Molecules*. 2020;25:564.
119. Xu G-L, Li G, Ma H-P, et al. Preventive effect of crocin in inflamed animals and in LPS-challenged RAW 264.7 cells *J Agric Food Chem*. 2009;57(18):8325–8330.
120. Umigai N, Takeda R, Mori A. Effect of crocetin on quality of sleep: A randomized, double-blind, placebo-controlled, crossover study. *Comp Ther Med*. 2018;41:47–51.
121. Easley T, Horne S. *The Modern Herbal Dispensary*. Berkeley, CA: North Atlantic Books; 2016. p. 297.
122. Abdullaev F. Biological properties and medicinal use of saffron (*Crocus sativus* L.). *Acta Hortic*. 2007;739:339–345.
123. Wichtl M. *Herbal Drugs and Phytopharmaceuticals: A Handbook for Practice on a Scientific Basis*, 3rd Edition. Boca Raton, FL: CRC Press; 2004.
124. Bensky D, Clavey S, Stoger E. *Chinese Herbal Medicine: Materia Medica*, 3rd edition. Seattle, WA: Eastland Press; 2004.
125. Gardner Z, McGuffin M, editors. *Botanical Safety Handbook*, 3rd edition. Boca Raton, FL: CRC Press; 2013. p. 274.
126. Dovrtelova G, Noskova K, Jurica J, et al. Can bioactive compounds of *Crocus sativus* L. Influence the metabolic activity of selected CYP enzymes in the rat? *Physiol Res*. 2015;64(Suppl 4): S453–S458.
127. Remadevi R, Surendran E, Kimura T. Turmeric in traditional medicine. In: PN Ravindran, K Nirmal Babu, K Sivaraman (Eds.), *Turmeric: The Genus Curcuma*. Boca Raton: CRC Press; 2007. pp. 409–436.
128. Sirajudeen MAA, Najeeb BM. *A Literary Review of Single Drug White Zedoary (Curcuma zedoria) Commonly Used in Indigenous Medicine*. Sri Lanka: National Research Symposium, Department of Ayurveda Basic Principles, Gampaha Wickramarachchi Ayurveda Institute, University of Kelaniya; 2016.
129. Kawasaki K, Muroyama K, Murosaki S. Effect of a water extract of *Curcuma longa* on emotional states in healthy participants. *Biosc Microbiota Food Health*. 2018;37:25–29.
130. Chakraborty PS, Ali SA, Kaushik S, et al. *Curcuma longa*- A multicentric clinical verification study. *Indian J Res Homeop*. 2011;5(1):19–27.
131. Lopresti AL, Maes M, Maker GL, et al. Curcumin for the treatment of major depression: A randomized, double-blind, placebo-controlled study. *J Affect Dis*. 2014;167:368–375.
132. Esmaily H, Sahebkar A, Iranshahi M, et al. An investigation of the effects of curcumin on anxiety and depression in obese individuals: A randomized controlled trial. *Chin J Integr Med*. 2015;21(5):332–338.
133. Asadi S, Gholami MS, Siassi F, et al. Beneficial effects of nano-curcumin supplement on depression and anxiety in diabetic patients with peripheral neuropathy: A randomized, double-blind, placebo-controlled clinical trial. *Phytother Res*. 2020;34(4):896–903.
134. Lobo R, Prabhu KS, Shirwaikar A, et al. *Curcuma zedoaria* Rosc. (white turmeric): A review of its chemical, pharmacological and ethnomedicinal properties. *JPP*. 2009;61:13–21.
135. Singh G, Kapoor IPS, Singh P, et al. Comparative study of chemical composition and antioxidant activity of fresh and dry rhizomes of turmeric (*Curcuma longa* Linn.) *Food Chem Toxicol*. 2010;48:1026–1031.
136. Ishola IO, Katola FO, Adeyemi OO. Involvement of GABAergic and nitrergic systems in the anxiolytic and hypnotic effects of *Curcuma longa*: Its interaction with anxiolytic-hypnotics. *Drug Metab Person Ther*. 2021;36(2):135–143.
137. Shoba G, Joy D, Joseph T, et al. Influence of piperine on the pharmacokinetics of curcumin in animals and human volunteers. *Planta Med*. 1998;64:353–356.

138. Aggarwal ML, Chacko KM, Kuruvilla BT. Systematic and comprehensive investigation of the toxicity of curcuminoid-essential oil complex: A bioavailable turmeric formulation. *Mole Med*. 2016;13(1):592–604.

139. Bensky D, Clavey S, Stoger E. *Chinese Herbal Medicine: Materia Medica*, 3rd edition. Seattle, WA: Eastland Press; 2004.

140. Chen JK, Chen TT. *Chinese Medical Herbology and Pharmacology*. City of Industry, CA: Art of Medicine Press; 2004.

141. Gardner Z, McGuffin M, editors. *Botanical Safety Handbook*, 3rd edition. Boca Raton, FL: CRC Press; 2013. p. 264.

142. Appiah-Opong R, Commandeur JNM, van Vugt-Lussenburg B, et al. Inhibition of human recombinant cytochrome P450s by curcumin and curcumin decomposition products. *Toxicology*. 2007;235:83–91.

143. Barrett B. Medicinal properties of echinacea: A critical review. *Phytomedicine*. 2003;10(1):66–86.

144. Haller J, Freund TF, Pelczer KG, et al. The anxiolytic potential and psychotropic side effects of an echinacea preparation in laboratory animals and healthy volunteers. *Phytother Res*. 2013;27(1):54–61.

145. Barnes J, Anderson LA, Gibbons S, et al. Echinacea species (*Echinacea angustifolia* (DC.) Hell., *Echinacea pallida* (Nutt.) Nutt., *Echinacea purpurea* (L.) Moench): A review of their chemistry, pharmacology and clinical properties. *J Pharm Pharmacol*. 2005;57:929–954.

146. Gertsch J, Leonti M, Raduner S, et al. Beta-caryophyllene is a dietary cannabinoid. *Proc Natl Acad Sci USA*. 2008;105:9099–9104.

147. Raduner S, Majewska A, Chen JZ, et al. Alkylamides from *Echinacea* are a new class of cannabinomimetics. Cannabinoid type 2 receptor-dependent and -independent immunomodulatory effects. *J Biol Chem*. 2006;281:14192–14206.

148. Zakari A, Kubmarawa D. Acute toxicity (LD50) studies using Swiss albino mice and brine shrimp lethality (LC50 and LC90) determination of the ethanol extract of stem bark of *Echinaceae angustifolia* DC. *Nat Prod Chem Res*. 2016;4(6):1–6.

149. Gardner Z, McGuffin M, editors. *Botanical Safety Handbook*, 3rd edition. Boca Raton, FL: CRC Press; 2013. p. 313.

150. Azizi H, Ghafari S, Ghods R, et al. A review study on pharmacological activities, chemical constituents, and traditional uses of *Echium amoenum*. *Phcog Rev*. 2018;12:208–213.

151. Sayyah M, Siahpoosh A, Khalili H, et al. A double-blind, placebo-controlled study of the aqueous extract of *Echium amoenum* for patients with general anxiety disorder. *Iran J Pharm Res*. 2012;11(2):697–701.

152. Sayyah M, Boostani H, Pakseresht S, et al. Efficacy of aqueous extract of *Echium amoenum* in treatment of obsessive-compulsive disorder. *Prog Neuropsychopharmacol Biol Psychiatry*. 2009;33(8):1513–1516.

153. Sayyaha M, Sayyah M, Kamalinejad M, et al. A preliminary randomized double-blind clinical trial on the efficacy of aqueous extract of *Echium amoenum* in the treatment of mild to moderate major depression. *Prog Neuropsychopharmacol Biol Psychiatry*. 2006;30(1):166–169.

154. Zarshenas M, Dabaghian F, Moein M. An overview on phytochemical and pharmacological aspects of *Echium amoenum*. *Nat Prod J*. 2016;6:285–291.

155. Farajdokht F, Vosoughi A, Ziaee M, et al. The role of hippocampal GABAA receptors on anxiolytic effects of *Echium amoenum* extract in a mice model of restraint stress. *Mol Biol Rep*. 2020;47:6487–6496.

156. Heidari MR, Azad EM, Mehrabani M. Evaluation of the analgesic effect of *Echium amoenum* Fisch & C.A. Mey. extract in mice: Possible mechanism involved. *J Ethnopharmacol*. 2006;103(3):345–349.

157. Zamansoltani F, Nassiri-Asl M, Karimi R, et al. Hepatotoxicity effects of aqueous extract of *Echium amoenum* in rats. *Pharmacology*. 2008;1:432–438.
158. Mehrabani M, Ghannadi A, Sajjadi SE, et al. Toxic pyrrolizidine alkaloids of *Echium amoenum* fish and Mey. *Daru*. 2006;14:122–127.
159. Mahsa K, Habibolah J. The antioxidant effect of *Echium Amoenum* to prevent teratogenic effects of lamotrigine on the skeletal system and fetal growth in mice. *J Pharmacol Clin Res*. 2017;3(4):555617.
160. Yan-Lin S, Lin-De L, Soon-Kwan H. *Eleutherococcus senticosus* as a crude medicine: Review of biological and pharmacological effects. *J Med Plant Res*. 2011;5(25):5946–5952.
161. Panossian AG. Adaptogens in mental and behavioral disorders. *Psychiat Clin N Am*. 2013;36:49–64.
162. Cicero AFG, Derosa G, Brillante R, et al. Effects of Siberian ginseng (*Eleutherococcus senticosus*) on elderly quality of life: A randomized trial. *Arch Gerontol Geriatr*. 2004;(Suppl 9):69–73.
163. Facchinetti F, Neri I, Tarabusi M, et al. *Eleutherococcus senticosus* reduces cardiovascular stress response in healthy subjects: A randomized, placebo-controlled trial. *Stress Health*. 2002;18(1):11–17.
164. Schaffler K, Wolf OT, Burkart M. No benefit adding *Eleutherococcus senticosus* to stress management training in stress-related fatigue/weakness, impaired work or concentration: A randomized controlled study. *Pharmacopsychiatry*. 2013;46(05):181–190.
165. Lee JM, Lee DG, Lee KH. Isolation and identification of phytochemical constituents from the fruits of *Acanthopanax senticosus*. *African J Pharm Pharmacol*. 2013;7(6):294–301.
166. Davydov M, Krikorian AD. *Eleutherococcus senticosus* (Rupr. & Maxim.) Maxim. (*Araliaceae*) as an adaptogen: A closer look. *J Ethnopharmacol*. 2000;72(3):345–393.
167. Yang H, Woo J, Pae AN, et al. alpha-Pinene, a major constituent of pine tree oils, enhances non-rapid eye movement sleep in mice through GABAA-benzodiazepine receptors. *Mol Pharmacol*. 2016;90:530–539.
168. Huang L, Zhao H, Huang B, et al. *Acanthopanax senticosus*: Review of botany, chemistry and pharmacology. *Pharmazie*. 2011;66:83–97.
169. Liu Y, Wang Z, Wang C, et al. Comprehensive phytochemical analysis and sedative-hypnotic activity of two Acanthopanax species leaves. *Food Function*. 2021;12(5):2292–2311.
170. Hartz AJ, Bentler S, Noyes R, et al. Randomized controlled trial of Siberian ginseng for chronic fatigue. *Psychol Med*. 2004;34:51–61.
171. Asano K, Takahashi T, Miyashita M, et al. Effect of *Eleutherococcus senticosus* extract on human physical working capacity. *Planta Med*. 1986;3:175–177.
172. Halstead BW, Hood LL. *Eleutherococcus senticosus/Siberian Ginseng: An Introduction to the Concept of Adaptogenic Medicine*. Long Beach, CA: Oriental Healing Arts Institute; 1984. p. 65.
173. Gardner Z, McGuffin M, editors. *Botanical Safety Handbook*, 3rd edition. Boca Raton, FL: CRC Press; 2013. p. 321.
174. Donovan JL, DeVane CL, Chavin KD, et al. Siberian ginseng (*Eleutheroccus senticosus*) effects on CYP2D6 and CYP3A4 activity in normal volunteers. *Drug Metab Dispos*. 2003;31(5):519–522.
175. Zampieron ER. Successful application of *Eschscholzia californica* to combat opioid addiction. *Int J Complement Alt Med*. 2018;11(4):228–229.
176. Hanus M, Lafon J, Mathieu M, et al. Double-blind, randomized, placebo-controlled study to evaluate the efficacy and safety of a fixed combination containing two plant extracts (*Crataegus oxyacantha* and *Eschscholzia californica*) and magnesium in mild-to-moderate anxiety disorders. *Curr Med Res Opin*. 200;20(1):63–71.

177. Schafer HL, Schäfer H, Schneider W, et al. Sedative action of extract combinations of *Eschscholzia californica* and *Corydalis cava. Arznei-Forschung.* 1995;45(2):124–126.
178. Beck MA, Haberlein H. Flavonol glycosides from *Eschscholzia californica. Phytochemistry* 1999;50(2):329–332.
179. Lim TK. Eschscholzia californica. In: *Edible Medicinal and Non Medicinal Plants.* Dordrecht: Springer; 2014. pp. 622–632.
180. Fedurco M, Gregorová J, Šebrlová K. Modulatory effects of *Eschscholzia californica* alkaloids on recombinant GABAA receptors. *Biochem Res Int.* 2015;2015.
181. Rolland A, Fleurentin J, Lanhers MC, et al. Neurophysiological effects of an extract of *Eschscholzia californica* Cham. (*Papaveraceae*). *Phytother Res.* 2001;15(5):377–381.
182. Hoffmann D. *Medical Herbalism: The Science and Practice of Herbal Medicine.* Rochester, VT: Healing Arts Press; 2003. p. 547.
183. Blumenthal M, Busse WR, Goldberg A, et al. *The Complete German Commission E Monographs.* Austin, TX: American Botanical Council; 1998. p. 389.
184. Gardner Z, McGuffin M, editors. *Botanical Safety Handbook*, 3rd edition. Boca Raton, FL: CRC Press; 2013. p. 339.
185. Bourin M, Bougerol T, Guiton B, et al. A combination of plant extracts in the treatment of outpatients with adjustment disorder with anxious mood: Controlled study versus placebo. *Fundam Clin Pharmacol.* 1997;11:127–132.
186. Carlson M, Thompson RD. Liquid chromatographic determination of methylxanthines and catechins in herbal preparations containing guaraná. *J AOAC Int.* 1998;81(4):691–701.
187. Adesanwo JK, Ogundele SB, Akinpelu DA, et al. Chemical analyses, antimicrobial and antioxidant activities of extracts from *Cola nitida* seed. *J Explor Res Pharmacol.* 2017;2(3):67–77.
188. Valli M, Paubert-Braquet M, Picot S, et al. Euphytose®, an association of plant extracts with anxiolytic activity: Investigation of its mechanism of action by an in vitro binding study. *Phytother Res.* 1991;5(6):241–244.
189. Bagheri H, Broué P, Lacroix I, et al. Fulminant hepatic failure after herbal medicine ingestion in children. *Thérapie* 1998;53:77–83.
190. Kathirvel B, Kalibulla SI, Shanmugam V, et al. A review on the pharmacological properties of *Evolvulus alsinoides* (Linn). *J Indian Sys Med.* 2021;9(3):153–160.
191. Nahata A, Patil UK, Dixit VK. Anxiolytic activity of *Evolvulus alsinoides* and *Convulvulus pluricaulis* in rodents. *Pharm Biol.* 2009;47(5):444–451.
192. Kumar D, Dhobi M. Screening antianxiety and antioxidant profile of stems and leaves of blue variety of *Clitoria ternatea* L. *Indian J Pharm Sci.* 2018;79(6):1022–1025.
193. Sethiya NK, Nahata A, Dixit VK. Anxiolytic activity of *Canscora decussata* in albino rats. *J Compliment Integr Med.* 2010;7(1):19.
194. Shamsi Y, Ahmad J, Khan AA, et al. A clinical study on the management of anxiety neurosis with *Sankhaholi. Indian J Tradit Know.* 2007;6(4):668–677.
195. Gupta P, Siripurapu KB, Ahmad A, et al. Anti-stress constituents of *Evolvulus alsinoides*: An Ayurvedic crude drug. *Chem Pharma Bull.* 2007;55(5):771–775.
196. Luo L, Sun T, Yang L, et al. Scopoletin ameliorates anxiety-like behaviors in complete Freund's adjuvant-induced mouse model. *Mol Brain.* 2020;13(1):1–3.
197. Jain G, Patil UK. Formulation, characterization and evaluation of behavioral effects of suspension and effervescent granules of *Evolvulus alsinoides* Linn. And *Convolvulus pluricaulis* Choisy. *Int J Pharma Invest.* 2020;10(4):460–465.
198. Balkrishna A, Thakur P, Varshney A. Phytochemical profile, pharmacological attributes and medicinal properties of *Convolvulus prostratus*—a cognitive enhancer herb for the management of neurodegenerative etiologies. *Front Pharmacol.* 2020;11:171.
199. Agarwala N, Dey CD. Behavioural and lethal effects of alcoholic extracts of *Evolvulus alsinoides* in albino mice. *Indian J Physiol Allied Sci.* 1977;31:81–85.

200. Gardner Z, McGuffin M, editors. *Botanical Safety Handbook*, 3rd edition. Boca Raton, FL: CRC Press; 2013. p. 355.
201. Badgujar SB, Patel VV, Bandivdekar AH. *Foeniculum vulgare* Mill: A review of its botany, phytochemistry, pharmacology, contemporary application, and toxicology. *BioMed Res internat*. 2014;2014: Article ID 842674.
202. Mendelson SD. *Herbal Treatment of Major Depression: Scientific Basis and Practical Use*. Boca Raton, FL: CRC Press; 2020. p. 149.
203. Kian RF, Bekhradi R, Rahimi R, et al. Evaluating the effect of fennel soft capsules on the quality of life and its different aspects in menopausal women: A randomized clinical trial. *Nurs Pract Today*. 2017;4(2):87–95.
204. Ghazanfarpour M, Mohammadzadeh F, Shokrollahi P, et al. Effect of *Foeniculum vulgare* (fennel) on symptoms of depression and anxiety in postmenopausal women: A double-blind randomised controlled trial. *J Obstet Gynaecol*. 2018;38(1):121–126.
205. Omidali F. The effect of Pilates exercise and consuming fennel on pre-menstrual syndrome symptoms in non-athletic girls. *CMJA*. 2015;5(2):1203–1213.
206. Pazoki H, Bolouri G, Farokhi F, et al. Comparing the effects of aerobic exercise and *Foeniculum vulgare* on pre-menstrual syndrome. *Middle East Fert Soc J*. 2016;21(1):61–64.
207. Delaram M, Kheiri S, Hodjati MR, et al. Comparing the effects of *Echinophora-platyloba*, fennel and placebo on pre-menstrual syndrome. *J Reprod Infertil*. 2011; 12(3):221–226.
208. Miguel MG, Cruz C, Faleiro L, et al. *Foeniculum vulgare* essential oils: Chemical composition, antioxidant and antimicrobial activities. *Nat Prod Commun*. 2010;5:319–328.
209. Pourabbas S, Kesmati M, Rasekh A. Study of the anxiolytic effects of fennel and possible roles of both gabaergic system and estrogen receptors in these effects in adult female rat. *Physiol Pharmacol*. 2011;15(1):134–143.
210. Bossé R, Di Paolo T. The modulation of brain dopamine and GABA A receptors by estradiol: A clue for CNS changes occurring at menopause. *Cell Mol Neurobiol*. 1996;16(2):199–212.
211. Blumenthal M, Busse WR, Goldberg A, et al. *The Complete German Commission E Monograph: Therapeutic Guide to Herbal Medicines*. Austin, TX: American Botanical Council; 1998. pp. 128–129.
212. Özbek H. Investigation of the level of the lethal dose 50 and the hypoglycemic effect of *Foeniculum vulgare* Mill. Fruit essential oil extract in healthy and diabetic mice. *Van Tip Dergisi*. 2002;9(4):98–103.
213. Gardner Z, McGuffin M, editors. *Botanical Safety Handbook*, 3rd edition. Boca Raton, FL: CRC Press; 2013. p. 361.
214. Zaidi SFH, Kadota S, Tezuka Y. Inhibition on human liver cytochrome P450 3A4 by constituents of fennel (*Foeniculum vulgare*): Identification and characterization of a mechanism-based inactivator. *J Agric Food Chem*. 2007;55(25):10162–10167.
215. Estrada E. *Jardin Botanico de Plantas Medicinales Maximino Martinez*. Mexico: Universidad Autonoma de Chapingo, Departamento de Fitotecnia; 1985. p. 15.
216. Romero-Cerecero O, Islas-Garduño AL, Zamilpa A, et al. Therapeutic effectiveness of *Galphimia glauca* in young people with social anxiety disorder: A pilot study. *Evid-Based Compl Alt*. 2018;2018: ID 1716939.
217. Herrera-Arellano A, Jiménez-Ferrer E, Zamilpa A, et al. Efficacy and tolerability of a standardized herbal product from *Galphimia glauca* on generalized anxiety disorder. A randomized double blind clinical trial controlled with lorazepam. *Planta Med*. 2007;73(8):713–717.
218. Sharma A, Angulo-Bejarano PI, Madariaga-Navarrete A, et al. Multidisciplinary investigations on *Galphimia glauca*: A Mexican medicinal plant with pharmacological potential. *Molecules*. 2018;23(11):2985–3007.

219. Garige BSR, Keshetti S, Vattikuti UMR. Assessment of antinociceptive and anti-inflammatory activities of *Galphimia glauca* stem methanol extract on noxious provocation induced pain and inflammation in in-vivo models. *J Chem Pharm Res.* 2016;8(4):1282–1289.

220. Sharma A, Angulo-Bejarano PI, Madariaga-Navarrete A, et al. Multidisciplinary investigations on *Galphimia glauca*: A Mexican medicinal plant with pharmacological potential. *Molecules.* 2018;23(11):2985–3007.

221. Khatian N, Aslam M. A review of *Ganoderma lucidum (Reishi)*: A miraculous medicinal mushroom. *Ethnopharmacology.* 2018;4:1–6.

222. Zhao H, Zhang Q, Zhao L, et al. Spore powder of *Ganoderma lucidum* improves cancer-related fatigue in breast cancer patients undergoing endocrine therapy: A pilot clinical trial. *eCAM.* 2012; Article ID 809614.

223. Pazzi F, Adsuar JC, Domínguez-Muñoz FJ, et al. *Ganoderma lucidum* effects on mood and health-related quality of life in women with fibromyalgia. *Healthcare.* 2020;8(4):520–531.

224. Wang G-H, Wang L, Wang C, et al. Spore powder of *Ganoderma lucidum* for the treatment of Alzheimer disease: A pilot study. *Medicine.* 2018;97(19):e0636.

225. Kikuchi T, Kanomi S, Kadota S, et al. Constituents of the fungus *Ganoderma lucidum* (FR.) KARST. I.: Structures of ganoderic acids C2, E, I, and K, lucidenic acid F and related compounds. *Chem Pharm Bull.* 1986;34(9):3695–3712.

226. Veljović S, Veljović M, Nikićević N, et al. Chemical composition, antiproliferative and antioxidant activity of differently processed *Ganoderma lucidum* ethanol extracts. *J Food Sci Technol.* 2017;54:1312–1320.

227. Sharma P, Tulsawani R, Agrawal U. Pharmacological effects of *Ganoderma lucidum* extract against high-altitude stressors and its subchronic toxicity assessment. *J Food Biochem.* 2019;43(12):e13081.

228. Mohammed A, Tanko Y, Mohammed KA, et al. Studies of analgesic and anti-inflammatory effects of aqueous extract of *Ganoderma Lucidum* in mice and Wister rats. *IOSR-JPBS.* 2012;4(4):54–57.

229. Tao J, Feng KY. Experimental and clinical studies on inhibitory effect of *Ganoderma lucidum* on platelet aggregation. *J Tongji Med Univ.* 1990;10:240–243.

230. Gill SK, Rieder MJ. Toxicity of a traditional Chinese medicine, *Ganoderma lucidum*, in children with cancer. *Can J Clin Pharmacol.* 2008;15(2):e275–285.

231. Gardner Z, McGuffin M, editors. *Botanical Safety Handbook*, 3rd edition. Boca Raton, FL: CRC Press; 2013. p. 379.

232. Chan P-O, Xia Q, Fu PP. *Ginkgo Biloba* leave extract: Biological, medicinal, and toxicological effects. *J Environ Sci Heal.* 2007;25:211–244.

233. Woelk H, Arnoldt KH, Kieser M, et al. *Ginkgo biloba* special extract EGb 761 in generalized anxiety disorder and adjustment disorder with anxious mood: A randomized, double-blind, placebo-controlled trial. *J Psych Res.* 2007;41:472–480.

234. Jezova D, Duncko R, Lassanova M, et al. Reduction of rise of in blood pressure and cortisol release during stress by *Ginkgo biloba* extract (EGB 761) in healthy volunteers. *J Physio Pharmacol.* 2002;53(3):337–348.

235. Xia S-H, Fang D-C. Pharmacological action and mechanisms of ginkgolide B. *Chinese Med J.* 2007;120(10):922–928.

236. Bai S, Zhang X, Chen Z, et al. Insight into the metabolic mechanism of Diterpene ginkgolides on antidepressant effects for attenuating behavioural deficits compared with venlafaxine. *Sci Rep.* 2017;7(1):1–4.

237. Kuribara H, Weintraub ST, Yoshihama T, et al. An anxiolytic-like effect of *Ginkgo biloba* extract and its constituent, ginkgolide-A, in mice. *J Nat Prod.* 2003;66(10):1333–1337.

238. Priyanka A, Sindhu G, Shyni GL, et al. Bilobalide abates inflammation, insulin resistance and secretion of angiogenic factors induced by hypoxia in 3T3-L1 adipocytes by controlling NF-κB and JNK activation. *Int Immunopharmacol.* 2017;42:209–217.

239. Blumenthal M, Busse WR, Goldberg A, et al. *The Complete German Commission E Monograph: Therapeutic Guide to Herbal Medicines.* Austin, TX: American Botanical Council; 1998. p. 138.
240. Naik SR, Panda VS. Antioxidant and hepatoprotective effects of *Ginkgo biloba* phytosomes in carbon tetrachloride-induced liver injury in rodents. *Liver Int.* 2007;27(3):393–399.
241. Diamond BJ, Bailey MR. *Ginkgo biloba*: Indications, mechanisms, and safety. *Psychiat Clin.* 2013;36(1):73–83.
242. Kupiec T, Raj V. Fatal seizures due to potential herb-drug interactions with *Ginkgo Biloba. J Analyt Toxicol.* 2005;29(7):755–758.
243. Biendl M, Pinzl C. *Hops and Health. Uses, Effects, History.* Wolznach: German Hop Museum Wolznach; 2008.
244. Franco L, Galán C, Bravo R, et al. Effect of non-alcohol beer on anxiety: Relationship of 5-HIAA. *Neurochem J.* 2015;9:149–152.
245. Kyrou I, Christou A, Panagiotakos D, et al. Effects of a hops (*Humulus lupulus* L.) dry extract supplement on self-reported depression, anxiety and stress levels in apparently healthy young adults: A randomized, placebo-controlled, double-blind, crossover pilot study. *Hormones.* 2017;16(2):171–180.
246. Almaguer C, Schönberger C, Gastl M, et al. *Humulus lupulus*—a story that begs to be told. A review. *J I Brewing.* 2014;120(4):289–314.
247. Benkherouf AY, Eerola K, Soini SL, et al. Humulone modulation of GABAA receptors and its role in hops sleep-promoting activity. *Front Neurosci.* 2020;14:594708.
248. Ceremuga TE, Johnson LA, Adams-Henderson JM, et al. Investigation of the anxiolytic effects of xanthohumol, a component of *Humulus lupulus* (Hops), in the male Sprague-Dawley rat. *AANA J.* 2013;81:193–198.
249. Benkherouf AY, Logrén N, Somborac T, et al. Hops compounds modulatory effects and 6-prenylnaringenin dual mode of action on GABAA receptors. *Eur J Pharmacol.* 2020;873:172962.
250. Marciano M, Vizniak NA. *Botanical Medicine.* Toronto: Prohealth; 2016. p. 225.
251. Hänsel R, Keller K, Rimpler H, *Hagers Handbuch der Pharmazeutische Praxis*, Hrsg. Berlin: Springer Verlag; 1993. pp. 447–458.
252. Gardner Z, McGuffin M, editors. *Botanical Safety Handbook*, 3rd edition. Boca Raton, FL: CRC Press; 2013. p. 439.
253. Yuan Y, Qiu X, Nikolić D, et al. Inhibition of human cytochrome P450 enzymes by hops (*Humulus lupulus*) and hop prenylphenols. *Eur J Pharm Sci.* 2014;53(12):55–61.
254. Pöldinger W. History of St. Johns wort. *Praxis.* 2000;89(50):2102–2109.
255. Lecrubier Y, Clerc G, Didi R, et al. Efficacy of St. John's wort extract WS® 5570 in major depression: A double-blind, placebo-controlled trial. *Am J Psychiatr.* 2002;159:1361–1366.
256. Volz HP. St John's wort extract (LI 160) in somatoform disorders: Results of a placebo-controlled trial. *Psychopharmacol.* 2002;164:294–300.
257. Davidson JRT, Connor KM. St. John's wort in generalized anxiety disorder: Three case reports. *J Clin Psychopharmacol.* 2001;21(6):635–636.
258. Kobak K, Taylor L, Warner G, et al. St. John's wort versus placebo in social phobia: Results from a placebo-controlled pilot study. *J Clin Psychopharmacol.* 2005;25:51–58.
259. Barnes J, Anderson LA, Phillipson JD. St John's wort (*Hypericum perforatum* L.): A review of its chemistry, pharmacology and clinical properties. *J Pharm Pharmacol.* 2001;53(5):583–600.
260. Zanoli P, Rivasi M, Baraldi C, et al. Pharmacological activity of hyperforin acetate in rats. *Behav Pharmacol.* 2002;13(8):645–651.
261. Müller WE, Singer A, Wonnemann M. Hyperforin-antidepressant activity by a novel mechanism of action. *Pharmacopsychiatry.* 2001;34(Suppl 1):98–102.

262. Vandenbogaerde A, Zandi P, Puia G, et al. Evidence that the total extract of *Hypericum perforatum* affects exploratory behaviour and exerts anxiolytic effects in rats. *Pharmacol Biochem Behav*. 2000;65:627–633.

263. Blumenthal M, Busse WR, Goldberg A, et al. *The Complete German Commission E Monographs*. Austin, TX: American Botanical Council; 1998. p. 215.

264. Bukahri I, Dar A, Khan R. Antinociceptive activity of methanolic extracts of St. John's wort (*Hypericum perforatum*) preparation. *Pak J Pharmaceut Sci*. 2004;17(2):13–19.

265. Schempp CM, Ludtke R, Winghofer B, et al. Effect of topical application of *Hypericum perforatum* extract (St John's wort) on skin sensitivity to solar simulated radiation. *Photodermatol. Photoimmunol. Photomed*. 2000;16:125–128.

266. Gardner Z, McGuffin M, editors. *Botanical Safety Handbook*, 3rd edition. Boca Raton, FL: CRC Press; 2013. p. 449.

267. Henderson L, Yue QY, Bergquist C, et al. St John's wort (*Hypericum perforatum*): Drug interactions and clinical outcomes *BJCP*. 2002;54(4):349–356.

268. Obach RS. Inhibition of human cytochrome P450 enzymes by constituents of St. John's wort, an herbal preparation used in the treatment of depression. *JPET*. 2000;294(1):88–95.

269. Rau T, Wohlleben G, Wuttke H. CYP2D6 genotype: Impact on adverse effects and non-response during treatment with antidepressants—a pilot study. *Clin Pharmacol Ther*. 2004;75:386–393.

270. Upson T. The taxonomy of the genus *Lavandula* L. In: M Lis-Balchin (Ed.), *Lavender, the Genus Lavandula. Medicinal and Aromatic Plants: Industrial Profiles*. London: Taylor and Francis; 2002. pp. 2–34.

271. Bradley BF, Brown SL, Chu S, et al. Effects of orally administered lavender essential oil on responses to anxiety-provoking film clips. *Hum Psychopharm*. 2009;24(4):319–330.

272. Woelka H, Schläfkeb S. A multi-center, double-blind, randomized study of the lavender oil preparation Silexan in comparison to Lorazepam for generalized anxiety disorder. *Phytomedicine*. 2009;17(2):94–99.

273. Kasper S, Gastpar M, Müller WE, et al. Lavender oil preparation Silexan is effective in generalized anxiety disorder—a randomized, double-blind comparison to placebo and paroxetine. *Int J Neuropsychopharmacol*. 2014;17(6):859–869.

274. Takahashia M, Satoua T, Ohashia M, et al. Interspecies comparison of chemical composition and anxiolytic-like effects of lavender oils upon inhalation. *NPC*. 2011;6(11):1769–1774.

275. Umezu T, Nagano K, Ito H, et al. Anticonflict effects of lavender oil and identification of its active constituents. *Pharmacol Biochem Behav*. 2006;85(4):713–721.

276. Hoffmann D. *Medical Herbalism: The Science and Practice of Herbal Medicine*. Rochester, VT: Healing Arts Press; 2003. p. 562.

277. Easley T, Horne S. *The Modern Herbal Dispensary*. Berkeley, CA: North Atlantic Books; 2016. p. 258.

278. Da Silva GL, Luft C, Lunardelli A, et al. Antioxidant, analgesic and anti-inflammatory effects of lavender essential oil. *An Acad Bras Ciên*. 2015;87(Suppl 2):1397–1408.

279. Basch E, Foppa I, Liebowitz R, et al. Lavender (*Lavandula angustifolia* Miller) *J Herb Pharmacother*. 2004;4(2):63–78.

280. Guillemain J, Rousseau A, Delaveau P. Neurodepressive effects of the essential oil of *Lavandula angustifolia* Mill. *Ann Pharm Fr*. 1989;47(6):337–343.

281. Doroshyenko O, Rokitta D, Zadoyan G, et al. Drug cocktail interaction study on the effect of the orally administered lavender oil preparation silexan on cytochrome P450 enzymes in healthy volunteers. *Drug Metab Dispo*. 2013;41(5):987–993.

282. Wojtyniak K, Szymański M, Matławska I. *Leonurus cardiaca* L. (Motherwort): A review of its phytochemistry and pharmacology. *Phytother Res*. 2013;27(8):1115–1120.

283. Baxter J. A successful treatment of hypertension. *Australian J Med Herb.*1996;8(3):83–87.
284. Shikov AN, Pozharitskaya ON, Makarov VG, et al. Effect of *Leonurus cardiaca* oil extract in patients with arterial hypertension accompanied by anxiety and sleep disorders. *Phytother Res.* 2001;25(4):540–543.
285. Ovanesov KB, Ovanesova IM, Arushanian EB. Effects of melatonin and motherwort tincture on the emotional state and visual functions in anxious subjects. *Eksp Klin Farmakol.* 2006;69(6):17–19.
286. Angeloni S, Spinozzi E, Maggi F, et al. Phytochemical profile and biological activities of crude and purified *Leonurus cardiaca* extracts. *Plants.* 2021 Feb;10(2):195–210.
287. Fierascu RC, Fierascu I, Ortan A, et al. *Leonurus cardiaca* L. as a source of bioactive compounds: An update of the european medicines agency assessment report. *BioMed Res Int.* 2019;17: 2019.
288. Blumenthal M, Busse WR, Goldberg A, et al. *The Complete German Commission E Monographs.* Austin, TX: American Botanical Council; 1998. p. 172.
289. Milkowska-Leyck K, Filipek B, Strzelecka H. Pharmacological effects of lavandulifolioside from *Leonurus cardiaca.* J *Ethnopharmacol.* 2002;80:85–90.
290. Gardner Z, McGuffin M, editors. *Botanical Safety Handbook*, 3rd edition. Boca Raton, FL: CRC Press; 2013. p. 504.
291. Muhammad I, Zhao J, Khan IA. Maca (*Lepidium meyenii*). In: P Coates, MR Blackman, G Cragg, M Levine, J Moss, J White (Eds.), *Encyclopedia of Dietary Supplement*, 2nd edition; New York: Marcel Dekker; 2005. pp. 522–531.
292. Brooks NA, Wilcox G, Walker KZ, et al. Beneficial effects of *Lepidium meyenii* (Maca) on psychological symptoms and measures of sexual dysfunction in post-menopausal women are not related to estrogen or androgen content. *Menopause.* 2008;15(6):1157–1162.
293. Meissner HO, Reich-Bilinska H, Mscisz A, et al. Therapeutic effects of pre-gelatinized organic maca (*Lepidium peruvanum* chacon) used as a nonhormonal alternative to HRT in perimenopausal women-clinical pilot study. *Int J Biomed Sci.* 2006;2:143–159.
294. Gonzales GF, Córdova A, Vega K, et al. Effect of *Lepidium meyenii* (MACA) on sexual desire and its absent relationship with serum testosterone levels in adult healthy men. *Andrologia.* 2002;34(6):367–372.
295. Edwards SE, da Costa Rocha I, Williamson EM, et al. *Lepidium meyenii* Walp. In: *Phytopharmacy: An Evidence-Based Guide to Herbal Medicinal Products.* West Sussex, UK: John Wiley & Sons; 2015 Apr 27.
296. Meissner HO, Mscisz A, Kedzia B, et al. Peruvian maca: Two scientific names *Lepidium meyenii* and *Lepidium peruvianum* Chacon—are they phytochemically-synonymous? *Int J Biomed Sci.* 2015;11(1):1–15.
297. Lee MS, Shin BC, Yang EJ, et al. Maca (*Lepidium meyenii*) for treatment of menopausal symptoms: A systematic review. *Maturitas.* 2011;70:227–233.
298. Gardner Z, McGuffin M, editors. *Botanical Safety Handbook*, 3rd edition. Boca Raton, FL: CRC Press; 2013. p. 508.
299. Okubo H, Hiramatsu M, Masuda JI, et al. New insight into *Lilium brownii* var. volchesteri. *Floricult Ornament Biol.* 2012;6(2):44–52.
300. Zhang LH, Yu X, Zhang S, et al. The clinical study of decoction of lily mind-tranquilizing on generalized anxiety disorder. *Shanxi J. of TCM.* 2008;24(9):14–15.
301. Hu Y, Zhang M, Zhang X, et al. Characters and comprehensive evaluation of nutrients and active components of 12 *Lilium* species. *Nat Prod Res Dev.* 2019;31(2):292–298.
302. Si Y, Wang L, Lan J, et al. *Lilium davidii* extract alleviates p-chlorophenylalanine-induced insomnia in rats through modification of the hypothalamic-related neurotransmitters, melatonin and homeostasis of the hypothalamic-pituitary-adrenal axis. *Pharm Biol.* 2020;58(1):915–924.

303. Gardner Z, McGuffin M, editors. *Botanical Safety Handbook*, 3rd edition. Boca Raton, FL: CRC Press; 2013. p. 514.
304. Bahramsoltani R, Rostamiasrabadi P, Shahpiri Z, et al. *Aloysia citrodora* Paláu (Lemon verbena): A review of phytochemistry and pharmacology. *J Ethnopharmacol.* 2018;222:34–51.
305. Martinez-Rodriguez A, Moya M, Vicente-Salar N, et al. Biochemical and psychological changes in university students performing aerobic exercise and consuming lemon verbena extracts. *Curr Top Nutraceut Res.* 2015;13(2):95–102.
306. Mohamadi SD, Sahaf R, Karimi M, et al. Assessment of *Lippia citriodora* oil effect on sleep disturbances in Ageing: A double blind randomized controlled trial. *Iran J Age.* 2020;15(1):54–67.
307. Fitsiou E, Mitropoulou G, Spyridopoulou K, et al. Chemical composition and evaluation of the biological properties of the essential oil of the dietary phytochemical *Lippia citriodora*. *Molecules.* 2018;23(1):123–136.
308. Skaltsa H, Shammas G. Flavonoids from *Lippia citriodora*. *Planta Medica*. 1988 Oct;54(05):465.
309. Makino Y, Kondo S, Nishimura Y, et al. Hastatoside and verbenalin are sleep-promoting components in *Verbena officinalis*. *Sleep Biol Rhyth.* 2009;7:211–217.
310. Rashidian A, Farhang F, Vahedi H, et al. Anticonvulsant effects of *Lippia citriodora* (*verbenaceae*) leaves ethanolic extract in mice: Role of GABAergic system. *Int J Prev Med.* 2016;7:97–97.
311. Miraj S, Kiani S. Study of pharmacological effect of *Verbena officinalis* Linn: A review. *Der Pharmacia Lettre.* 2016;8(9):321–325.
312. Bonyani A, Sajjadi SE, Rabbani M. Anxiolytic effects of *Lippia citriodora* in a mouse model of anxiety. *Res Pharm Sci.* 2018;13(3):205–212.
313. Gardner Z, McGuffin M, editors. *Botanical Safety Handbook*, 3rd edition. Boca Raton, FL: CRC Press; 2013. p. 50.
314. Luo H, Wu H, Yu X, et al. A review of the phytochemistry and pharmacological activities of *Magnoliae officinalis* cortex. *J Ethnopharmacol.* 2019;236:412–442.
315. Kalman DS, Feldman S, Feldman R, et al. Effect of a proprietary *Magnolia* and *Phellodendron* extract on stress levels in healthy women: A pilot, double-blind, placebo-controlled clinical trial. *Nutr J.* 2008;7:11.
316. Talbott SM, Talbott JA, Pugh M. Effect of *Magnolia officinalis* and *Phellodendron amurense* (Relora®) on cortisol and psychological mood state in moderately stressed subjects. *J Int Soc Sports Nutr.* 2013;10:37.
317. Wu J-Y. Chemical constituents in leaves of *Magnolia officinalis* var. biloba. *Chinese Trad Herb Drug.* 2013;24:2965–2968.
318. Hu H, Wang Z, Hua W, et al. Effect of chemical profiling change of processed *Magnolia officinalis* on the pharmacokinetic profiling of honokiol and magnolol in rats. *J Chromatograph Sci.* 2016;54(7):1201–1212.
319. Borgonetti V, Governa P, Biagi M, et al. Novel therapeutic approach for the management of mood disorders: In vivo and in vitro effect of a combination of l-theanine, *Melissa officinalis* L. And *Magnolia officinalis*. *Nutrients.* 2020;12(6):1803–1818.
320. Ai J, Wang X, Nielsen M. Honokiol and magnolol selectively interact with GABAA receptor subtypes in vitro. *Pharmacology.* 2001;63(1):34–41.
321. Sokkar NM, Rabeh MA, Ghazal G, et al. Determination of flavonoids in stamen, gynoecium, and petals of Magnolia grandiflora L. And their associated antioxidant and hepatoprotection activities. *Quim Nova.* 2014;37(4):667–671.
322. Bensky D, Clavey S, Stoger E. *Chinese Herbal Medicine: Materia Medica*, 3rd edition. Seattle, WA: Eastland Press; 2004.
323. Chen JK, Chen TT. *Chinese Medical Herbology and Pharmacology*. City of Industry, CA: Art of Medicine Press; 2004.

324. Gardner Z, McGuffin M, editors. *Botanical Safety Handbook*, 3rd edition. Boca Raton, FL: CRC Press; 2013. pp. 531–533.

325. Joo J, Liu KH. Inhibitory effect of honokiol and magnolol on cytochrome P450 enzyme activities in human liver microsomes. *Mass Spec Lett*. 2013;4(2):34–37.

326. Grieve MA. *Modern Herbal*. New York: Harcourt, Brace & Company; 1931. p. 185.

327. Amsterdam JD, Li Y, Soeller I, et al. A randomized, double-blind, placebo-controlled trial of oral *Matricaria recutita* (Chamomile) extract therapy of generalized anxiety disorder. *J Clin Psychopharmacol*. 2009;29(4):378–382.

328. Mao JJ, Xie SX, Keefe JR, et al. Long-term chamomile (*Matricaria chamomilla* L.) treatment for generalized anxiety disorder: A randomized clinical trial. *Phytomedicine*. 2016;23(14):1735–1742.

329. Keefe JR, Mao JJ, Soeller I, et al. Short-term open-label chamomile (*Matricaria chamomilla* L.) therapy of moderate to severe generalized anxiety disorder. *Phytomedicine*. 2016;23(14):1699–1705.

330. Amsterdam JD, Shults J, Soeller I, et al. Chamomile (*Matricaria recutita*) may have antidepressant activity in anxious depressed humans—an exploratory study. *Altern Ther Health Med*. 2012;18(5):44–49.

331. Gupta V, Mittal P, Bansal P, et al. Pharmacological potential of *Matricaria recutita*-a review. *Int J Pharm Sci Drug Res*. 2010;2(1):12–16.

332. Tabari MA, Tehrani MAB. Evidence for the involvement of the GABAergic, but not serotonergic transmission in the anxiolytic-like effect of bisabolol in the mouse elevated plus maze. *N-S Arch Pharmacol*. 2017;390:1041–1046.

333. Granger RE, Campbell EL, Johnston GAR. (+)- And (–)-borneol: Efficacious positive modulators of GABA action at human recombinant α1β2γ2L GABAA receptors. *Biochem Pharmacol*. 2005;69(7):1101–1111.

334. Hoffmann D. *Medical Herbalism: The Science and Practice of Herbal Medicine*. Rochester, VT: Healing Arts Press; 2003. p. 566.

335. Sebai H, Jabri MA, Souli A, et al. Antidiarrheal and antioxidant activities of chamomile (*Matricaria recutita* L.) decoction extract in rats. *J Ethnopharmacol*. 2014;152:327–332.

336. Hajjaj G, Bounihi A, Tajani M, et al. Evaluation of CNS activities of *Matricaria chamomilla* L. essential oil in experimental animals from Morocco. *Int J Pharm Pharm Sci*. 2013;5(2):530–534.

337. Al-Ramahi R, Jaradat N, Adawi D, et al. Use of herbal medicines during pregnancy in a group of Palestinian women. *J Ethnopharmacol*. 2013;150(1):79–84.

338. Gardner Z, McGuffin M, editors. *Botanical Safety Handbook*, 3rd edition. Boca Raton, FL: CRC Press; 2013. p. 541.

339. Ganzera M, Schneider P, Stuppner H. Inhibitory effects of the essential oil of chamomile (*Matricaria recutita* L.) and its major constituents on human cytochrome P450 enzymes. *Life Sci*. 2006;78(8):856–861.

340. Grieve MA. *Modern Herbal*. New York: Harcourt, Brace & Company; 1931. p. 76.

341. Cases J, Ibarra A, Feuillère N, et al. Pilot trial of *Melissa officinalis* L. Leaf extract in the treatment of volunteers suffering from mild-to-moderate anxiety disorders and sleep disturbances. *Mediterr J Nutr Metab*. 2011;4(3):211–218.

342. Soltanpour A, Alijaniha F, Naseri M, et al. Effects of *Melissa officinalis* on anxiety and sleep quality in patients undergoing coronary artery bypass surgery: A double-blind randomized placebo-controlled trial. *Eur J Integr Med*. 2019;28:27–32.

343. Nurzyńska-Wierdak R, Bogucka-Kocka A, Szymczak G. Volatile constituents of *Melissa officinalis* leaves determined by plant age. *NPC*. 2014;9(5):703–706.

344. Awad R, Muhammad A, Durst T, et al. Bioassay-guided fractionation of lemon balm (*Melissa officinalis* L.) using an in vitro measure of GABA transaminase activity. *Phytother Res*. 2009;23(8):1075–1081.

345. López V, Martín S, Gómez-Serranillos MP, et al. Neuroprotective and neurological properties of *Melissa officinalis*. *Neurochem Res*. 2009;34:1955–1961.

346. Hoffmann D. *Medical Herbalism: The Science and Practice of Herbal Medicine.* Rochester, VT: Healing Arts Press; 2003. p. 567.
347. Namjoo A, MirVakili M, Faghani M, et al. Biochemical, liver and renal toxicities of *Melissa officinals* hydroalcoholic extract on balb/C mice. *J HerbMed Pharmacol.* 2013;2(2):35–40.
348. Gardner Z, McGuffin M, editors. *Botanical Safety Handbook*, 3rd edition. Boca Raton, FL: CRC Press; 2013. p. 550.
349. Mahendran G, Rahman LU. Ethnomedicinal, phytochemical and pharmacological updates on Peppermint (*Mentha× piperita* L.)—a review. *Phytother Res.* 2020 Sep;34(9):2088–2139.
350. Blumenthal M, Busse WR, Goldberg A, et al. *The Complete German Commission E Monographs.* Austin, TX: American Botanical Council; 1998. p. 180.
351. Abdelhalim AR. The effect of *Mentha piperita* L. on the mental health issues of university students: A pilot study. *J Pharm Pharmacog Res.* 2021;9(1):49–57.
352. Sun Z, Wang H, Wang J, et al. Chemical composition and anti-inflammatory, cytotoxic and antioxidant activities of essential oil from leaves of *Mentha piperita* grown in China. *PloS One.* 2014;9(12):e114767.
353. Hoffmann BG, Lunder LT. Flavonoids from *Mentha piperita* leaves. *Planta Medica.* 1984;50(04):361.
354. Hall AC, Turcotte CM, Betts BA, et al. Modulation of human GABAA and glycine receptor currents by menthol and related monoterpenoids. *Eur J Pharmacol.* 2004;506(1):9–16.
355. Albishi FM, Albeshi SM, Alotaibi K. The effect of menthol on anxiety and related behaviors in mice. *Bahrain Med Bull.* 2020;42(4):277–282.
356. Blumenthal M, Busse WR, Goldberg A, et al. *The Complete German Commission E Monographs.* Austin, TX: American Botanical Council; 1998. p. 1280.
357. Gardner Z, McGuffin M, editors. *Botanical Safety Handbook*, 3rd edition. Boca Raton, FL: CRC Press; 2013. p. 554.
358. Cornara L, Ambu G, Trombetta D, et al. Comparative and functional screening of three species traditionally used as antidepressants: *Valeriana officinalis* L., *Valeriana jatamansi* Jones ex Roxb. And *Nardostachys jatamansi* (D. Don) DC. *Plants.* 2020 Aug;9(8):994–1021.
359. Shahinfar J, Hossein Z, Saeid S. The efficacy of *Nardostachys Jatamansi* root on preoperative anxiety in orthopedic surgery. *J Neyshabur Univ Med Sci.* 2016;4(3):56–64.
360. Purnima BM, Kothiyal P. A review article on phytochemistry and pharmacological profiles of *Nardostachys jatamansi* DC-medicinal herb. *J Pharmacog Phytochem.* 2015;3(5):102–106.
361. Takemoto H, Ito M, Asada Y. Inhalation administration of the sesquiterpenoid aristolen-1 (10)-en-9-ol from *Nardostachys chinensis* has a sedative effect via the GABAergic system. *Planta Medica.* 2015;81(5):343–347.
362. Chen YP, Ying SS, Zheng HH, et al. Novel serotonin transporter regulators: Natural aristolane-and nardosinane-types of sesquiterpenoids from *Nardostachys chinensis. Batal. Sci Rep.* 2017;7(1):1–2.
363. Prashith Kekuda TR, Chinmaya A, Valleesha NC, et al. Central nervous system (CNS) depressant and analgesic activity of methanolic extracts of *Nardostachys jatamansi* DC. And *Coscinium fenestratum* Colebr. in experimental animal model. *J Pharm Res.* 2009;2(11):1716–1719.
364. Gardner Z, McGuffin M, editors. *Botanical Safety Handbook*, 3rd edition. Boca Raton, FL: CRC Press; 2013. p. 585.
365. Verma S. Chemical constituents and pharmacological action of *Ocimum sanctum* (Indian holy basil-*Tulsi*) *J Phytopharmacol.* 2016;5(5):205–207.
366. Bhattacharyya D, Sur TK, Jana U, et al. Controlled programmed trial of *Ocimum sanctum* leaf on generalized anxiety disorders. *Nepal Med Coll J.* 2008;10(3):176–179.

367. Sampath S, Mahapatra SC, Padhi MM, et al. Holy basil (*Ocimum sanctum* Linn.) leaf extract enhances specific cognitive parameters in healthy adult volunteers: A placebo controlled study. *Indian J Physiol Pharmacol.* 2015;59(1):69–77.
368. Bano N, Ahmed A, Tanveer M, et al. Pharmacological evaluation of *Ocimum sanctum*. *J Bioequiv Availab.* 2017;9(3):387–392.
369. Mediratta PK, Sharma KK, Singh S. Evaluation of immunomodulatory potential of *Ocimum sanctum* seed oil and its possible mechanism of action. *J Ethnopharmacol.* 2002;80:15–20.
370. Ismail M. Central properties and chemical composition of *Ocimum basilicum*. Essential oil. *Pharm Biol.* 2006;44(8):619–626.
371. Chen JK, Chen TT. *Chinese Medical Herbology and Pharmacology*. City of Industry, CA: Art of Medicine Press; 2004.
372. Gardner Z, McGuffin M, editors. *Botanical Safety Handbook*, 3rd edition. Boca Raton, FL: CRC Press; 2013. p. 591.
373. Kom DH. Chemical diversity of *Panax ginseng, Panax quinquifolium*, and *Panax notoginseng*. *J Ginseng Res.* 2012;36(1):1–15.
374. Wiklund I, Karlberg J, Lund B, et al. A double-blind comparison of the effect on quality of life of a combination of vital substances including standardized ginseng G115 and placebo. *Curr Ther Res.* 1994;55:32–42.
375. Infante B. Double-blind study of a multivitamin complex supplemented with ginseng extract. *Drug Exp Clin Res.* 1995;22(6):323–329.
376. Wiklund IK, Mattsson LA, Lindgren R, et al. Effects of a standardized ginseng extract on quality of life and physiological parameters in symptomatic postmenopausal women: A double-blind, placebo-controlled trial. *Int J Clin Pharm Res.* 1999;19:89–99.
377. Ellis JM, Reddy P. Effects of *Panax ginseng* on quality of life. *Ann Pharmacother.* 2002;36:375–379.
378. Cardinal BJ, Engles HJ. Ginseng does not enhance psychological well-being in healthy, young adults: Results of a double-blind, placebo-controlled, randomized clinical trial. *J Am Diet Assoc.* 2001;101:655–660.
379. Leung KW, Wong AS. Pharmacology of ginsenosides: A literature review. *Chinese Med.* 2010;5: Article 20.
380. Choi S-E, Choi S, Lee J-H, et al. Effects of ginsenosides on GABA$_A$ receptor channels expressed in xenopus oocytes. *Arch Pharm Res.* 2003;26(1):28–33.
381. Kimura T, Saunders PA, Kim HS, et al. Interactions of ginsenosides with ligand-bindings of GABA (A) and GABA (B) receptors. *Gen Pharmacol.* 1994;25(1):193–199.
382. Drake RG, Davis LL, Cates ME, et al. Baclofen treatment for chronic posttraumatic stress disorder. *Ann Pharmacother.* 2003;37(9):1177–1181.
383. Hoffmann D. *Medical Herbalism: The Science and Practice of Herbal Medicine*. Rochester, VT: Healing Arts Press; 2003. p. 570.
384. Brekham II, Dardymov IV. New substances of plant origin, which increase non-specific resistance. *Ann Rev Pharmacol.* 1969;9:419–430.
385. Chuang CH, Doyle P, Wang JD, et al. Herbal medicines used during the first trimester and major congenital malformations: An analysis of data from a pregnancy cohort study. *Drug Safety.* 2006;29(6):537–548.
386. Chin R. Ginseng and common pregnancy disorders. *Asia Oceania J Obstet Gynaecol.* 1991;17(4):379–380.
387. Janetsky K, Morreale A. Probable interaction between warfarin and ginseng. *Am J Health-Syst Pharm.* 1997;54:692–693.
388. Jiang X, Williams KM, Liauw WS, et al. Effect of St John's wort and ginseng on the pharmacokinetics and pharmacodynamics of warfarin in healthy subjects. *BJCP.* 2004;57(5):592–599.
389. Malati CY, Robertson SM, Hunt JD, et al. Influence of *Panax ginseng* on cytochrome P450 (CYP)3A and P-glycoprotein (P-gp) activity in healthy participants. *J Clin Pharm.* 2012;52(6):932–939.

390. Patel SS, Saleem TM, Ravi V, et al. *Passiflora incarnata* Linn: A phytopharmacological review. *Int J Green Pharm.* 2009;3(4):277–280.
391. Grieve MA. *Modern Herbal.* New York: Harcourt, Brace & Company; 1931. p. 618.
392. Akhondzadeh S, Naghavi HR, Vazirian M, et al. Passionflower in the treatment of generalized anxiety: A pilot double-blind randomized controlled trial with oxazepam. *J Clin Pharm Therap.* 2001;26(5):363–367.
393. Movafegh A, Alizadeh R, Hajimohamadi F, et al. Preoperative oral *Passiflora incarnata* reduces anxiety in ambulatory surgery patients: A double-blind, placebo-controlled study. *Anesth Analg.* 2008;106(6):1728–1732.
394. Kaviani N, Tavakoli M, Tabanmehr MR, et al. The efficacy of *Passiflora Incarnata* Linnaeus in reducing dental anxiety in patients undergoing periodontal treatment. *J Dent* (Shiraz). 2013;14(2):68–72.
395. Patel SS, Verma NK, Gauthaman K. *Passiflora Incarnata* Linn: A review on morphology, phytochemistry and pharmacological aspects. *Pharmacog Rev.* 2009;3(5):175–181.
396. Grundmann O, Wang J, McGregor GP, et al. Anxiolytic activity of a phytochemically characterized *Passiflora incarnata* extract is mediated via the GABAergic system. *Planta medica.* 2008;74(15):1769–1773.
397. Hoffmann D. *Medical Herbalism: The Science and Practice of Herbal Medicine.* Rochester, VT: Healing Arts Press; 2003. p. 571.
398. Aoyagi N, Kimura R, Murata T. Studies on *Passiflora incarnata* dry extract. I. Isolation of maltol and pharmacological action of maltol and ethyl maltol. *Chem Pharm Bull.* 1974;22(5):1008–1013.
399. Sopranzi N, De Feo G, Mazzanti G, et al. Biological and electroencephalographic parameters in rats in relation to *Passiflora incarnata* L. *La Clinica Terapeutica.* 1990;132(5):329–333.
400. Gardner Z, McGuffin M, editors. *Botanical Safety Handbook*, 3rd edition. Boca Raton, FL: CRC Press; 2013. p. 621.
401. Hirakawa T, Suzuki T, Sano Y, et al. Reproductive studies of *P. incarnata* extract teratological study. *Kiso To Rinsho.* 1981;15:3431–3451.
402. Patel SS, Verma NK, Gauthaman K. *Passiflora Incarnata* Linn: A review on morphology, phytochemistry and pharmacological aspects. *Phcog Rev.* 2009;3(5):175–181.
403. Pepping J. Kava: *Piper methysticum. Am J Health-Syst Ph.* 1999;56(10):957–958.
404. Pittler MH, Ernst E. Kava extract for treating anxiety. *Cochrane Database Syst Rev.* 2003;(1):CD003383.
405. Sarris J, LaPorte E, Schweitzer I. Kava: A comprehensive review of efficacy, safety, and psychopharmacology. *Aust N Z J Psychiatry.* 2011;45(1):27–35.
406. Sarris J, Stough C, Bousman CA, et al. Kava in the treatment of generalized anxiety disorder a double-blind, randomized, placebo-controlled study. *J Clin Psychopharmacol.* 2013;33(5):643–648.
407. Jussofie A, Schmiz A, Hiemke C. Kavapyrone enriched extract from *Piper methysticum* as modulator of the GABA binding site in different regions of rat brain. *Psychopharmacology.* 1994;116:469–474.
408. Prinsloo D, Van Dyk S, Petzer A, et al. Monoamine oxidase inhibition by kavalactones from kava (*piper methysticum*). *Planta Medica.* 2019;85(14/15):1136–1142.
409. Baum SS, Hill R, Rommelspacher H. Effect of kava extract and individual kavapyrones on neurotransmitter levels in the nucleus accumbens of rats. *Prog Neuropsychopharmacol Biol Psychiatry.* 1998;22:1105–1120.
410. Seitz U, Schule A, Gleitz J. [3H]-monoamine uptake inhibition properties of kava pyrones. *Planta Med.* 1997;63:548–549.
411. Ligresti A, Villano R, Allarà M, et al. Kavalactones and the endocannabinoid system: The plant-derived yangonin is a novel CB1 receptor ligand. *Pharmacol Res.* 2012;66(2):163–169.

412. Garrett KM, Basmadjian G, Khan IA, et al. Extracts of kava (*Piper methysticum*) induce acute anxiolytic-like behavioral changes in mice. *Psychopharmacology.* 2003;170:33–41.
413. Mendelson SD. *Herbal Treatment of Major Depression: Scientific Basis and Practical Use.* Boca Raton, FL: CRC Press; 2020. p. 236.
414. Abenavoli L, Capasso R, Milic N, et al. Milk thistle in liver diseases: Past, present and future. *Phytother Res.* 2010;24(10):1423–1432.
415. Kiefer P, Vogt J, Radermacher P. From mucolytic to antioxidant and liver protection: New aspects in the intensive care unit career of N-acetylcysteine. *Crit Care Med.* 2000;28(12):3935–3936.
416. Gardner Z, McGuffin M, editors. *Botanical Safety Handbook*, 3rd edition. Boca Raton, FL: CRC Press; 2013. p. 658.
417. García-Suástegui WA, Ramos-Chávez LA, Rubio-Osornio M, et al. The role of CYP2E1 in the drug metabolism or bioactivation in the brain. *Oxi Med Cell Longev.* 2017;2017: Article ID 4680732.
418. Wang YZ, Zhang J, Zhao YL, et al. Mycology, cultivation, traditional uses, phytochemistry and pharmacology of *Wolfiporia cocos* (Schwein.) Ryvarden et Gilb.: A review. *J Ethnopharmacol.* 2013;147(2):265–276.
419. Li Z, Lei QF, Liu HY, et al. Clinical evaluation of Wuling capsule in anxiety disorder. *New Med.* 2010;41(1):10–13.
420. Wang X, Li J, Zou Q, et al. *Wuling* capsule for climacteric patients with depression and anxiety state: A randomized, positive parallel controlled trial. *J Chin Integr Med.* 2009;7(11):1042–1046.
421. Ríos JL. Chemical constituents and pharmacological properties of *Poria cocos. Planta Medica.* 2011;77(07):681–691.
422. Shah VK, Choi JJ, Han JY, et al. Pachymic acid enhances pentobarbital-induced sleeping behaviors via GABAA-ergic systems in mice. *Biomol Ther.* 2014 Jul;22(4):314–320.
423. Gao Y, Yan H, Jin R, Lei P. Antiepileptic activity of total triterpenes isolated from *Poria cocos* is mediated by suppression of aspartic and glutamic acids in the brain. *Pharm Biol.* 2016 Nov 1;54(11):2528–2535.
424. Lee JH, Lee YJ, Shin JK, et al. Effects of triterpenoids from *Poria cocos* Wolf on the serotonin type 3A receptor-mediated ion current in Xenopus oocytes. *Eur J Pharmacol.* 2009 Aug 1;615(1–3):27–32.
425. Huang YJ, Hsu NY, Lu K, et al. *Poria cocos* water extract ameliorates the behavioral deficits induced by unpredictable chronic mild stress in rats by down-regulating inflammation. *J Ethnopharmacol.* 2020;258:112566.
426. Yin J, Gun LG. *Modern Research and Clinical Applications of Chinese Materia Medica.* Beijing: Academic Publishing; 1993. pp. 489–492.
427. Dong HY, Shao JW, Chen JF, et al. Transcriptional regulation of cytochrome P450 3A4 by four kinds of traditional Chinese medicines. *J Chinese Mat Med.* 2008;33(9):1014–1017.
428. van der Weide K, van der Weide J. The influence of the CYP3A4*22 polymorphism and CYP2D6 polymorphisms on serum concentrations of aripiprazole, haloperidol, pimozide, and risperidone in psychiatric patients. *J Clin Psychopharmacol.* 2015;35(3):228–236.
429. Haduch A, Wójcikowski J, Daniel WA. The effect of tricyclic antidepressants, selective serotonin reuptake inhibitors (SSRIs) and newer antidepressant drugs on the activity and level of rat CYP3A. *Eur Neuropsychopharm.* 2006;16(3):178–186.
430. Freye E. The mushroom psilocybin with psychedelic properties. In: *Pharmacology and Abuse of Cocaine, Amphetamines, Ecstasy and Related Designer Drugs.* Dordrecht: Springer; 2009.
431. Carhart-Harris RL, Bolstridge M, Day CMJ, et al. Psilocybin with psychological support for treatment-resistant depression: Six-month follow-up. *Psychopharmacol.* 2018;235(2):399–408.

432. Griffiths R. A single dose of psilocybin produces substantial and enduring decreases in anxiety and depression in patients with a life-threatening cancer diagnosis: A randomized double-blind trial. *Neuropsychopharmacol.* 2015;40:S90–S91.

433. Moreno FA, Wiegand CB, Taitano EK, et al. Safety, tolerability, and efficacy of psilocybin in 9 patients with obsessive-compulsive disorder. *J Clin Psychiatry.* 2006;67:1735–1740.

434. Bird CIV, Modlin NL, Rucker JJH. Psilocybin and MDMA for the treatment of trauma-related psychopathology. *Int Rev Psychiat.* 2021;33:3, 229–249.

435. Anderson T, Petranker R, Rosenbaum D, et al. Microdosing psychedelics: Personality, mental health, and creativity differences in microdosers. *Psychopharmacol (Berl).* 2019;236(2):731–740.

436. Johnstad PG. Powerful substances in tiny amounts: An interview study of psychedelic microdosing. *Nordic Stud Alco Drug.* 2018;35(1):39–51.

437. van Elk M, Fejer G, Lempe P, et al. Effects of psilocybin microdosing on awe and aesthetic experiences: A preregistered field and lab-based study. *Psychopharmacol.* 2021. https://doi.org/10.1007/s00213-021-05857-0.

438. Szigeti B, Kartner L, Blemings A, et al. Self-blinding citizen science to explore psychedelic microdosing. *Elife.* 2021;10:e62878.

439. Risca HI. *Preclinical Behavioral Assessment of Chronic, Intermittent Low-Dose Psilocybin in Rodent Models of Depression and Anxiety.* Dissertations. 3770, Western Michigan University; 2021.

440. Lowe H, Toyang N, Steele B, et al. The therapeutic potential of psilocybin. *Molecules.* 2021;26(10):2948.

441. Coutinho JF, Fernandesl SV, Soares JM, et al. Default mode network dissociation in depressive and anxiety states. *Brain Imaging Behav.* 2016;10:147–157.

442. Kraehenmann R, Schmidt A, Friston K, et al. The mixed serotonin receptor agonist psilocybin reduces threat-induced modulation of amygdala connectivity. *Neuroimage Clin.* 2016;11:53–60.

443. Gawliński D, Smaga I, Zaniewska M, et al. Adaptive mechanisms following antidepressant drugs: Focus on serotonin 5-HT2A receptors. *Pharmacol Rep.* 2019;71(6):994–1000.

444. Carbonaro TM, Bradstreet MP, Barrett FS, et al. Survey study of challenging experiences after ingesting psilocybin mushrooms: Acute and enduring positive and negative consequences. *J Psychopharmacol.* 2016;30(12):1268–1278.

445. Rumack BH, Spoerke DG. *Handbook of Mushroom Poisoning: Diagnosis and Treatment.* Boca Raton, FL: Taylor & Francis; 1994.

446. Bigwood J, Beug MW. Variation of psilocybin and psilocin levels with repeated flushes (harvests) of mature sporocarps of *psilocybe cubensis* (Earle) singer. *J Enthopharmacol.* 1982;5:287–291.

447. Novitaloka OS, Bhima SKL, Dhanardhonob T. *Pengaruh pemberian ekstrak jamur Psilocybe cubensis dosis bertingkat terhadap aktivitas motorik miencit Swiss Webster dengan metode rotarod manual.* Undergraduate Thesis, Faculty of Medicine Diponegoro University; 2013.

448. Lebedev AV, Lövdén M, Rosenthal GA, et al. Finding the self by losing the self: Neural correlates of ego-dissolution under psilocybin. *Hum Brain Mapp.* 2015;36:3137–3153.

449. Law FCP, Poon G, Chui YC. 14C-Psilocin tissue distribution in pregnant rats after intravenous administration. *Funct Food Health Dis.* 2014;4(6):232–244.

450. Brown RP, Gerbarg PL, Ramazanov Z. *Rhodiola rosea.* A phytomedicinal overview. *HerbalGram.* 2002;56:40–52.

451. Bystritsky A, Kerwin L, Feusner JD. A pilot study of *Rhodiola rosea* (Rhodax) for generalized anxiety disorder (GAD). *J Altern Complement Med.* 2008;14:175–180.

452. Cropley M, Banks AP, Boyle J. The effects of *Rhodiola rosea* L. Extract on anxiety, stress, cognition and other mood symptoms. *Phytother Res.* 2015;29(12):1934–1939.

453. Spasov AA, Wikman GK, Mandrikov VB, et al. A double-blind, placebo-controlled pilot study of the stimulating and adaptogenic effect of *Rhodiola rosea* SHR-5 extract on the fatigue of students caused by stress during an examination period with a repeated low-dose regimen. *Phytomedicine*. 2000;7(2):85–89.
454. Darbinyan V, Aslanyan G, Amroyan E, et al. Clinical trial of *Rhodiola rosea* L. Extract SHR-5 in the treatment of mild to moderate depression. *Nord J Psychiatry*. 2007;61(5):343–348.
455. Mao JJ, Xie SX, Zee J, et al. *Rhodiola rosea* versus sertraline for major depressive disorder: A randomized placebo-controlled trial. *Phytomedicine*. 2015;22(3):394–399.
456. Panossian A, Wikman G, Sarris J. Rosenroot (*Rhodiola rosea*): Traditional use, chemical composition, pharmacology and clinical efficacy. *Phytomedicine*. 2010;17(7):481–493.
457. Cayer C, Ahmed F, Filion V, et al. Characterization of the anxiolytic activity of Nunavik *Rhodiola rosea*. *Planta Medica*. 2013;79(15):1385–1391.
458. Palmeri A, Mammana L, Tropea MR. Salidroside, a bioactive compound of *Rhodiola Rosea*, ameliorates memory and emotional behavior in adult mice. *J Alzheimers Dis*. 2016;52(1):65–75.
459. Zhong Z, Han J, Zhang J, et al. Pharmacological activities, mechanisms of action, and safety of salidroside in the central nervous system. *Drug Des Devel Ther*. 2018;12:1479–1489.
460. Van Diermen D, Marston A, Bravo J, et al. Monoamine oxidase inhibition by *Rhodiola rosea* L. Roots. *J Ethnopharmacol*. 2009;122(2):397–401.
461. Mendelson S. *Herbal Treatment of Major Depression: Scientific Basis and Practical Use*. CRC Press; 2019. p. 257.
462. Marciano M, Vizniak NA. *Botanical Medicine*. Toronto: Prohealth; 2016. p. 297.
463. Kurkin V, Zapesochnaya G. Chemical composition and pharmacological characteristics of *Rhodiola rosea*. *J Med Plants*. 1985:1231–1445.
464. Kennedy DA, Lupattelli A, Koren G. Safety classification of herbal medicines used in pregnancy in a multinational study. *BMC Compl Alt Med*. 2016;16:102.
465. Hellum BH, Tosse A, Hoybakk K, et al. Potent inhibition of CYP3A4 and P-glycoprotein by *Rhodiola rosea*. *Planta Med*. 2010;76(4):331–338.
466. Gerbarg PL, Brown RP. Integrating rhodiola rosea in clinical practice. In: PL Gerbarg, PR Muskin, RP Brown (Eds.), *Complimentary and Intergrative Treatments in Psychiatric Practice*. Arlington, VA: American Psychiatric Association Publishing; 2017. pp. 135–141.
467. Begum A, Sandhya S, Vinod KR, et al. An in-depth review on the medicinal flora *Rosmarinus officinalis* (Lamiaceae). *Acta Sci Pol Technol Aliment*. 2013;12(1):61–73.
468. Grieve MA. *Modern Herbal*. New York: Harcourt, Brace & Company; 1931. p. 682.
469. Nematolahi P, Mehrabani M, Karami-Mohajeri S, et al. Effects of *Rosmarinus officinalis* L. on memory performance, anxiety, depression, and sleep quality in university students: A randomized clinical trial. *Complement Ther Clin*. 2018;30:24–28.
470. Achour M, Ben Salem I, Ferdousi F, et al. Rosemary tea consumption alters peripheral anxiety and depression biomarkers: A pilot study in limited healthy volunteers. *J Am Coll Nutr*. 2021;1:1–10.
471. Araki R, Sasaki K, Onda H, et al. Effects of continuous intake of rosemary extracts on mental health in working generation healthy Japanese men: Post-Hoc testing of a randomized controlled trial. *Nutrients*. 2020;12(11):3551–3562.
472. Özcan MM, Chalchat JC. Chemical composition and antifungal activity of rosemary (*Rosmarinus officinalis* L.) oil from Turkey. *Int J Food Sci Nutr*. 2008;59(7–8):691–698.
473. Pereira P, Tysca D, Oliveira P, et al. Neurobehavioral and genotoxic aspects of rosmarinic acid. *Pharmacol Res*. 2005;52(3):199–203.
474. Wang CC, Hsieh PW, Kuo JR, et al. Rosmarinic acid, a bioactive phenolic compound, inhibits glutamate release from rat cerebrocortical synaptosomes through GABAA receptor activation. *Biomolecules*. 2021 Jul;11(7):1029.

475. Abdelhalim A, Karim N, Chebib M, et al. Antidepressant, anxiolytic and antinociceptive activities of constituents from *Rosmarinus officinalis*. *J Pharm Pharmaceut Sci*. 2015;18(4):448–459.

476. Hoffmann D. *Medical Herbalism: The Science and Practice of Herbal Medicine*. Rochester, VT: Healing Arts Press; 2003. p. 567.

477. Alnamer R, Alaoui K, Bouidida EH, et al. Psychostimulants activity of *Rosmarinus officinalis* L. Methanolic and aqueous extracts. *J Med Plants Res*. 2012;6(10):1860–1865.

478. Dipe de Faria LR, Lima CS, Perazzo FF, et al. Anti-inflammatory and antinociceptive activities of the essential oil from *Rosmarinus officinalis* L. *Int J Pharmaceut Sci Rev Res*. 2011;7(2): Article-001.

479. Gardner Z, McGuffin M, editors. *Botanical Safety Handbook*, 3rd edition. Boca Raton, FL: CRC Press; 2013. p. 740.

480. Debersac P, Heydel J-M, Amiot M-J, et al. Induction of cytochrome P450 and/or detoxication enzymes by various extracts of rosemary: Description of specific patterns. *Food Chem Toxicol*. 2001;39(9):907–918.

481. Turpeinen M, Raunio H, Pelkonen O. The functional role of CYP2B6 in human drug metabolism: Substrates and inhibitors in vitro, in vivo and in silico. *Curr Drug Metab*. 2006;7(7):705–714.

482. Sharma Y, Fagan J, Schaefer J. Ethnobotany, phytochemistry, cultivation and medicinal properties of garden sage (*Salvia officinalis* L.). *J Pharmacogn Phytochem*. 2019;8:3139–3148.

483. Kennedy DO, Pace S, Haskell C, et al. Effects of cholinesterase inhibiting sage (*Salvia officinalis*) on mood, anxiety and performance on a psychological stressor battery. *Neuropsychopharmacol*. 2006;31(4):845–852.

484. Tildesley NTJ, Kennedy DO, Perry EK, et al. Positive modulation of mood and cognitive performance following administration of acute doses of *Salvia lavandulaefolia* essential oil to healthy young volunteers. *Physiol Behav*. 2005;83(5):699–709.

485. Zeidabadi A, Yazdanpanahi Z, Dabbaghmanesh MH, et al. The effect of *Salvia officinalis* extract on symptoms of flushing, night sweat, sleep disorders, and score of forgetfulness in postmenopausal women. *J Family Med Prim Care*. 2020;9(2):1086–1092.

486. Khedher MR, Khedher SB, Chaieb I, et al. Chemical composition and biological activities of *Salvia officinalis* essential oil from Tunisia. *EXCLI J*. 2017;16:160–173.

487. Kavvadias D, Monschein V, Sand P, et al. Constituents of sage (*Salvia officinalis*) with in vitro affinity to human brain benzodiazepine receptor. *Planta Medica*. 2003;69(02):113–117.

488. Zuccarini P, Soldani G. Camphor: Benefits and risks of a widely used natural product. *Acta Biologica Szegediensis*. 2009;53(2):77–82.

489. Höld KM, Sirisoma NS, Ikeda T, et al. α-Thujone (the active component of absinthe): γ-aminobutyric acid type A receptor modulation and metabolic detoxification. *P Natl Acad Sci*. 2000;97(8):3826–3831.

490. Al-Barazanjy R, Dizaye K, Al-Asadye A. Cytotoxic and cytogenetic effects of *Salvia officinalis* on different tumor cell lines. *Middle East J Int Med*. 2013;13:15–25.

491. Blumenthal M, Busse WR, Goldberg A, et al. *The Complete German Commission E Monographs*. Austin, TX: American Botanical Council; 1998. p. 198.

492. Gardner Z, McGuffin M, editors. *Botanical Safety Handbook*, 3rd edition. Boca Raton, FL: CRC Press; 2013. p. 764.

493. Panossian AG. Pharmacology of *Schisandra chinensis* Bail.: An overview of Russian research and uses in medicine. *J Ethnopharmacol*. 2008;118(2):183–212.

494. Belluzzi A, Lembke P, Marasco G, et al. The effect of supplementing a novel n-3 polyunsaturated fatty acids formulation containing *Schisandra chinensis* extract and vitamin D3 to a group of elite sport athletes on competition related stress, anxiety and self-confidence. *Ann Appl Sport Sci*. 2020;8(1).

495. Chen X, Zhang Y, Zu Y, et al. Chemical composition and antioxidant activity of the essential oil of *Schisandra chinensis* fruits. *Nat Prod Res*. 2012;26(9):842–849.
496. Mocan A, Crişan G, Vlase L, et al. Comparative studies on polyphenolic composition, antioxidant and antimicrobial activities of *Schisandra chinensis* leaves and fruits. *Molecules*. 2014;19(9):15162–15179.
497. Wang BL, Hu JP, Tan W, et al. Simultaneous quantification of four active schisandra lignans from a traditional Chinese medicine *Schisandra chinensis* (Wuweizi) in rat plasma using liquid chromatography/mass spectrometry. *J Chromatogr B*. 2008;865(1–2):114–120.
498. Li N, Liu J, Wang M, et al. Sedative and hypnotic effects of Schisandrin B through increasing GABA/Glu ratio and upregulating the expression of GABAA in mice and rats. *Biomed Pharmacother*. 2018;103:509–516.
499. Lin Q, Qin X, Shi M, et al. Schisandrin B inhibits LPS-induced inflammatory response in human umbilical vein endothelial cells by activating Nrf2. *Int Immunopharmacol*. 2017;49:142–147.
500. Panossian A, Amsterdam JD. Adaptogens in psychiatric practice. In: PL Gerbarg, PR Muskin, RP Brown (Eds.), *Complementary and Integrative Treatments in Psychiatric Practice*, vol. 21. Arlington, VA: American Psychiatric Association Publishing; 2017. pp. 113–134.
501. Bensky D, Gamble A. *Chinese Herbal Medicine: Materia Medica*, Revised edition. Seattle, WA: Eastland Press; 1993.
502. Pan SY, Yu ZL, Dong H, et al. Ethanol extract of *fructus schisandrae* decreases hepatic triglyceride level in mice fed with a high fat/cholesterol diet, with attention to acute toxicity. *eCAM*. 2011:729412.
503. Ryu SN. Acute toxicity of fruit pigment and seed oil of *Schizandra chinensis* in mice. *J Korean Soc Int Agric*. 1998;10:37–41.
504. Gaistruk A, Taranovskij K. The treatment of arterial hypotension in pregnant women using *Schisandra chinensis*. *Urb Prob Obstet Gynecol*. 1968;1:183–186.
505. Trifinova A. Stimulation of labor activity using *Schizandra chinensis*. *Obstet Gynecol*. 1954;4:19–22.
506. Cao Y-F, Zhang Y-Y, Li J, et al. CYP3A catalyses schizandrin biotransformation in human, minipig and rat liver microsomes. *Xenobiotica*. 2010;40(1):38–47.
507. van der Weide K, van der Weide J. The Influence of the CYP3A422 polymorphism and CYP2D6 polymorphisms on serum concentrations of aripiprazole, haloperidol, pimozide, and risperidone in psychiatric patients. *J Clin Psychopharmacol*. 2015;35(3):228–236.
508. Haduch A, Wójcikowski J, Daniel WA. The effect of tricyclic antidepressants, selective serotonin reuptake inhibitors (SSRIs) and newer antidepressant drugs on the activity and level of rat CYP3A. *Eur Neuropsychopharm*. 2006;16(3):178–186.
509. Cole IB, Cao J, Alan AR, et al. Comparisons of *Scutellaria baialensis, Scutellaria laterflora*, and *Scutellaria racemosa*: Genome size, antioxidant potential and phytochemistry. *Planta*. 2007;74:1–8.
510. Grieve MA. *Modern Herbal*. New York: Harcourt, Brace & Company; 1931. p. 723.
511. Wolfson P, Hoffmann DL. An investigation into the efficacy of *Scutellaria lateriflora* in healthy volunteers. *Altern Ther Health M*. 2003;9:74–78.
512. Brock C, Whitehouse J, Tewfik I, et al. American skullcap (*Scutellaria lateriflora*): A randomised, double-blind placebo-controlled crossover study of its effects on mood in healthy volunteers. *Phytother Res*. 2014;28:692–698.
513. Olennikov DN, Chirikova NK, Tankhaeva LM. Phenolic compounds of *Scutellaria baicalensis* Georgi. *Russ J Bioorg Chem*. 2010;36(7):816–824.
514. Hui KM, Huen MS, Wang HY, et al. Anxiolytic effect of wogonin, a benzodiazepine receptor ligand isolated from *Scutellaria baicalensis* Georgi. *Biochem Pharmacol*. 2002;64(9):1415–1424.

515. Park HG, Yoon SY, Choi JY, et al. Anticonvulsant effect of wogonin isolated from *Scutellaria baicalensis*. *Eur J Pharmacol*. 2007;574(2–3):112–119.
516. de Carvalho RS, Duarte FS, de Lima TC. Involvement of GABAergic non-benzodiazepine sites in the anxiolytic-like and sedative effects of the flavonoid baicalein in mice. *Behav Brain Res*. 2011;221(1):75–82.
517. Easley T, Horne S. *The Modern Herbal Dispensary*. Berkeley, CA: North Atlantic Books; 2016. p. 301.
518. Lee J-W, Jung Y, Jung T, et al. Mouse single oral dose toxicity test of *Scutellariae Radix* aqueous extracts. *Korean J Orient Int Med*. 2013;34(1):46–58.
519. Melchart D, Hager S, Albrecht S, et al. Herbal traditional Chinese medicine and suspected liver injury: A prospective study. *World J Hepatol*. 2017;9(29):1141–1157.
520. Chen JK, Chen TT. *Chinese Medical Herbology and Pharmacology*. City of Industry, CA: Art of Medicine Press; 2004.
521. Mo SL, Liu WF, Chen Y, et al. Ligand- and protein-based modeling studies of the inhibitors of human cytochrome P450 2D6 and a virtual screening for potential inhibitors from the Chinese herbal medicine, *Scutellaria baicalensis* (Huangqin, Baikal Skullcap). *Comb Chem High Throughput Screen*. 2012;15(1):36–80.
522. Bertilsson L, Dahl ML, Dalén P, et al. Molecular genetics of CYP2D6: Clinical relevance with focus on psychotropic drugs. *BJCP*. 2002;53(2):111–122.
523. Pepping J. Milk thistle: *Silybum marianum*. *Amer J Health-Syst Ph*. 1999;56(12): 1195–1197.
524. Blumenthal M, Busse WR, editors. *The Complete German Commission E Monographs: Therapeutic Guide to Herbal Medicines*. Austin, TX: American Botanical Council; 1998.
525. Sayyah M, Boostani H, Pakseresht S, et al. Comparison of *Silybum marianum* (L.) Gaertn. with fluoxetine in the treatment of obsessive–compulsive disorder. *Prog Neuropsychopharmacol Biol Psychiatry*. 2010;34(2):362–365.
526. Grant JE, Odlaug BL. Silymarin treatment of obsessive-compulsive spectrum disorders. *J Clin Psychopharmacol*. 2015;35(3):340–342.
527. Padma M, Ganesan S, Jayaseelan T, et al. Phytochemical screening and GC—MS analysis of bioactive compounds present in ethanolic leaves extract of *Silybum marianum* (L). *J Drug Del Thera*. 2019;9(1):85–89.
528. Kvasnička F, Bıba B, Ševčík R, et al. Analysis of the active components of silymarin. *J Chromatogr A*. 2003;990(1–2):239–245.
529. Malaguarnera G, Bertino G, Chisari G, et al. Silybin supplementation during HCV therapy with pegylated interferon-α plus ribavirin reduces depression and anxiety and increases work ability. *BMC Psychiatry*. 2016;16(1):1–10.
530. Blumenthal M, Busse WR, Goldberg A, et al. *The Complete German Commission E Monographs*. Austin, TX: American Botanical Council; 1998. p. 170.
531. Lecomte J. Pharmacologic properties of silybin and silymarin. *Rev Med Liege*. 1975;30:110–114.
532. Gonzalez M, Reyes H, Ribalta J, et al. Effect of sylimarin on pruritus of cholestasis. *Hepatology*. 1988;8(5):1356.
533. Hahn G, Lehmann HD, Kürten M. On the pharmacology and toxicology of silymarin, an antihepatotoxic active principle from *Silybum marianum* (L.) Gaertn). *Arznei-Forschung*. 1968;18(6):698–704.
534. Gardner Z, McGuffin M, editors. *Botanical Safety Handbook*, 3rd edition. Boca Raton, FL: CRC Press; 2013. p. 807.
535. Doehmer J, Weiss G, McGregor GP, et al. Assessment of a dry extract from milk thistle (*Silybum marianum*) for interference with human liver cytochrome-P450 activities. *Toxicol in Vitro*. 2011;25(1):21–27.

536. Sinha K, Mishra NP, Singh J, et al. *Tinospora cordifolia (Guduchi)*: A reservoir plant for therapeutic applications: A review. *Indian J Trad Know.* 2004;3:257–270.
537. Vishal G, Shetty S, Vishal S. A comparative study on *guduchi vati* and *mandookaparni vati* in the management of *chittodvega* (generalized anxiety disorder). *IAMJ.* 2015;3(7):2030–2040.
538. Biswas P, Saha A, Maity LN. Antistress activity of *Tinospora Cordifolia* with application of yoga. *Int J Ayurvedic Med.* 2015;6(3):220–224.
539. Sharma P, Dwivedee BP, Bisht D, et al. The chemical constituents and diverse pharmacological importance of *Tinospora cordifolia*. *Heliyon.* 2019;5(9):e02437.
540. Sharma A, Kalotra S, Bajaj P, et al. Butanol extract of *Tinospora cordifolia* ameliorates cognitive deficits associated with glutamate-induced excitotoxicity: A mechanistic study using hippocampal neurons. *Neuromol Med.* 2020;22(1):81–99.
541. Peng WH, Wu CR, Chen CS, et al. Anxiolytic effect of berberine on exploratory activity of the mouse in two experimental anxiety models: Interaction with drugs acting at 5-HT receptors. *Life Sci.* 2004;75(20):2451–2462.
542. Dhingra D, Bhankher A. Behavioral and biochemical evidences for antidepressant-like activity of palmatine in mice subjected to chronic unpredictable mild stress. *Pharmacol Rep.* 2014;66(1):1–9.
543. Salve BA, Tripathi RK, Petare AU, et al. Effect of *Tinospora cordifolia* on physical and cardiovascular performance induced by physical stress in healthy human volunteers. *Ayu.* 2015;36(3):265–270.
544. Madhuri S, Pandey G, Khanna A. Studies on phytochemistry and toxicities of *Tinospora cordiofolia* (giloe). *Anusandhan.* 2011;5:64–68.
545. Gardner Z, McGuffin M, editors. *Botanical Safety Handbook*, 3rd edition. Boca Raton, FL: CRC Press; 2013. p. 562.
546. Sabudak T, Guler N. *Trifolium* L.—a review on its phytochemical and pharmacological profile. *Phytother Res.* 2009;23(3):439–446.
547. Coon JT, Pittler MH, Ernst E. *Trifolium pratense* isoflavones in the treatment of menopausal hot flushes: A systematic review and meta-analysis. *Phytomedicine.* 2007;14(2–3):153–159.
548. Lipovac M, Chedraui P, Gruenhut C, et al. Improvement of postmenopausal depressive and anxiety symptoms after treatment with isoflavones derived from red clover extracts. *Maturitas.* 2010;65:258–261.
549. Hidalgo LA, Chedraui PA, Morocho N, et al. The effect of red clover isoflavones on menopausal symptoms, lipids and vaginal cytology in menopausal women: A randomized, double-blind, placebo-controlled study. *Gynecol Endocrinol.* 2005;21:257–264.
550. Kanadys WS, Barańska A, Błaszczuk A, et al. Evaluation of clinical meaningfulness of red clover (*Trifolium pratense* L.) extract to relieve hot flushes and menopausal symptoms in peri- and post-menopausal women: A systematic review and meta-analysis of randomized controlled trials. *Nutrients.* 2021;13(4):1258.
551. Tice JA, Ettinger B, Ensrud K, et al. Phytoestrogen supplements for the treatment of hot flashes: The isoflavone clover extract (ICE) Study: A randomized controlled trial. *JAMA.* 2003;290:207–214.
552. Geller SE, Shulman LP, Van Breemen RB, et al. Safety and efficacy of black cohosh and red clover for the management of vasomotor symptoms: A randomized controlled trial. *Menopause.* 2009;16:1156–1166.
553. Beck V, Rohr U, Jungbauer A. Phytoestrogens derived from red clover: An alternative to estrogen replacement therapy? *J Steroid Biochem Mol Biol.* 2005;94(5):499–518.
554. Tava A, Pecio Ł, Stochmal A, et al. Clovamide and flavonoids from leaves of *Trifolium pratense* and *T. pratense* subsp. Nivale grown in Italy. *Nat Prod Commun.* 2015;10:933–936.

555. Nissan HP, Lu J, Booth NL, et al. A red clover (*Trifolium pratense*) phase II clinical extract possesses opiate activity. *J Ethnopharmacol.* 2007;112(1):207–210.
556. Bakirel T, Keles O, Bozkurt HH, et al. The effect of *Trifolium pratense* on spermatogenesis and its acute toxicity (LD_{50}) in mice. *Turk J Vet Anim Sci.* 2002;26:555–559.
557. Gardner Z, McGuffin M, editors. *Botanical Safety Handbook*, 3rd edition. Boca Raton, FL: CRC Press; 2013. p. 869.
558. Jugran A, Rawat S, Dauthal P, et al. Association of ISSR markers with some biochemical traits of *Valeriana jatamansi* Jones. *Ind Crop Prod.* 2013;44:671–676.
559. Sharma S, Dutt A, Katwal S. Clinical evaluation of *tagra* (*Valeriana jatamansi* Jones) as a premedication agent in dissociative anesthesia. *World J Pharm Res.* 2019;8(4):843–851.
560. Wang R, Shi S, Tan Y, et al. Chemical constituents from *Valeriana jatamansi*. *Biochem Syst Ecol.* 2021;94:104177.
561. Wang S-N, Yao Z-W, Zhao C-B, et al. Discovery and proteomics analysis of effective compounds in *Valeriana jatamansi* jones for the treatment of anxiety. *J Ethnopharmacol.* 2021;265:113452.
562. Vishwakarma S, Goyal R, Gupta V et al. GABAergic effect of valeric acid from *Valeriana wallichii* in amelioration of ICV STZ induced dementia in rats. *Rev Bras Farmacogn.* 2016;26(4):484–489.
563. You JS, Peng M, Shi JL, et al. Evaluation of anxiolytic activity of compound *Valeriana jatamansi* Jones in mice. *BMC Complem Altern M.* 2012;12(1):1–9.
564. Joseph L, Puthallath RE, Rao SN. Acute and chronic toxicity study of *Valeriana wallichii* rhizome hydro-ethanolic extract in Swiss albino mice. *Asian J Med Sci.* 2016;7:13326.
565. Gardner Z, McGuffin M, editors. *Botanical Safety Handbook*, 3rd edition. Boca Raton, FL: CRC Press; 2013. p. 903.
566. Gurley BJ, Gardner SF, Hubbard MA, et al. In vivo effects of goldenseal, kava kava, black cohosh, and valerian on human cytochrome P450 1A2, 2D6, 2E1, and 3A4 phenotypes. *Clin Pharmacol Ther.* 2005;77(5):415–426.
567. Murti K, Kaushik M, Sangwan Y, et al. Pharmacological properties of *Valeriana officinalis*-a review. *Pharmacology.* 2011;3:641–646.
568. Andreatini R, Sartori VA, Seabra ML, et al. Effect of valepotriates (valerian extract) in generalized anxiety disorder: A randomized placebo-controlled pilot study. *Phytother Res.* 2002;16(7):650–654.
569. Pakseresht S, Boostani H, Sayyah M. Extract of valerian root (*Valeriana officinalis* L.) vs. placebo in treatment of obsessive-compulsive disorder: A randomized double-blind study. *J Complement Integr Med.* 2011;8(10)1553.
570. Vorbach EU, Gortelmeyer R, Bruning J. Therapy of insomnia. The efficacy and tolerability of valerian. *Psychopharmakotherapie.* 1996;3:109–115.
571. Leathwood PD, Chauffard F. Aqueous extract of valerian reduces latency to fall asleep in man. *Planta Med.* 1985;51:144–148.
572. Ziegler G, Ploch M, Miettinen-Baumann A, et al. Efficacy and tolerability of valerian extract LI 156 compared with oxazepam in the treatment of non-organic insomnia, a randomized double blind comparative clinical study. *Euro J Med Res.* 2002;7:480–486.
573. Patočka J, Jakl J. Biomedically relevant chemical constituents of *Valeriana officinalis*. *J Appl Biomed.* 2010;8(1):11–18.
574. Cavadas C, Araujo I, Cotrim MD, et al. In vitro study on the interaction of *Valeriana officinalis* L. Extracts and their amino acids on GABAA receptor in rat brain. *Arznei-Forschung.* 1995 Jul 1;45(7):753–755.
575. Khom S, Baburin I, Timin E, et al. Valerenic acid potentiates and inhibits GABAA receptors: Molecular mechanism and subunit specificity. *Neuropharmacology.* 2007;53(1):178–187.

576. Benke D, Barberis A, Kopp S, et al. GABAA receptors as in vivo substrate for the anxiolytic action of valerenic acid, a major constituent of valerian root extracts. *Neuropharmacology*. 2009;56(1):174–181.

577. Blumenthal M, Busse WR, Goldberg A, et al. *The Complete German Commission E Monographs*. Austin, TX: American Botanical Council; 1998. p. 227.

578. Atmojo DD, Wijayahadi N. *Acute Toxicity Test LD50 Value of Valerian (Valeriana Officinalis) in Balb/c Mice*. Doctoral Dissertation, Fakultas Kedokteran Universitas Diponegroro, Semarang, Indonesia; 2009.

579. Van Die MD, Burger HG, Teede HJ, et al. *Vitex agnus-castus* (Chaste-Tree/Berry) in the treatment of menopause-related complaints. *J Altern Complement Med*. 2009;15(8):853–862.

580. Lucks BC, Sørensen J, Veal L. *Vitex agnus-castus* essential oil and menopausal balance: A self-care survey. *Complement Ther Nurs Midwifery*. 2002;8:148–154.

581. Propping D, Bohnert KJ, Peeters M. *Vitex agnus castus*. The treatment of gynaecological syndromes. *Therapeutikon*. 1991;5:581–585.

582. Lauritzen CH, Reuter HD, Repges R, et al. Treatment of premenstrual tension syndrome with *Vitex agnus castus*: Controlled, double-blind study versus pyridoxine. *Phytomedicine*. 1997;4:183–189.

583. Loch EG, Selle H, Boblitz N. Treatment of premenstrual syndrome with a phytopharmaceutical formulation containing *Vitex agnus castus*. *J Womens Health Gend Based Med*. 2000;9:315–320.

584. Berger D, Schaffner W, Schrader E, et al. Efficacy of *Vitex agnus castus* L. extract Ze 440 in patients with pre-menstrual syndrome (PMS). *Arch Gynecol Obstet*. 2000;264:150–153.

585. Schellenberg R. Treatment for the premenstrual syndrome with *Vitex agnus castus* fruit extract: Prospective, randomised, placebo-controlled study. *BMJ*. 2001;322:134–137.

586. Atmaca M, Kumru S, Tezcan E. Fluoxetine versus *Vitex agnus castus* extract in the treatment of premenstrual dysphoric disorder. *Hum Psychopharmacol*. 2003;18:191–195.

587. Momoeda M, Sasaki H, Tagashira E, et al. Efficacy and Safety of *Vitex agnus-castus* extract for treatment of premenstrual syndrome in Japanese patients: A prospective, open-label study. *Adv Ther*. 2014;31(3):362–373.

588. Khalilzadeh E, Saiah GV, Hasannejad H, et al. Antinociceptive effects, acute toxicity and chemical composition of *Vitex agnus-castus* essential oil. *Avicenna J Phytomed*. 2015;5(3):218–230.

589. Abbasi E, Nassiri-Asl M, Shafeei M, et al. Neuroprotective effects of vitexin, a flavonoid, on pentylenetetrazole-induced seizure in rats. *Chem Biol Drug Des*. 2012;80(2):274–278.

590. Jarry H, Spengler B, Porzel A, et al. Evidence for estrogen receptor β-selective activity of *Vitex agnus-castus* and isolated flavones. *Planta medica*. 2003;69(10):945–947.

591. Wuttke W, Gorkow CH, Jarry H. Dopaminergic compounds in Vitex agnus castus. In: *Phytopharmaka in Forschung und klinischer Anwendung*. Heidelberg, GR: Steinkopff; 1995. pp. 81–91.

592. Webster DE, Lu J, Chen SN, et al. Activation of the μ-opiate receptor by *Vitex agnus-castus* methanol extracts: Implication for its use in PMS. *J Ethnopharmacol*. 2006;106(2):216–221.

593. Dericks-Tan JS, Schwinn P, Hildt C. Dose-dependent stimulation of melatonin secretion after administration of Agnus castus. *Exp Clin Endocrinol Diabetes*. 2003;111(01):44–46.

594. Hoffmann D. *Medical Herbalism: The Science and Practice of Herbal Medicine*. Rochester, VT: Healing Arts Press; 2003. p. 596.

595. Khalilzadeh E, Saiah GV, Hasannejad H, et al. Antinociceptive effects, acute toxicity and chemical composition of *Vitex agnus-castus* essential oil. *Avicenna J Phytomed.* 2015;5(3):218–230.

596. Daniele C, Coon JT, Pittler MH, et al. *Vitex agnus castus*: A systematic review of adverse events. *Drug Safety.* 2005;28:319–332.

597. Blumenthal M, Busse WR, Goldberg A, et al. *The Complete German Commission E Monographs.* Austin, TX: American Botanical Council; 1998. p. 108.

598. Gardner Z, McGuffin M, editors. *Botanical Safety Handbook*, 3rd edition. Boca Raton, FL: CRC Press; 2013. p. 923.

599. Mukherjee PK, Banerjee S, Biswas S, et al. *Withania somnifera* (L.) Dunal-Modern perspectives of an ancient *Rasayana* from Ayurveda. *J Ethnopharmacol.* 2021;264:113157.

600. Andrade C, Aswath A, Chaturvedi SK, et al. A double-blind, placebo-controlled evaluation of the anxiolytic efficacy of an ethanolic extract of *Withania somnifera. Indian J Psychiatry.* 2000;42:295–301.

601. Abedon B, Auddy B, Hazra J, et al. A standardized *Withania somnifera* extract significantly reduces stress-related parameters in chronically stressed humans: A double-blind, randomized, placebo-controlled study. *JANA.* 2008;11:50–56.

602. Chandrasekhar K, Kapoor J, Anishetty S. A prospective, randomized double-blind, placebo controlled study of safety and efficacy of a high concentration full-spectrum extract of *Ashwagandha* root in reducing stress and anxiety in adults. *Indian J Psych Med.* 2012;34(3):255–262.

603. Lee I. *Stress & Anxiety Improvements with Ashwagandha and B-vitamins.* Master's Thesis. University of Delaware, Department of Behavioral Health and Nutrition.

604. Langade D, Kanchi S, Salve J, et al. Efficacy and safety of ashwagandha (*Withania somnifera*) root extract in insomnia and anxiety: A double-blind, randomized, placebo-controlled study. *Cureus.* 2019;11(9):e5797.

605. Dhanani T, Shah S, Gajbhiye NA, et al. Effect of extraction methods on yield, phytochemical constituents and antioxidant activity of *Withania somnifera. Arab J Chem.* 2017;10(1):S1193–S1199.

606. Kumar A, Kalonia H. Effect of *Withania somnifera* on sleep-wake cycle in sleep-disturbed rats: Possible GABAergic mechanism. *Indian J Pharm Sci.* 2008;70(6):806–810.

607. Khan ZA, Ghosh AR. Withaferin-A displays enhanced anxiolytic efficacy without tolerance in rats following sub chronic administration. *African J Biotech.* 2011;10(60):12973–12978.

608. Candelario M, Cuellar E, Reyes-Ruiz JM, et al. Direct evidence for GABAergic activity of *Withania somnifera* on mammalian ionotropic GABAA and GABAρ receptors. *J Ethnopharmacol.* 2015;171:264–272.

609. Sonar VP, Fois B, Distinto S, et al. Ferulic acid esters and withanolides: In search of *Withania somnifera* GABAA receptor modulators. *J Nat Prod.* 2019;82(5):1250–1257.

610. Umadevi M, Rajeswari R, Rahale CS, et al. Traditional and medicinal uses of *Withania somnifera. Pharma Innovation.* 2012;1(9, Part A):102.

611. Bhattacharya SK, Muruganandam AV. Adaptogenic activity of *Withania somnifera*: An experimental study using a rat model of chronic stress. *Pharmacol Biochem Behav.* 2003;75(3):547–555.

612. Singh B, Saxena AK, Chandan BK, et al. Adaptogenic activity of a novel, withanolide-free aqueous fraction from the roots of *Withania somnifera* Dun. *Phytother Res.* 2001;15(4):311–318.

613. Sharada AC, Solomon FE, Devi PU. Toxicity of *Withania Somnifera* root extract in rats and mice. *Int J Pharmacog.* 1993;31(3):205–212.

614. Easley T, Horne S. *The Modern Herbal Dispensary.* Berkeley, CA: North Atlantic Books; 2016. p. 178.

615. Gardner Z, McGuffin M, editors. *Botanical Safety Handbook*, 3rd edition. Boca Raton, FL: CRC Press; 2013. p. 274.
616. Savai J, Varghese A, Pandita N, et al. Investigation of CYP3A4 and CYP2D6 interactions of *Withania somnifera* and *Centella asiatica* in human liver microsomes. *Phytotherapy Res.* 2015;29(5):785–790.
617. Ji X, Peng Q, Yuan Y, et al. Isolation, structures and bioactivities of the polysaccharides from jujuba fruit (*Zizyphus jujuba* Mill.): A review. *Food Chem.* 2017;227:349–357.
618. Zou J-S. The control research about sour jujuba soup in the treatment of generalized anxiety disorder. https://en.cnki.com.cn/Article_en/CJFDTotal-ZMYX200616042.html.
619. Cheng G, Bai Y, Zhao Y, et al. Flavonoids from *Zizyphus jujuba* Mill var. spinosa. *Tetrahedron.* 2000;56(45):8915–8920.
620. Han HS, Ma YA, Eun JS, et al. Anxiolytic-like effects of methanol extract of *Zizyphi Spinosi Semen* in mice. *Biomol Ther.* 2007;15(3):175–181.
621. Tabassum S, Misrani A, Tang BL, et al. Jujuboside A prevents sleep loss-induced disturbance of hippocampal neuronal excitability and memory impairment in young APP/PS1 mice. *Sci Rep.* 2019 Mar 14;9(1):1–3.
622. You ZL, Xia Q, Liang FR, et al. Effects on the expression of GABAA receptor subunits by jujuboside a treatment in rat hippocampal neurons. *J Ethnopharmacol.* 2010;128(2):419–423.
623. Zhang M, Ning G, Shou C, et al. Inhibitory effect of jujuboside A on glutamate-mediated excitatory signal pathway in hippocampus. *Planta Medica.* 2003;69(08):692–695.
624. Yang B, Zhang A, Sun H, et al. Metabolomic study of insomnia and intervention effects of *Suanzaoren* decoction using ultra-performance liquid-chromatography/electrospray-ionization synapt high-definition mass spectrometry. *J Pharmaceut Biomed.* 2012;58:113–124.
625. Chen CY, Chen YF, Wu CH, et al. What is the effective component in *suanzaoren* decoction for curing insomnia? Discovery by virtual screening and molecular dynamic simulation. *J Biomol Struct.* 2008;26(1):57–64.
626. Hovaneţ MV, Ancuceanu RV, Dinu M, et al. Toxicity and anti-inflammatory activity of *Zizyphus jujuba* mill. *Leaves Farmacia.* 2016;64(5):802–808.
627. Gardner Z, McGuffin M, editors. *Botanical Safety Handbook*, 3rd edition. Boca Raton, FL: CRC Press; 2013. p. 946.
628. Einerson LS. *A Delphi Study on Herbs Used to Address Depression and Anxiety According to Master Herbalists*. Lubbock: Texas Tech University; 2017.
629. Asadi-Samani M, Bahmani M, Rafieian-Kopaei M. The chemical composition, botanical characteristic and biological activities of *Borago officinalis*: A review. *Asian Pac J Trop Med.* 2014;7:S22–28.
630. Karimi E, Oskoueian E, Karimi A, et al. *Borago officinalis* L. flower: A comprehensive study on bioactive compounds and its health-promoting properties. *J Food Meas Charact.* 2018;12(2):826–838.
631. Komaki A, Rasouli B, Shahidi S. Anxiolytic effect of *Borago officinalis* (Boraginaceae) extract in male rats. *Avicenna J Neuropsychophysiol.* 2015;2(1):34–38.
632. Rabiei Z, Lorigooini Z, Rafieian-Kopaei M. Effects of hydroalcoholic extract of *Borago officinalis* on naloxone-precipitated withdrawal syndrome in morphine-dependent mice. *Bangladesh J Pharmacol.* 2016;11(4):824–829.
633. Khatri S, Yadav S, Sharma V. Importance of γ-linolenic acid in clinical indications. *Int J Ther Appl.* 2012;2:33–42.
634. Khare CP. *Indian Herbal Remedies*. Berlin, Heidelberg: Springer; 2004. pp. 277–295.
635. Wesołowska A, Nikiforuk A, Michalska K, et al. Analgesic and sedative activities of lactucin and some lactucin-like guaianolides in mice. *J Ethnopharmacol.* 2006;107(2):254–258.

636. Harsha SN, Anilakumar KR. Effects of *Lactuca sativa* extract on exploratory behavior pattern, locomotor activity and anxiety in mice. *Asian Pac J Trop Med.* 2012;2(Suppl 1):S475–S479.

637. Kim HW, Suh HJ, Choi HS, et al. Effectiveness of the sleep enhancement by green romaine lettuce (*Lactuca sativa*) in a rodent model. *Biol Pharm Bull.* 2019;42(10):1726–1732.

638. Besharat S, Besharat M, Jabbari A. Wild lettuce (*Lactuca virosa*) toxicity. *Case Reports.* 2009;2009:bcr0620080134.

639. Ahmad H, Sehgal S, Mishra A, et al. *Mimosa pudica* L.(Laajvanti): An overview. *Pharmacogn Rev.* 2012;6(12):115–124.

640. Zhang J, Yuan K, Zhou WL, et al. Studies on the active components and antioxidant activities of the extracts of *Mimosa pudica* Linn. from southern China. *Pharmacog Mag.* 2011;7(25):35–39.

641. Shaikh Z, Roy SP, Patel P, et al. Medicinal value of *Mimosa pudica* as an anxiolytic and antidepressant: A comprehensive review. *World J Pharm Pharm Sci.* 2016;5:420–432.

642. Ayissi Mbomo R, Gartside S, Ngo Bum E, et al. Effect of *Mimosa pudica* (Linn.) extract on anxiety behaviour and GABAergic regulation of 5-HT neuronal activity in the mouse. *J Psychopharmacol.* 2012;26(4):575–583.

643. Aćimović M, Zeremski T, Kiprovski B, et al. *Nepeta cataria*—cultivation, chemical composition and biological activity. *JATEM.* 2021;4(4):620–634.

644. Aydin S, Beis R, Ozturk Y, et al. Nepetalactone: A new opioid analgesic from *Nepeta caesarea* Boiss. *J Pharm Pharmacol.* 1998;50:813–817.

645. Massoco CO, Silva MR, Gorniak SL. Behavioral effects of acute and long-term administration of catnip (*Nepeta cataria*) in mice. *Vet Hum Toxicol.* 1995;37(6):530–533.

646. Rabbani M, Sajjadi SE, Mohammadi A. Evaluation of the anxiolytic effect of *Nepeta persica* Boiss. in mice. *eCAM.* 2008;5(2):181–186.

647. Bernardi MM, Kirsten TB, Salzgeber SA, et al. Antidepressant-like effects of an apolar extract and chow enriched with *Nepeta cataria* (catnip) in mice. *Psych Neurosci.* 2010;3(2):251–258.

648. Hosseini A, Forouzanfar F, Rakhshandeh H. Hypnotic effect of *Nepeta glomerulosa* on pentobarbital-induced sleep in mice. *Jundishapur J Nat Pharm Prod.* 2016;11(1).

649. Russell A, Eaczka EA. Fish poisons from *Ichthyomethia Piscipula*. I. *J Am Chem Soc.* 1944;66(4):548–550.

650. Auxence EG. A pharmacognostic study of *Piscidia Erythrina*. *Econ Bot.* 1953;7:270–284.

651. Ingham JL, Tahara S, Shibaki S, et al. Isoflavonoids from the root bark of *Piscidia erythrina* and a note on the structure of piscidone. *Z Naturforsch.* 1989;44(11–12):905–913.

652. Kapoor AL. *Isolation and Chemistry of the Active Principles of Piscidia Erythrina* L. Doctoral Dissertation, ETH Zurich; 1957.

653. Hamilton W. On the medical properties of the *Piscidia Erythrina*, or Jamaica Dogwood. *London Med Phys J.* 1832;13(75):177–183.

654. Evelyn N. Death with dignity: The role of herbal medicine. *Aust J Herb Med.* 1996;8(2):40–44.

655. Cannon JR, Tapias V, Na HM, et al. A highly reproducible rotenone model of Parkinson's disease. *Neurobiol Dis.* 2009;34(2):279–290.

656. Schütz K, Carle R, Schieber A, *Taraxacum*—A review on its phytochemical and pharmacological profile. *J Ethnopharmacol.* 2006;107(3):313–323.

657. Kunneman BPAM, Albers MRJ. Linden trees (*Tilia* spp.). In: YPS Bajaj (Eds.), *Trees III. Biotechnology in Agriculture and Forestry.* vol 16. Berlin, Heidelberg: Springer; 1991.

658. Kıvrak Ş, Göktürk T, Kıvrak İ. Determination of phenolic composition of *Tilia Tomentosa* flowers using UPLC-ESI-MS/MS. *Int J Second.* 2017;4(3) (Sppl1):249–256.

659. Viola H, Wolfman C, Levi de Stein M, et al. Isolation of pharmacologically active benzodiazepine receptor ligands from *Tilia tomentosa* (*Tiliaceae*). *J Ethnopharmacol.* 1994;44(1):47–53.

660. Noguerón-Merino MC, Jiménez-Ferrer E, Román-Ramos R, et al. Interactions of a standardized flavonoid fraction from *Tilia americana* with Serotoninergic drugs in elevated plus maze. *J Ethnopharmacol.* 2015;164:319–327.

661. Allio A, Calorio C, Franchino C, et al. Bud extracts from *Tilia tomentosa* Moench inhibit hippocampal neuronal firing through GABAA and benzodiazepine receptors activation. *J Ethnopharmacol.* 2015;172:288–296.

7 Chinese Herbal Treatment of Anxiety

In Western medicine, the brain is seen as the source of thought, sensation, and emotion. The mind itself, though mysterious and ill defined, is thought to reside in the brain and to be entirely dependent on brain activity. Thus, psychiatric illness is thought to arise from disturbances in the chemistry of the brain or, in some cases, simply in how we use our brains. Because the brain is made of living neurons, Western medicine understands that the function of those brain cells can also be disturbed by abnormalities in the body such as nutritional or hormonal imbalances, inadequate blood flow, poor oxygenation, inflammation, toxins, or even invasive bacterial or viral infections. But these problems are often seen as having only indirect effects on the mind and brain.

In traditional Chinese medicine, the mind is not thought to be merely the product of the brain. Rather, our thoughts, sensations, and emotions are said to arise from manifestations of *Qi*, a universal energy that circulates throughout the body.[1] In the Chinese view, each organ system in the body uniquely contributes to the quality and characteristics of *qi*. It must be emphasized that Western notions of the internal organs—their anatomy, functions, and relationships to other organs—are quite different from how traditional Chinese medicine conceives of them. In Chinese thought, the organs don't merely digest, absorb, metabolize, transform, and transport substances. Rather, the movement of *Qi* through the organ systems of the body, through pathways called meridians, is thought to lend it special qualities. Five so-called spirits are created by *Qi* in the organs of the body. These are the *Hun, Po, Zhi, Yi*, and *Shen*. These five qualities of *Qi* created by the organs have special importance in psychiatric disorders. Disturbances in emotion, thought, and sensation are thought to be due to disharmonies in the Five Spirits.

Hun is associated with the liver *Qi*. *Hun* is not dependent upon physical being and is thought to continue after death. In some ways, it might be thought of as the soul. From *Hun* comes benevolence, empathy, compassion, and tolerance. Disharmonies of *Hun* may lead to anger, frustration, resentment, unkindness, and feeling "cut off" from the meaning of life. *Po* is associated with lung *Qi*. *Po* animates the body and is responsible for sensations and emotional and physical responses to the environment. From *Po* comes justice and fairness. Disharmonies of *Po* lead to persistent grief, sadness, apathy, or hypersensitivity. *Zhi* is the will, and it derives from kidney *Qi*. *Zhi* gives rise to motivation and self-determination. However, it also is the basis for trust and faith in the unknown. Disharmony of *Zhi* is thought to lead to illogical fears or reckless behaviors. *Yi* is essentially rational thought or intellect. *Yi* is associated with the spleen, and disharmonies give rise to worry and overthinking. *Shen* is associated with the heart *Qi*, and it may be considered

DOI: 10.1201/9781003300281-7

as self-awareness. *Shen* is the mind, where thoughts and feelings are experienced. Disharmonies of *Shen* may lead to edginess, shyness, social awkwardness, or, in extreme cases, agitation and delusions. As yet another layer of complexity, the Five Spirits carry the additional qualities of *yin* and *yang*. *Yin* and *yang* themselves are constellations of complimentary characteristics that include female and male but also many other characteristics such as cold and hot, soft and hard, dark and light, and other pairs of opposites.

The organ systems and the Five Spirits of *Qi* they generate are seen as flowing into one another and affecting the activities of each other. *Hun*, the soul, is thought to control the "comings and goings" of *Shen*, the mind. Deficiency or stagnation of *Hun* thus deflates and limits the activity of the mind, leading to withdrawal, lack of motivation, and lack of enjoyment of life all around. *Yi*, of the spleen, is affected by disharmonies of *Hun*, *Shen*, and *Po*. Disturbances in *Yi* are, in turn, seen as leading to disharmonies of *Po*, *Zhi*, and *Shen*. Thus, the organ systems and the energies they create affect each other in complex circles of interaction and transformation. In traditional Chinese medicine, aberrations of spleen *Qi* are seen as particularly important in anxiety states.[2] However, the circles of interaction among the various energies in the body lead to the understanding that a single set of symptoms—for example, what may be diagnosed as GAD in Western medicine—may arise from quite different patterns of disharmony from the Chinese perspective.[3]

Among the various Chinese diagnoses that might be given the same Western diagnoses of GAD are:

Spleen *Qi* deficiency
Heart *yin*/blood deficiency
Heart fire
Liver *Qi* stagnation
Liver fire
Liver *yin*/blood deficiency
Liver *yang* rising
Lung *Qi* deficiency
Kidney *yin* deficiency
Kidney-heart disharmony
Kidney *yin* failing to nourish heart *yin*
Heart fire failing to nourish kidney *yang*

What Western medicine sees as a specific psychiatric disorder is never seen by traditional Chinese medicine as a single illness to be treated by a specific treatment. Rather, the treatments may be quite different depending upon which of many types of disharmonies among the Five Spirits are found by the diagnostic techniques of Chinese medicine to be responsible for the signs and symptoms of the presenting illness. Thus, what would be seen as a single, specific illness by Western psychiatry—for example, GAD or major depression—might be treated in many different ways in different individuals or circumstances.

7.1 TRADITIONAL CHINESE TREATMENTS OF ANXIETY

In treating a patient with an anxiety disorder, Western psychiatrists might not only prescribe medication but also treat contributory medical conditions, such as low thyroid levels, vitamin deficiencies, or sleep apnea. They are likely to recommend psychotherapy, seeking spiritual peace, improvements in diet, getting more exercise, and establishing regular sleeping habits. Chinese physicians have a similarly wide range of treatments to address disorders. Among the treatment modalities of traditional Chinese medicine are acupuncture, cupping, herbs, massage, movement and concentration exercises such as tai chi and *Qi-gong*, improvement of diet, and spiritual exercises. Although quite different from one another in how they are applied to the body, the goal of each of these modalities of Chinese medicine is the same—that is, to restore the proper flow and quality of *Qi* through the organs systems and bring the body back into balance.[4]

In their classic English-language treatise, *Chinese Herbal Medicine: Formulas and Strategies*, Scheid et al. explain the underlying philosophy beneath all approaches to treating anxiety and other disorders of "Spirit." They write,

> Like all other disorders in Chinese medicine, those of the spirit can be sorted into two types, deficiency and excess. Here, these refer both to the branch (manifestations) and to the root. Manifestations of deficiency include palpitations with anxiety, forgetfulness, disorientation, and insomnia. Generally, such patterns are due to deficiency or constraint of *Qi* or blood, preventing the expression of the spirit and thereby causing it to become agitated. The method of treating this type of disorder is tonify and harmonize the *Qi* and blood. Manifestations of excess include a feeling of being overstressed, manic behavior, bad temper, and agitation. Such patterns are due to excess heat uncontrolled *yang*, blood stagnation, phlegm, and severe *Qi* stagnation. The strategy for treating this type of disturbance is to sedate and calm the spirit.[5]

7.2 HERBAL TREATMENT IN TRADITIONAL CHINESE MEDICINE

A cornerstone of traditional Chinese medicine is the use of herbs. The herbal remedies of Chinese medicine are thousands of years old. The processes of discovery of the thousands of medical herbs are lost to antiquity. In Western herbal medicine, the so-called Doctrine of Signatures guided herbalists in choosing herbs for use in treatment of specific ailments. By that doctrine, if the leaf of a plant was kidney shaped, it was thought likely to help in treatment of urinary conditions. If the leaves were heart shaped, the herb might be tried in treatment of heart conditions. A far more complicated and elaborate system of relationships guided the ancient Chinese herbalists. In the larger philosophical view of the Chinese, all things were seen as arising from the Five Elements: fire, earth, metal, water, and wood. Each of the Five Elements had unique qualities and relationships to the organs and Five Spirits, as well as to emotion, taste, color, season, direction, and even weather. Thus, the physical characteristics of plants, such as flavor, size, color, the environment in which it grows, the season of the year in which the plant thrives, the temperature, and the region in which the plant grows all tie the herb to the Five Elements and their corresponding organ systems and manifestations of Qi. These ties with specific organs then allowed the essences of the herbs to flow through the corresponding energy meridians of the body and resolve imbalances in Qi.[6]

An important characteristic of traditional Chinese medicine is that most of the ancient Chinese treatments of anxiety, depression, and other conditions are combinations of herbs. Indeed, in traditional Chinese medical theory, every herb in a Chinese medicine formula is essential and plays its own necessary role. This is defined according to the principle of *jun chen zuo shi*, or "monarch, minister, assistant and envoy."[7] The Chinese herbalists long recognized that one herb in a combination, the "monarch," may provide the primary benefits. However, others in the combination are necessary to prepare the body, block adverse effects, improve general health, or regulate activity in pathways that supply or receive Qi from the system primarily targeted. This philosophy is quite at odds with mainstream Western medicine in which the ideal treatment is a single, potent medication that solves the problem with as few collateral effects as possible. Indeed, the use of combinations of herbs might be seen as a form of the much maligned "polypharmacy." Yet, in many respects, the *jun chen zuo shi* approach is quite insightful. Problematic side effects, such as weight gain, sexual dysfunction, nausea, or disturbed sleep, can be addressed. This leads to more successful treatment.

Each of the various Chinese diagnoses that might present like a specific Western anxiety disorder—perhaps GAD—require their own combination of herbs as treatment as determined by Chinese diagnostic methods. Most of the ancient herbal formulas to treat symptoms consistent with anxiety have not been proven in clinical trials. Nonetheless, some of the classical combinations, or at least variations of those formulas, have been tested clinically, and some are discussed in the following. In reviewing these remedies, it should be noted that the terms *san*, *wan*, and *tang* that frequently appear refer to powder, pill, and tea or soup.

The position of this book is that the effects of herbs of traditional Chinese medicine, either alone or in combination, are manifested through actions of their constituent phytochemicals upon known physiological systems of the brain and body. Thus, there is every reason to assume that these herbs can be effective in contexts entirely divorced from Chinese medicine. Many recent research papers out of China concerning psychiatric effects of herbal medicines include not only discussions of Qi; *yin* and *yang*; and heart, spleen, or kidney meridians but also discussions of effects on neuronal activity, neurotransmitters, cell signaling systems, cytokines, and other physiological processes that form the basis of the modern Western understanding of brain processes and neuropharmacology. Nonetheless, this position is not at odds with the likelihood that the underlying philosophy, nosology, and diagnostics methods of traditional Chinese medicine have generated means to select effective herbal treatments of specific psychiatric conditions.

7.2.1 *BAI ZI YANG XIN TANG* WITH *SHU GAN NING SHEN SAN*

Bai zi yang xin tang, translated as "arborvitae seed to nourish the heart," is an ancient formula intended to treat symptoms of palpitations, chronic anxiety, insomnia, memory loss, and recurring nightmares. Classically, it is thought to act by nourishing heart blood, cooling the blood, strengthening heart *yin*, and calming the *Shen*. Its ingredients include *semen Platycladus orientalis* (arborvitae), *Poria cocos sclerotium*, *radix Astragalus membranaceous*, *Ligusticum wallichii*, *radix Angelica sinensis*, *rhizoma Pinellia ternata*, *radix Codonopsis pilosula*, *radix Polygala tenuifolia*, *cortex Cinnamomum cassia*, *radix Glycyrrhizae inflata*, *semen Zizyphus jujuba*, and *Schisandra chinensis*. It is not uncommon for one or more herbs to be added to address special conditions of anxiety by calming the liver or strengthening the kidney. *Shu gan ning shen san* is a formula almost identical to *bai zi yang xin tang*, but with the addition of the herbs *Prunella vulgaris* and *Eleutherococcus gracilistylus*.

In a Chinese study, *bai zi yang xin tang* was combined with *shu gan ning shen san* in the treatment of patients diagnosed with GAD.[8] Patients received either the *bai zi yang xin* and *shu gan ning shen san* combination or the Western prescription antidepressant medication escitalopram. Data were gathered using the Hamilton Anxiety Rating Scale, and by the end of the study, those who received the herbal combination were significantly more improved than those who received the escitalopram. Over the following months, the recurrence of anxiety among those treated with the herbal remedies was also significantly less likely than in those who received the Western antidepressant.

7.2.2 *BAN XIA HOU PU*

Ban xia hou pu is an ancient herbal formula composed of *rhizoma Pinellia ternata*, *cortex Magnoliae officinalis*, *fructus Citri sarcodactylis*, *Poria cocos*, *Perilla frutescens*, and *Zingiber officinale*. It has been employed for hundreds of years by practitioners of traditional Chinese medicine in the treatment of various psychiatric disorders, including major depression, anxiety, and even schizophrenia.

A classical syndrome of severe anxiety is a panicked feeling of a "lump in the throat" when, in fact, there is nothing there. In traditional Chinese medicine, this malady is called "imagined plum pit in the throat." In Western medicine, this complaint has long been known as globus hystericus, and it is often treated with benzodiazepines. In a Chinese study, the effects of *ban xia hou pu* were tested on patients experiencing persistent globus hystericus over the previous 12 months.[9] *Ban xia hou pu* was given three times a day for 3 weeks, and its effects were compared with those of the Chinese herbal formula *man yan shu ning*, or "Granules for clearing the throat." Along with the relief from the globus hystericus, the degrees of anxiety and depression of the patients were also measured. The *ban xia hou pu* formula not only resolved the symptoms of globus hystericus in most of the patients but also significantly reduced the severity of both anxiety and depression.

In another study, *ban xia hou pu* was evaluated for the treatment of persistent indigestion secondary to anxiety.[10] After 4 weeks of daily treatment, *ban xia hou pu* improved indigestion more effectively than domperidone, a standard treatment of Western medicine. In addition, the herbal combination significantly reduced both anxiety and symptoms of depression as measured by the Hamilton Anxiety Rating Scale and Hamilton Depression Rating Scale, respectively.

7.2.3 BAO SHEN

Bao shen decoction is a formula often used to treat kidney ailments. However, in traditional Chinese medicine, deficiency of kidney *Qi* may be a cause of anxiety and worry. *Bu shen yang xue wan* and *suan zao ren tang* are examples of treatments that both nourish the kidney and relieve anxiety. *Bao shen* is described as containing *radix Salvia miltiorrhiza, radix Codonopsis pilosula, radix Polygala tenuifolia, Amomum cardamomum, Poria cocos*, ground oyster shell, peel of *Citri reticulatae*, dried immature *fructus Citrus aurantium, herba Lycopi hirti, Crataegus pinnatifida, semen Zizyphus jujuba, semen Psoralea corylifolia*, and *semen Perillae argutae*.

In a Chinese study, patients diagnosed with GAD were given either *bao shen* decoction three times a day or a daily dose of 20 to 40mg of the Western antidepressant medicine paroxetine once daily for 6 weeks.[11] Paroxetine is commonly used by Western doctors to treat both major depression and GAD. The effects of the two treatments were evaluated by the Hamilton Anxiety Rating Scale and Hamilton Depression Rating Scale. The effectiveness of the *bao shen* decoction, with a response rate of 88%, was equal to that of paroxetine, which had a response rate of 92%. Fewer side effects were noted among the patients receiving *bao shen* versus paroxetine, with rates of 14% and 64%, respectively. Unlike the herbal treatment, one of the most common side effects of antidepressants like paroxetine is sexual dysfunction.

7.2.4 GENG NI AN CHUN

Geng ni an chun is a traditional Chinese medicine composed of 11 herbs: *radix Rehmannia glutinosa, rhizoma Coptis chinensis, radix Paeonia alba, Anemarrhena asphodeloides, Cistanche salsa, radix Morinda officinalis, Poria cocos, Epimedium brevicornum, cortex Phellodendron chinense, fructus Lycium barbarum*, and *semen Cuscuta chinensis*. It also contains the unusual ingredient of tortoise shell. These ingredients can be difficult to find but may be available individually or in the prepared combination in large cities at Chinese herbal pharmacies.

In a randomized, placebo-controlled study, postmenopausal women suffering symptoms as measured by the standard Kupperman Index were treated with *geng ni an chun* for 12 weeks.[12] The herbal formula reduced hot flashes as well as significantly reduced scores on both the Hamilton Depression Rating Scale and Hamilton Anxiety Rating Scale. Surprisingly, no differences were noted in sleep quality. The authors noted that there were no adverse effects.

7.2.5 GUI PI TANG

Gui pi tang is likely the herbal combination most commonly used in traditional Chinese medicine for the treatment of anxiety and insomnia. The name is roughly translated as "restore the spleen decoction," and it is a formula often recommended to help treat heart and spleen deficiency. References to this formula date back at least 500 years. The principal ingredients of *gui pi tang* are *Panax ginseng, Astragalus radix, Atractylodes rhizomes*, and *Glycyrrhiza glabra*. The "helper" components include *Dimocarpus longan* (dried fruit), *Angelica sinensis, Poria cocos, Polygala tenuifolia, Saussurea lappa, Zingiber officinale,* and *Zizyphus jujuba* (fruit and seed). Scheid et al. include the dried root of *Aucklandia lappa* in the formula and note that *radix Codonopsis pilosula* is often substituted for *Panax ginseng.* They further note that the formula is often used for treatment of anxiety, phobias, forgetfulness, palpitations, insomnia, nightmares, and feverishness.[13]

There is little in the Western literature to establish efficacy for *gui pi tang* in the treatment of anxiety. A doctoral dissertation from China has reviewed the use of *gui pi tang* in insomnia and described studies showing its effectiveness.[14] Certainly, many treatments that help insomnia also help reduce anxiety, often acting by the same mechanisms.

7.2.6 *Jiu wei zhen xin*

The herbal combination *jiu wei zhen xin* has long been used in traditional Chinese medicine as a treatment for what Western medicine would diagnose as GAD. This ancient formula contains nine herbs: *Panax ginseng, semen Zizyphus jujuba, Schisandra chinensis, Poria cocos,* root of *Polygala tenuifolia, Corydalis yanhusuo tuber, radix Asparagus cochinchinensis, radix Rehmannia glutinosa,* and *Cinnamomum cassia.*

Jiu wei zhen xin appears to be one of the most thoroughly studied herbal treatments of anxiety. Whereas many combinations may have one or two reports of clinical effectiveness, there are perhaps a dozen of more reports of successful treatment of anxiety with this formula. A review of 14 such studies has recently been published. The conclusion of the authors of that review was that *jiu wei zhen xin* is a safe and effective treatment of GAD. While not quite as effective as SSRI antidepressants, it is far more tolerable and causes fewer adverse side effects. The herbal combination was also seen as at least as effective as azapirones—an example being buspirone—that are commonly prescribed in Western medicine as treatment for GAD.[15]

7.2.7 *Kami-shoyo-san* and *Hange-koboku-to*

While not a formal study, a Japanese group has reported four cases using two herbal combinations, *kami-shoyo-san* and *hange-koboku-to,* to treat previously unresponsive anxiety and panic disorder.[16] In all four cases, the diagnoses were made by psychiatrists according to criteria in the American Psychiatric Association's *Diagnostic and Statistical Manual.* Both of the herbal combinations are prescribed by practitioners of *Kampo,* the traditional Japanese school of medicine. However, they each contain herbs commonly used in traditional Chinese medicine formulas. *Kami-shoyo-san* contains *radix Bupleurum chinense, radix Paeonia lactiflora, Atractylodes lancea, radix Angelica sinensis, Poria cocos, fructus Gardenia jasminoides, cortex Paeonia suffruticosa, radix Glycyrrhiza uralensis, Zingiber officinale,* and *Mentha haplocalyx. Hange-koboku-to* consists of *rhizoma Pinellia ternate, Poria cocos, cortex Magnolia officinalis,* and *Zingiber officinale.*

In the first case, a woman had suffered panic disorder with agoraphobia for years despite treatment with benzodiazepines. She had reached the point where she could not leave the house alone. *Hange-koboku-to* had been ineffective, and instead *kami shoyo san* was added to her Western tranquilizers. After 8 weeks of daily treatment, the panic attacks disappeared and did not return. Another woman suffered panic disorder for 10 years despite conventional Western therapy, which included benzodiazepines and antidepressants. The daily addition of *kami-shoyo-san* to her Western medicines over 10 weeks reduced the attacks of fear, palpitation, dizziness, trembling, sweating, and nausea by 90%. After stopping the *kami-shoyo-san* therapy, the panic attacks returned, and the combination was readministered with good effect.

In another case, a woman had developed panic attacks with choking, shortness of breath, palpitation, nausea, and numbness of the fingers, with secondary anticipatory anxiety and agoraphobia. In her case, *kami-shoyo-san* therapy for 4 weeks failed to improve her attacks. However, her symptoms abated after 12 weeks of treatment with *hange-koboku-to*. Another successful use of *hange-koboku-to* involved a 45-year-old woman who had suffered panic disorder with agoraphobia for 7 years, despite treatment with Western benzodiazepines. In that case, the *kami-shoyo-san* had failed to relieve the panic attacks, consisting of palpitation, shortness of breath, numbness, sweating, and fear of dying. *Hange-koboku-to* was then added to the benzodiazepine, and after 2 weeks, the panic attacks disappeared. When the herbal combination was stopped, the panic returned. The combination was restarted, and the woman went an additional 2 years without symptoms.

7.2.8 RIKKUNSHINTO

Western medicine recognizes the role that anxiety and emotional disturbance can play in producing physical symptoms. Some illness, such as high blood pressure, irritable bowel disease, and various digestive disorders, are often caused or exacerbated by anxiety and other psychiatric issues. The branch of Western medicine that addresses these relationships is often referred to as psychosomatic medicine. However, Eastern approaches to healing have long recognized this relationship and do not so clearly distinguish emotional, mental, and physical presentations. Japanese *Kampo* physicians used the herbal treatment *rikkunshinto* to treat dyspepsia—that is, severe and persistent indigestion—in the context of chronic anxiety. *Rikkunshinto* is an herbal remedy frequently prescribed in *Kampo* medicine. It consists of eight herbs commonly used in traditional Chinese medicine: *radix Glycyrrhiza uralensis*, *Zingiber officinale*, *rhizoma Atractylodis lanceae*, *Zizyphus jujuba*, aged *Citri reticulatae Pericarpium*, *Panax ginseng*, *rhizoma Pinelliae ternata*, and *Poria cocos*.

Patients diagnosed with dyspepsia, anxiety, and depression were treated with *rikkunshinto* twice daily for 8 weeks. At the end of the study, those who received the herbal combination had significant improvement both in their dyspepsia and in symptoms of anxiety in comparison with those who received placebo capsules. The significant decreases in symptoms of anxiety were measured by the Hamilton Depression Rating Scale and Hamilton Anxiety Rating Scale.[17]

7.2.9 SHEN QI WU WEI ZI

Examinations can cause a great deal of anxiety for college students. A study evaluated the anxiolytic effects of the herbal combination *shen qi wu wei zi* on students preparing to take college entrance examinations.[18] *Shen qi wu wei zi* is an ancient combination thought to strengthen *Qi*, invigorate the spleen, nourish the Heart, and calm the *shen*. The combination is usually composed of *radix Codonopsis pilosula*, an adaptogenic herb native to Asia; *radix Astragalus membranaceous*; and *Schisandra chinensis*. In some cases, the combination may include *Kadsura longipedunculata* and *Zizyphus jujuba*, a common ingredient in combinations intended to calm the mind. It was found that administration of the combination three times a day over 6 weeks significantly reduced anxiety as measured by the Hamilton Anxiety Rating Scale, Clinical Global Impression test, and Self-Rating Anxiety Scale. It was as effective as treatment with 0.5mg of the Western anxiolytic medication alprazolam three times a day over the same period of time. My experience tells me this was a significant dosing of alprazolam, perhaps better known as Xanax. The effects of the alprazolam, which can be almost immediate, appeared much sooner than those of *shen qi wu wei zi*. The anxiolytic effects of the herbal combination were apparent after 2 weeks of treatment. An interesting study showed that no adverse effects were seen in mice treated with a dose 200 times the standard human dose of that combination.

7.2.10 *Shen Song Yang Xin*

Shen song yang xin is a traditional Chinese herbal formula composed of *Panax ginseng*, *Ophiopogonis japonicus radix*, *Cornus mas*, *radix Salvia miltiorrhiza*, *Zizyphus jujuba*, *Taxillus chinensis*, *Paeoniae radix rubra*, the dried body of the female *Eupolyphaga sinensis* beetle, *Nardostachys jatamansi*, *Coptis chinensis*, *fructus Schisandra chinensis*, and fossilized bone. The combination, unusual by Western standards, is thought to tonify *Qi*, nourish *yin*, and promote blood circulation to remove meridian obstruction to clear away heart fire and calm the mind.

A study compared the combined treatment of *shen song yang xin* plus electroacupuncture against 0.4 to 1.6mg a day of the Western drug alprazolam.[19] After 6 weeks, the herb and electroacupuncture treatment was equally effective as alprazolam as measured by the Hamilton Anxiety Rating Scale. Of course, it is not possible to determine to what degree the herbs, versus the acupuncture, contributed to the anxiolytic effect.

7.2.11 *Suan Zao Ren Tang* in Combination with *Zhi Zi Chi Tang*

Suan zao ren tang and *zhi zi chi tang* have been used separately to treat anxiety and insomnia for centuries. They were first documented by Zhong-jing Zhang in approximately 210 CE in the classic Chinese text *Synopsis of Prescriptions of the Golden Chamber*. *Suan zao ren* refers specifically to the seed of *Zizyphus jujuba*. When the seed alone is used, it is sometimes referred to as *Zizyphus spinosa* or *semen Zizyphus jujuba*. However, *suan zao ren*, as the monarch in the combination, gives a commonly used herbal formula its name, *suan zao ren tang*. This formula is often a blend of five medicinal Chinese herbs: *Zizyphus jujuba*, *Poria cocos*, *rhizoma Ligusticum chuanxiong*, *Anemarrhena asphodeloides*, and *radix Glycyrrhiza uralensis*. *Zhi zi chi tang* is a combination of *Gardenia jasminoides* and fermented soybeans. According to classic theory, *suan zao ren tang* is beneficial for the replenishment of liver *yin* and kidney *yin*, while *zhi zi chi tang* aids in eliminating internal fire.

In one study, *suan zao ren tang* was modified by adding *Gardenia jasminoides*, fermented soybean, and ground shell of the cicada insect. The modified *suan zao ren tang* was given to patients who were also being given the Western drug paroxetine for treatment of GAD. Paroxetine itself can relieve symptoms of anxiety, but its effect rarely begins before 3 or 4 weeks of treatment. The purpose of the study was to see if the herbal formula could hasten the anxiolytic effect of the paroxetine. Indeed, it was found that addition of the herbal combination to paroxetine gave relief from anxiety 2 weeks earlier than paroxetine alone. After 4 weeks of treatment, 90% of patients getting both the herbs and paroxetine experienced significant relief from anxiety whereas only 74% of those receiving paroxetine alone achieved relief. In fact, the study also showed that the herbal treatment was as effective as adding the Western drug diazepam to the paroxetine. Results were analyzed by the standard Hamilton Anxiety Rating Scale and Self-Rating Anxiety Scale.[20]

In another evaluation, the same modified *suan zao ren tang* formula, described as "*suan zao ren tang* in combination with *zhi zi chi tang*," was used to treat insomnia secondary to GAD, and its effects were compared against those of 0.5mg of the standard Western anxiolytic benzodiazepine drug lorazepam. After 4 weeks of twice daily treatment, the herbal formula was found to be significantly more effective than the lorazepam in improving sleep, per the Insomnia Severity Index; improving the quality of sleep, per the Pittsburgh Sleep Quality Index; improving sleep architecture, per polysomnography; and reducing anxiety, per the Self-Rating Anxiety Scale.[21] Other studies have shown that the anxiolytic and sleep-inducing effects of *suan zao ren tang* are due in part to stimulation of GABA receptors in the brain.[22]

7.2.12 WEN DAN TANG

Wen dan tang, also called warm gallbladder decoction, is one of the classical Chinese herb formulas for psychiatric illnesses. It has even been used for severe illnesses such as schizophrenia. It is an ancient remedy, first recorded about 1,500 years ago in *Yao's Collection of Effective Prescriptions*. In that writing, it was considered as a remedy to "dry dampness and transform phlegm." According to Scheid et al.,[23] the indications for using *wen dan* include dizziness, vertigo, insomnia, sleep disturbed by strange dreams, palpitations, and anxiety. However, they also include symptoms such as nausea or vomiting, gnawing hunger, and bitter taste in the mouth. Unlike many other formulas that are directed toward balancing the heart, spleen, liver, and kidney, the purpose of *wen dan* is to restore harmony between the gallbladder and stomach. This is indicative of the wide range of disharmonies that the Chinese see as leading to symptoms of anxiety.

The *wen dan* formula consists of *rhizoma Pinellia ternate*, *Bambusae caulis*, dried unripe *Citrus aurantium*, *Poria cocos*, *Zingiber officinale*, *Ziziphus jujuba*, and *radix Glycyrrhiza uralensis*. *Wen dan tang* is a time-honored formulation available premade in many outlets, including the internet.

There are few clinical trials of *wen dan tang*, and in one study, the formula was evaluated in patients suffering the lung disease COPD, exacerbated by anxiety and depression. In this study, all patients were given the inhaled steroid budesonide over 4 weeks. One group also received the *wen dan tang* herbal combination over that time. In the group that also received *wen dan tang*, the anxiety and depression scores, as measured by the Hamilton Anxiety Rating Scale and Hamilton Depression Rating Scale, were significantly reduced from baseline and even in comparison to those who had their respiratory symptoms relieved by the steroid.[24]

7.2.13 XIAO YAO SAN

Xiao yao san is a well-known traditional Chinese medicine formula that has been most frequently used to treat depression. Clinical trials have established the antidepressant effect of the herbal formulation. In fact, *xiao yao* is translated into the charming English name, "free and easy wanderer." According to tradition, it acts by unblocking and soothing the liver, strengthening the spleen, and nourishing the blood. The herbs contained in *xiao yao san* are *Poria cocos, radix Paeonia alba, radix Glycyrrhiza uralensis, radix Bupleurum chinense, radix Angelica sinensis, Atractylodis macrocephalae, Mentha haplocalyx,* and *Zingiber officinale.* It is one of the Chinese herbal formulas that is premade and available for purchase in many outlets.

A study showed that 6 weeks of treatment with *xiao yao san* relieved anxiety and insomnia in patients suffering what was referred to as insomnia due to persistent psychological stress. This treatment significantly reduced scores on the Self-Rating Anxiety Scale and appeared to enhance the anxiolytic effects of the Western drug estazolam.[25] Other reports have confirmed that *xiao yao* can help relieve insomnia.[26]

7.2.14 XIN WEI TANG

Xin wei tang is a traditional Chinese herbal formula consisting of *radix Bupleurum chinense, Trichosanthes kirilowii,* and *Lilium brownii.* These are common ingredients in Chinese herbal formulas, but among them only *Lilium brownii* has been clinically tested and found to have anxiolytic effects on its own. There is at least one clinical study of *xin wei tang* in regard to anxiety and depression.[27] In this case, its effects were evaluated in patients suffering dyspepsia—that is, persistent indigestion—thought to be secondary to the emotional disturbance. The subjects of the study received daily treatments of either the standard Western medication domperidone, the *xin wei tang* combination, or simply placebo over 8 weeks. Before and after treatment, all subjects were evaluated with the Hamilton Depression Rating Scale and Hamilton Anxiety Rating Scale. Surprisingly, the *xin wei tang* formula was more effective than domperidone in relieving the dyspepsia. The herbal combination also significantly relieved symptoms of anxiety and depression, with substantial relief being reported by 70% of patients.

7.2.15 YANG XIN TANG

Yang xin tang is an ancient herbal formula to "nourish the heart." The formula blends multiple herbs, including *radix Astragalus membranaceous, Panax ginseng,*

Poria cocos, Angelica sinensis, Ligusticum chuanxiong, Zizyphus jujuba, semen Platycladus orientalis, Schisandra chinensis, radix Zingiber officinale, Zizyphus jujuba, Citri reticulatae pericarpium, rhizoma Pinellia ternata, Polygala tenuifolia, radix Glycyrrhiza uralensis, and *Cinnamomum cassia.* In modern Chinese herbal medicine, this formula is often used to treat heart conditions, including anginal pain cause by poor blood flow in the heart muscle. However, traditional Chinese medicine sees an influence of heart *Qi* upon states of anxiety, with symptoms arising from what has been called heart *yin*/blood deficiency, heart fire, kidney-heart disharmony, kidney *yin* failing to nourish heart *yin*, and heart fire failing to nourish kidney *yang.* Regardless of the theoretical foundation for using this formula, there are many phyto-chemicals, such as flavonoids, terpenes, and steroid-like molecules, contained in the constituent herbs that very well might affect brain activity thought to mediate anxiety.

In a study of the anxiolytic effects of *yang xin tang,* patients diagnosed with GAD were given a strong tea made from the herbal combination twice a day for 6 weeks, and the effects of the treatment were compared against the effects of daily treat-ment with the Western drug, Deaxit.[28] Deanxit, while no longer used in Western medicine, is itself a combination of an antipsychotic tranquilizer and antidepressant. The response rates to the two treatments, measured by reductions in scores in the Hamilton Anxiety Rating Scale and Hamilton Depression Rating Scale, were 89% for *yang xin tang* and 91% for Deanxit. Sleep was also reported to be significantly improved in each group.

7.2.16 *YI GAN SAN*

Chinese herbal medicines were first introduced into Japan around the 5th century. Japan embraced the Chinese use of herbal medicine and further developed it as the traditional healing practice of *Kampo.* There have been studies performed in Japan of the effects of the traditional Chinese herbal formula *yi gan san* (known in Japan as *yokukansan*) on anxiety states in the elderly with dementia and in young, emotionally disturbed patients. *Yi gan san* contains the herbs *rhizoma Atractylodes lancea, Poria cocos, rhizoma Cnidii monnieri, Uncaria sinensis, radix Angelica sinensis, radix Bupleurum chinense,* and *radix Glycyrrhiza uralensis,* all of which are common ingredients in Chinese herbal treatments of anxiety and other emotional disorders.

In one such study, *yi gan san* was tested for benefits in reducing anxiety and agi-tation in elderly patients diagnosed with Alzheimer's dementia.[29] Patients received daily doses of the herbal combination over 4 weeks. Emotional states, including lev-els of anxiety, were assessed with the standard Neuropsychiatric Inventory. At the end of treatment, *yi gan san* was found to significantly improve anxiety, irritability, depression, and mood lability, as well as delusions, hallucinations, agitation, and aggression. No serious adverse reactions were observed.

In a similar evaluation of *yi gan san* in elderly patients with Alzheimer's dementia, the herbal combination improved Neuropsychiatric Inventory scores for delusions, hallucinations, agitation/aggression, anxiety, and irritability/lability.[30] Evaluation using the Pittsburgh Sleep Quality Index also revealed increases in total sleep time, sleep efficiency, stage 2 sleep, and decreases in the number of arousals and periodic limb movements. Subjective sleep quality was also improved. Interestingly, scores remained unchanged in the Mini-Mental Status Exam, a standard test of cognitive function. No adverse effects of the herbal treatment were observed.

Yi gan san was also found to be effective in a very different population of patients: young women diagnosed with borderline personality disorder. Borderline personality disorder causes severe instability in mood, interpersonal relationships, self-image, and behavior. The condition is notoriously difficult to treat, and there are no specific medications in Western psychiatry to apply to the condition. Female patients diagnosed with borderline personality disorder, according to criteria in the American Psychiatric Association's *DSM-IV*, received 12 weeks of daily dosage of 2.5 to 7.5g of *yi gan san*. Data were gathered using the Brief Psychiatric Rating Scale, Hamilton Depression Rating Scale, Global Assessment of Functioning, Clinical Global Impression scale, and Aggression Questionnaire. At the end of treatment, there were significant improvements in anxiety, tension, depressive mood, hostility, suspiciousness, motor retardation, uncooperativeness, and excitement subscale.[31]

7.2.17 *YI QI YANG XIN*

The Chinese herbal combination *yi qi yang xin* is one of many intended to "relieve heat, strengthen the spleen and tonify blood, clear away the heat-evil and phlegm, and promote the circulation of blood to remove blood stasis."[32] It has thus been seen as useful as a means of addressing syndromal anxiety.[33,34]

The *yi qi yang xin* combination consists of *Panax quinquefolius, Panax ginseng, Scutellaria baicalensis, radix Asparagus cochinchinensis, Lilium brownii, fructus Schisandra chinensis, radix Salvia miltiorrhiza, Panax notoginseng, rhizoma Acorus calamus, radix Polygala tenuifolia, Gardenia jasminoides*, fermented soybean, amber, and *Zizyphus spinosa*. This combination is available ready-made in Chinese markets and on the internet.

In one study, patients diagnosed with GAD were randomized into an active control group treated with paroxetine titrated to 20 to 60mg per day or a group treated with the *yi qi yang xin* herbal combination in twice daily dosing of 10g. Members of each group also underwent cognitive behavioral therapy every 2 weeks for the 6 months of treatment. Hamilton Anxiety Rating Scale and Zung Self-Rating Anxiety Scale scores were obtained at baseline and after 3 months and 6 months of treatment. The same tests were also administered 6 months after treatment was discontinued. After 3 and 6 months of treatment, both groups exhibited significant improvement in Hamilton Anxiety Rating Scale and Zung Self-Rating Anxiety Scale scores. The benefits of the paroxetine and cognitive behavioral therapy did not differ from those obtained by the group that received *yi qi yang xin* plus cognitive behavioral therapy. Improvements persisted in both groups 6 months after treatments were withdrawn. However, the rate of recurrence of symptoms of anxiety were significantly higher among members of the paroxetine control group.[35]

7.2.18 *YUKGUNJA* AND *BANHABAKCHULCHUNMA* DECOCTIONS

A report from Korea, a country that has shared the knowledge of traditional Chinese medicine, has described the use of the herbal treatment *yukgunja* decoction in one patient and *banhabakchulchunma* decoction in another for the treatment of anxiety in the context of gastrointestinal symptoms.[36] This situation is not uncommon, with patients complaining that anxiety worsens their gastrointestinal symptoms that in turn make their anxiety worse. Sometimes it is difficult to determine which condition comes first. Although this was not a complete study, these two patients were formally diagnosed as suffering GAD according to criteria in the *DSM-V* diagnostic manual, and changes in symptoms were monitored using a standard method—that is, the Beck Anxiety Inventory. Both patients received acupuncture. One received three daily dosings of the *yukgunja* combination consisting of *Pinellia ternate*, *Atractylodes macrocephala*, *Citri reticulatae pericarpium*, *Poria cocos*, *Panax ginseng*, *radix Glycyrrhiza uralensis*, *Zingiber officinale*, and *Zizyphus jujuba*. The other patient received three daily dosings of *banhabakchulchunma* decoction consisting of *Pinellia ternate*, dried *Citri reticulatae pericarpium*, germinated *Hordeum vulgare*, *radix Atractylodes macrocephala*, *Panax ginseng*, *radix Astragalus membranaceous*, *rhizoma Gastrodia elata*, *Poria cocos*, *rhizoma Alisma orientalis*, *Zingiber officinale*, *cortex Phellodendron chinense*, and *Zizyphus jujuba*. The formula also contains *Massa Medicata Fermentata*, which requires some explanation. *Massa Medicata Fermentata* is a product composed of wheat flour, wheat bran, rice bean powder, and bitter apricot seed powder, all of which is added to the water extract of the herbs *Artemisia vulgaris*, *Persicaria hydropiper*, and *Xanthium strumarium*. The resulting dough-like substance is then allowed to ferment. Some of the benefits of *Massa Medicata Fermentata* may be to restore healthy gut bacteria. Indeed, recent Western studies suggest that chronic use of probiotics can reduce symptoms of GAD. Neither of the patients in the Korean report had responded to Western medications prescribed by their Korean doctors. However, by the end of treatment, each patient had substantial relief from anxiety and was completely free of gastrointestinal symptoms.

7.3 TRADITIONAL BUT UNTESTED ANXIOLYTIC CHINESE HERBAL FORMULAS

Along with the formulas discussed prior that have been evaluated for use as treatment for GAD, many traditional Chinese herbal formulas used to treat various manifestations of anxiety, irritability, "hysteria," and insomnia have not been clinically tested. There is a class of formulas in traditional Chinese medicine known as *zhen jing ji*, or sedative formulas. In their English-language book, *Commonly Used Chinese Herbal Formulas*, Hsu and Hsu discuss some such formulas.[37]

Gan cao tang is simply *radix Glycyrrhiza glabra*, or licorice root. *Glycyrrhiza glabra* is a constituent of most of these sedating formulas. Another formula, simple in containing only three ingredients, is *gan mai da zao tang*. It consists of *radix Glycyrrhiza glabra*, *fructus Zizyphus jujuba*, and *fructus Triticum aestivum*, or common wheat berries. *Yi gan san jia chen pi ban xia* contains *Uncaria sinensis*, *radix Bupleurum chinense*, *radix Angelica sinensis*, *rhizoma Cnidium monnieri*, *Poria cocos*, *rhizoma Atractylodis macrocephalae*, *radix Glycyrrhiza glabra*, *Citrus* peel, and *Pinellia ternata* tuber. Beyond that, the formulas tend to contain variations of the same, with some minor addition and deletions. One of the more complicated formulas, *chai hu jia long gu mu li tang*, includes *radix Bupleurum chinense*, *Poria cocos*, and *Pinellia ternata* but also *radix Scutellariae baicalensis*, *Cinnamomum aromaticum*, *Zingiber officinale*, *rhizoma Rheum officinale*, *radix Panax ginseng*, and *fructus Zizyphus jujuba*. There are others in the class somewhat similar to *chai hu jia long gu mu li tang*. *Gui zhi jia long gu mu li tang* contains *Cinnamomum aromaticum*, *fructus Zizyphus jujuba*, *Zingiber officinale*, *radix Glycyrrhiza glabra*, and the addition of *radix Paeoniae Alba*. *Gui zhi qu shao yao jia shu qi long gu mu li tang* consists of *Cinnamomum aromaticum*, *Zingiber officinale*, *Glycyrrhiza glabra*, *fructus Zizyphus jujuba*, and *Dichroa febrifuga*. Of note, one sedative formula consists only of fossilized bone and oyster shell and is thus a rich source of calcium. Those two ingredients are often added to other sedative formulas.

In *Chinese Herbal Medicine: Formulas and Strategies*, Scheid et al. discuss other such remedies in the chapter "Formulas That Nourish the Heart (Blood and Yin) and Calm the Spirit."[38] *Tian wang bu xin dan*, or "Emperor of Heaven's Special Pill to Tonify the Heart," consists of *radix Rehmannia Glutinosa*, *radix Panax ginseng*, *radix Asparagus cochinchinensis*, *radix Ophiopogon japonicus*, *radix Scrophularia ningpoensis*, *radix Salvia miltiorrhizae*, *Poria cocos*, *radix Polygala tenuifolia*, *radix Angelica sinensis*, *fructus Schisandrae chinensis*, *semen et radix Platycladus orientalis*, *Zizyphus spinosae*, and cinnabar. It is recommended that the latter, a mineral rich in mercury, not be included. This formula is an elaboration of *yang xin tang*, or "Nourish the Heart Decoction," that is included in the chapter by Scheid et al., but also discussed prior among those formulas that have been clinically tested.

Ding zhi wan, or "Settle the Emotions Pill," consists of *radix Panax ginseng*, *Poria cocos*, *rhizoma Acorus tatarinowii*, and *radix Polygala tenuifolia*. It is intended to improve deficiency of heart *Qi*. Scheid et al. noted the indications to include, "feeling apprehensive, easily frightened, worried, disheartened, or incessant laughter or glee, together with fright, palpitations and forgetfulness." They also note several variations of *ding zhi wan*, with a substitution or two in recognition of contribution from an excess or deficiency in an organ system.

Another somewhat unique combination discussed by Scheid et al. is *long chi qing hun san*, or "Dragon Tooth Powder to Clear the Ethereal Soul." The indications seem more severe than others and suggest mania as a component. These include palpitations, restlessness, and laughing and crying uncontrollably. This formula includes fossilized mastodon tooth, from which it derives its name, and likely its calcium. Aside from that, the combination consists of *Poria cocos*, *radix Polygala tenuifolia*, *radix Panax ginseng*, *radix Angelica sinensis*, *radix Ophiopogon japonicus*, *cortex Cinnamomum aromaticum*, *radix Glycyrrhiza glabra*, *rhizoma Corydalis yanhuso*, and *radix et rhizoma Asarum sieboldii*.

Miao xiang san, or "Marvelously Fragrant Powder," consists of *radix Panax ginseng*, *rhizoma Dioscorea polystachya*, *radix Astragalus membranaceus*, *Poria cocos*, *radix Polygala tenuifolia*, *radix Aucklandia lappa*, *radix Platycladus orientalis*, and *radix Glycyrrhiza glabra*. It also contains dried musk gland of *Moschus moschiferus* and cinnabar, which should not be used due to its mercury content. It is considered useful for severe restlessness arising from a general deficiency of *Qi*.

The formula *jiao tai wan*, or "Grand Communication Pill," consists simply of *cortex Cinnamomum aromaticum* and *rhizoma Coptis chinensis*. It is intended to resolve Disharmony between the Heart and Kidneys, and its indications are irritability, restlessness, palpitations, and insomnia.

An unusual formula contains iron filings and cinnabar, as well as some less often used herbs. For example, the combination includes *Arisaema heterophyllum* mixed with the bile of ox. There are indications this herb may be toxic, and perhaps the bile tempers it in some way. In any case, it is suggested that it be used only under the guidance of an expert. It further contains *bulbus Fritillariae cirrhosae, radix Scrophularia ningpoensis, radix Asparagus cochinchinensis, radix Ophiopogon japonicus, fructus Forsythia suspensa, Uncaria rhynchophylla, radix Salvia miltiorrhizae, Poria cocos, pericarpus Citrus reticulata, rhizoma Acorus tatarinowii,* and *radix Polygala tenuifolia.* Among the indications for this formula are restlessness, agitation, bad temper, emotional instability, mania, shouting at people for no reason, headache, and insomnia.

For a flavor of the range of ingredients that may go into some traditional Chinese formulas, it is also worth noting *zhen zhu mu wan,* or "Mother of Pearl Pill." The indications for this formula are irritability, restless sleep, anxiety, palpitations, and dizziness. This formula includes ground conch shell, fossilized mastodon tooth, powdered water buffalo horn, *radix Angelica sinensis, radix Rehmannia glutinosa, radix Panax ginseng, Zizyphus spinosae, radix Platycladus orientalis, Poria cocos,* and *Aquilaria agallocha.*

7.4   THE MAINSTAYS OF CHINESE HERBAL TREATMENTS

The complexities of traditional Chinese medicine cannot be explained in a few pages of a book. It certainly cannot be given the dignity and respect it deserves in a few paragraphs. It must also be noted that it is an ancient, deep, and holistic approach to health that cannot be separated from general health, diet, lifestyle, or even society itself. Perhaps most important is that diagnosis in traditional Chinese medicine is not based merely on symptoms, as is often the case in Western medicine. Diagnoses arise from identification of specific patterns of deficits or overabundance of energy, or *Qi*, as it flows throughout the body. The outward manifestation of illness is less important than the underlying weakness of liver *Qi*, poor flow of energy from heart to spleen, or any of a number of other imbalances that may simply manifest as anxiety. Each of these imbalances may receive a different diagnosis and require different treatment.

Given that there are so many different underlying conditions that can present as anxiety, one might suspect that there would be an equal number of different combinations of herbs used to address each specific type of problem. To some extent this is true. A review of herbal treatments used by practitioners of traditional Chinese and Korean medicine to treat anxiety was recently published by Chan-Young Kwon in the Department of Korean Medicine at the Kyung Hee University in Seoul.[39] Kwon wrote that in the hundreds of papers he reviewed, 138 different herbs were mentioned as being used in the treatment of the varieties of conditions that Western psychiatrists would simply refer to as GAD. One or another herb would be added to a standard formula to address some specific deficit, blockage, or overabundance of *Qi* in a meridian or organ system in the body. With the addition or subtraction of a few herbs, the names of classical formulas are changed, making it appear that entirely different formulas are being used. Nonetheless, despite the seemingly wide variety of herbs that are at times used, Kwon noted that there were only a dozen or so herbs that formed the foundation of herbal treatment of anxiety. Those same herbs tend to appear in various combinations regardless of the specific problem with *Qi* that is determined by Chinese diagnostic techniques.

The herbs most commonly used by Chinese and Korean medical herbalists to treat what Western psychiatrists might categorize as GAD are—in order of frequency of use—*Poria cocos, Glycyrrhiza uralensis, Zizyphus jujuba, Bupleurum chinense, Paeonia lactiflora, Polygala tenuifolia, Angelicae gigantis, Curcuma wenyujin, Pinellia ternata, Schisandra chinensis,* and *Cnidium officinale.* Other herbs that often appear in combinations to treat anxiety, though somewhat less frequently, include *Acorus gramineus, Coptis chinensis, Albizia julibrissin, Polygonum multiflorum, Rehmannia glutinosa, Polyrachis* ants (yes, ants, the insects), *Ganoderma lucidum, Panax ginseng,* and *Cynomorium songaricum.*

Several of these individual herbs have been evaluated in human clinical studies and are discussed in Chapter 6. However, most of these herbs have not been so evaluated. In the following are discussions of existing animal data showing evidence of anxiolytic-like effects of those herbs, as well as consideration of bioactivities of some of their constituent phytochemicals.

7.4.1 *ACORUS GRAMINEUS*

The dry rhizome of *Acorus gramineus* is listed officially in the *Chinese Pharmacopoeia* and has been used in oriental medicines for hundreds of years primarily to treat neurological disorders. The herb is thought to protect from excitotoxic neuronal death and to ameliorate learning and memory deficits. Indeed, it is stated that among 75 of the most famous Chinese herbal formulas characterized as improving intelligence, more than half contain *Acorus gramineus.*[40]

It must be noted that the volatile oil of *Acorus gramineus* contains high concentrations of β-asarone and α-asarone.[41] Both alpha and beta asarones have anxiolytic and antidepressant effects in laboratory animals. Unfortunately, the asarones have also been shown capable of inducing liver toxicity, including hepatomas and hepatic carcinogenicity.[42] Use of the related species *Acorus calamus* has been banned by the FDA for use in the United States.

7.4.2 *ALBIZZIA JULIBRISSIN*

The bark of *Albizia julibrissin* has been used in traditional Chinese and Persian schools of herbal medicine to improve mood and treat insomnia. Modern studies have tended to confirm antidepressant- and anxiolytic-like effects.[43] An aqueous extract of *Albizia julibrissin* produced an anxiolytic-like effect in rats in the elevated plus maze. This effect was abolished by pretreatment with pindolol, a beta-adrenergic and 5-HT1A/1B receptor antagonist.[44] In another study, administration of julibroside C1, a saponin-containing compound isolated from *Albizzia julibrissin,* had an anxiolytic-like effect in mice in the elevated plus maze. The anxiolytic-like effect was attenuated by flumazenil, as well as by the 5-HT1A antagonist WAY-100635 and the GABA antagonist bicuculline.[45]

7.4.3 ANGELICAE GIGANTIS

Angelicae gigantis, also known as *Angelica sinensis* or *dong quai*, has been used for thousands of years in traditional Chinese, Korean, and Japanese medicines. It was first discussed in the classical text *Shennong Bencao Jing* from 200–300 CE. It is predominantly known for its use in the treatment of a wide variety of gynecological conditions and is sometimes referred to as "female ginseng."[46]

The essential oil of *Angelicae gigantis* showed anxiolytic activity in mice in the elevated plus maze.[47] A methylenechloride extraction of the herb enhanced pentobarbital-induced sleep, and that effect was reversed by flumazenil.[48] The plant's chemical constituents include phytosterols, polysaccharides, ligustilide, butylphthalide, cnidilide, isoenidilide, p-cymene, ferulate, and various flavonoids.[49] In the study of the methylenechloride extraction noted prior, the specific phytochemical constituents of *Angelicae gigantis*, ligustilide and butylidenephthalide, were each shown to enhance pentobarbital-induced sleep in rats by GABAergic mechanisms. Oral administration of decursinol angelate, a coumarin derivative extracted from *Angelicae gigantis*, was shown to augment pentobarbital-induced sleeping behaviors in rats through enhancement of GABA-A-ergic systems. Treatment increased both density of GABA-A receptors and expression of glutamic acid decarboxylase, the enzyme that synthesizes GABA from glutamate.[50]

7.4.4 BUPLEURUM CHINENSE

Radix Bupleuri chinense has been used as a traditional medicine for more than 2,000 years in China, Japan, Korea, and other Asian countries. It is referred to as *chaihu* in Chinese and is derived from the dried roots of *Bupleurum chinense* and *Bupleurum scorzonerifolium*. *Bupleurum chinense* itself has not been evaluated for anxiolytic effects. However, anxiolytic effects were seen in chronically stressed rodents in the elevated plus maze after treatment with extract of the related species *Bupleurum falcatum*. Treatment with the extract also blocked increase in tyrosine hydroxylase expression in the locus coeruleus of treated rats that experienced chronic stress. It was thus suggested that the anxiolytic effects were mediated in part by buffering central adrenergic activity.[51] A decoction of *Bupleurum chinense* and *Scutellaria baicalensis* conveyed anxiolytic-like effects in chronically stress rats in the open box paradigm, and these effects were accompanied by increases of GABA concentration in the hippocampus.[52]

More than 74 different phytochemicals have been identified in *Bupleurum chinense*, including essential oils, triterpenoid saponins, polyacetylenes, flavonoids, lignans, fatty acids, and sterols. Among those phytochemicals are the volatiles hexanal, furan-2-carbaldehyde, and heptanal; a variety of steroid-like triterpenoid saikosaponins; and flavonoids and flavonoid glycosides quercetin, isorhamnetin, isorhamnetin-3-O-glucoside, puerarin, rutin, narcissin, eugenin, saikochrome A, saikochromic acid, 7,4'-dihydroxy-isoflavone-7-O-β-D-glucoside, saikochromoside A (50), and saikoisoflavonoside A.[53] As discussed in a previous chapter, quercetin has been found to exert anxiolytic-like effects in rodents. Rutin, a glycoside of quercetin, is found in bupleurum and also shows anxiolytic effects in rats. Interestingly, these effects were not affected by flumazenil and only partially reversed by picrotoxin, suggesting some involvement of GABA-A receptors through a non-benzodiazepine mechanism.[54] Puerarin, the 8-C-glucoside of the isoflavone daidzein, also has anxiolytic-like effects in several anxiety paradigms. It attenuated the anxiety-like behavior induced either by alcohol withdrawal or administration of benzodiazepine inverse agonists.[55] In another study, puerarin's anxiolytic-like effects in mice were accompanied by increases of allopregnanolone and serotonin in the prefrontal cortex and hippocampus.[56]

Total saikosaponins extracted from *Bupleurum yinchowense* produced antidepressant-like and anxiolytic effects in mice that were accompanied by increases in synaptic proteins expression and attributed to induction of α-amino-3-hydroxy-5-methyl-4-isoxazolepropionic acid receptor (AMPA) and subsequent enhancement of the mammalian target of rapamycin (mTOR) signaling pathway.[57]

7.4.5 CNIDIUM OFFICINALE

Cnidium officinale is a flowering plant widely cultivated in China, Korea, and Japan. The herb is often used to attenuate pain and increase stamina. It is also known to have anti-inflammatory effects.[58] *Cnidium officinale* contains active phthalides, including butylidenephthalide, ligustilide, cnidilide, and senkyunolide. Butylidenephthalide and ligustilide are also found in *Angelica sinensis*. As noted prior, those substances each enhance pentobarbital-induced sleep through flumazenil-reversible mechanisms. Ligustilide, cnidilide, and senkyunolide were each found to have muscle-relaxant effects in rats thought to be central in action.[59]

7.4.6 COPTIS CHINENSIS

Coptis chinensis is another of the 50 fundamental herbs used in traditional Chinese medicine. The herb is notable for containing isoquinoline alkaloids, including berberine, coptisine, palmatine, epiberberine, and jatrorrhizine, that are thought responsible for its most important medicinal properties.[60] It also contains significant quantities of phenolic compounds and flavonoids.

The herb itself has not been evaluated for anxiolytic effects in humans or animals. However, at least one of its constituent alkaloids has been tested. Berberine increased time spent in the open arms of the elevated plus maze. These anxiolytic-like effects were accompanied by decreased serotonergic system activity via activation of somatodendritic 5-HT1A autoreceptors and inhibition of postsynaptic 5-HT1A and 5-HT2 receptors.[61]

In another study, jatrorrhizine isolated from a methanol extract of *Coptis chinensis* was shown to inhibit MAO-A and MAO-B from rat brain mitochondria with the IC50 values of 4 and 62μM, respectively.[62] Thus, it is likely that *Coptis chinensis* could contribute to anxiolytic effects of combinations of Chinese herbs by modulating monoaminergic activity that might synergize with enhancement of GABAergic activity.

7.4.7 CURCUMA WENYUJIN

In traditional Chinese medicine, *Curcuma wenyujin* is "cold-natured" and acts upon liver, heart, and lung energies to treat mental or gastrointestinal symptoms caused by "dampness-heat of liver and gallbladder." The herb is often included in combinations used to treat major depression and anxiety.[63] The medicinal properties of the herb are attributed to its sesquiterpenes, diarylheptanoids, and diarylpentanoids.[64] Curcumin is a diarylheptanoid contained in *Curcuma wenyujin*, and it has been found to exert anxiolytic effects in both humans and rodents on its own. Although *Curcuma wenyujin* itself has not been tested for anxiolytic effects in humans or animals, it shares many of the same phytochemical constituents with the closely related species *Curcuma longa*, which has been so tested, albeit with mixed results. For further details, see the section on *Curcuma longa* in Chapter 6.

7.4.8 CYNOMORIUM SONGARICUM

Cynomorium songaricum is a medicinal and food plant of North Africa, Europe, and Asia. It has been widely used in folk medicines to treat sexual dysfunction of various kinds as well as digestive complaints.[65] The are no studies of anxiolytic effects of *Cynomorium songaricum* in humans or animals. However, investigations into the phytochemical components of the herb show it to contain substances known to exert anxiolytic effects by various mechanisms. Among these anxiolytic phytochemicals— some of which are discussed in Chapter 5—are luteolin-7-O-glucoside, naringenin, epicatechin-3-O-gallate, rutin, isoquercetin, ursolic acid, β-sitosterol, campesterol, and other flavonoids, terpenoids, steroids and phenolic compounds.[66] Extracts of *Cynomorium songaricum* decrease uptake of GABA and serotonin in cultured hamster ovary cells, suggesting possible anxiolytic effects mediated by those two systems.[67]

7.4.9 GANODERMA LUCIDUM

Ganoderma lucidum, commonly known as the *reishi* fungus, is one of the few herbs in this group to have undergone human trials for evaluation of anxiolytic effects. Although none of the participants in those trials suffered any formal anxiety disorder, tests revealed decreases in feelings of anxiety and improvement in sense of well-being. It appears to act through enhancement of GABAergic activity and anti-inflammatory effects. See Chapter 6.

7.4.10 GLYCYRRHIZA URALENSIS

Glycyrrhiza uralensis, also known as Chinese licorice, is a flowering plant native to Asia. It is considered to be one of the 50 fundamental herbs used in traditional Chinese medicine.[68] It has several relatives, including *Glycyrrhiza glabra*, that are used for medicinal and confectionary purposes. Extract of *Glycyrrhiza glabra*, a close relative of *Glycyrrhiza uralensis* with a similar range of constituent phytochemicals, has anxiolytic-like effects in mice in the elevated plus maze test.[69] The extract of *radix Glycyrrhiza uralensis* is rich in saponins, flavonoids, isoflavones, coumarins, and stilbenoids.[70] Among its phytochemical constituents are glycyrrhizin, liquiritic acid, liquiritin, isoliquiritin, isotrifoliol, glisoflavanone, glabridin, galbrene, glabrone, shinpterocarpin, licoisoflavones A and B, formononetin, glyzarin, kumatakenin, liqcoumarin, glabrocoumarones, herniarin, umbelliferon, and dihydrostilbenes.

Several phytochemicals in species of *Glycyrrhiza* have been found to exert anxiolytic-like effects in laboratory animals. Herniarin, a derivative of coumarin, showed anxiolytic-like effects in rats in the open-box test, as well as antidepressant like-effects in the forced swim test.[71] A similar substance, umbelliferone, produced an antidepressant-like effect in a mouse model of PTSD.[72] Formononetin, an isoflavone in *Glycyrrhiza* species, produced an anxiolytic effect in mice through the inhibition of NMDA receptors and regulation of cAMP response element-binding protein, as well as anti-inflammatory actions.[73] The flavonoid glabridin from *Glycyrrhiza uralensis* potentiates GABA-A receptor evoked current. It acts through a flumazenil-insensitive mechanism.[74]

7.4.11 PAEONIA LACTIFLORA

Paeonia lactiflora is a species of perennial flowering plant in the family *Paeoniaceae*, native to central and eastern Asia from eastern Tibet across northern China to eastern Siberia. The roots of two peony species, *Paeonia lactiflora* and *Paeonia veitchii*, are often referred to as rubra (red) or alba (white). *Radix Paeonia rubra* is the dried root of *Paeonia lactiflora* or *Paeonia veitchii*, most often found in the wild. *Radix Paeonia alba* is the dried root of *Paeonia lactiflora* but after boiling and peeling and before drying. The herb has been used in Chinese medicine to treat menstrual disorders, pain, skin conditions, and inflammation.[75] Among the flavonoids and glycosides isolated from the herb are peonidin 3,5-di-O-glucoside, kaempferol di-hexoside, quercetin-3-O-galactoside, luteolin-7-O-glucoside, and isorhamnetin-3-O-glucoside.[76] Some of the constituent flavonoids have been found to exert anxiolytic effects and are noted in Chapter 5. A variety of monoterpenes and triterpenes have also been isolated from the roots of *Paeonia* species.[77]

In a somewhat tenuous rat model of premenstrual dysphoric disorder, sub-chronic treatment with extract of *Paeonia lactiflora* reduced anxiety-like behavior of female rats in the open field test. That effect was associated with increases in estrogen receptor β and tryptophan hydroxylase-2 but decreases in density of serotonin transporters.[78]

One of the herb's principal components, paeoniflorin, was found to exert an anxiolytic-like effect in a rat model of PTSD. Those effects were associated with modulation of the hypothalamic-pituitary-adrenal axis and 5-HT system activation.[79] Paeoniflorin is also seen as neuroprotective, and it offered antidepressant-like effects in rat model of poststroke depression. Ostensibly, this was largely due to potent anti-inflammatory effects.[80]

7.4.12 PANAX GINSENG

Panax ginseng is another of the herbs in this group to have undergone human trials for evaluation of anxiolytic effects. Although none of the participants in those trials suffered any formal anxiety disorder, tests revealed improvement in mood and increased relaxation, which would suggest a decrease in anxiety. It appears to act through enhancement of GABAergic activity and as an adaptogen. Though ginseng may be useful to enhance general health and well-being, it does not seem to be a strong or reliable treatment for significant anxiety on its own. It might best be added to more effective treatments to help build resiliency and restore health. See Chapter 6.

7.4.13 PINELLIA TERNATA

Pinellia ternata is one of the most commonly used herbs in traditional Chinese medical science. It contains a variety of phytochemicals including phenylpropanoids,[81] phytosterols,[82] and purine alkaloids, thought to be synthesized by endophytic bacteria.[83] One study evaluated the effects of an ethanolic extract of *Pinellia ternata* on pentobarbital-induced sleeping and nikethamide-induced convulsions. The extract enhanced sleep and ameliorated convulsions. Each effect was reversed by flumazenil, suggesting mediation by benzodiazepine receptors.[84]

Many phenylpropanoids, such as are found in *Pinellia ternata*, exert anxiolytic effects in rodents.[85] Some of the phytosterol components of *Pinellia ternata*—for example, β-sitosterol—also have anxiolytic-like effects in rodents.[86] Finally, there is evidence that the purines uniquely abundant in *Pinellia ternata* may play a role in any anxiolytic effects of the herb.[87]

7.4.14 POLYGALA TENUIFOLIA

Polygala tenuifolia is one of the 50 fundamental herbs used in traditional Chinese medicine and is frequently used in combinations to treat anxiety. Various species of *Polygala* have been used to treat wounds, inflammation, and cardiovascular and central nervous system disorders. Phytochemical studies showed that they contain triterpene saponins, triterpenes, terpenoids, xanthones, flavonoids, coumarins, oligosaccharide esters, styryl-pyrones, benzophenones, and polysaccharides.[88] There are no published studies of anxiolytic effects of *Polygala tenuifolia* in humans. However, there are several studies demonstrating anxiolytic effects of the herb and its components in laboratory animals.

The daily administration of extract of *Polygala tenuifolia* to chronically stressed mice increased open-arm exploration in an elevated plus maze and the total number of line crossings in an open field test. These anxiolytic-like effects were accompanied by normalization of central noradrenergic system, upregulation of BDNF expression in the hippocampus, and buffering of serum corticosterone levels.[89] In another study, acute administration of aqueous extract of *Polygala tenuifolia* produced anxiolytic effects in mice in the elevated plus maze and hole board apparatus. These effects were blocked by the 5-HT1A receptor antagonist WAY-100635 but not by flumazenil.[90]

Several specific components of *Polygala tenuifolia* have also been found to exert anxiolytic-like effects in rodents. Acute administration of steroid-like saponins extracted from the root of the herb produced an anxiolytic-like effect in mice.[91] The phenylpropanoid 3,4,5-trimethoxycinnamic acid, from the roots of *Polygala tenuifolia*, both prolongs hexobarbital-induced sleeping time and ameliorates cold-induced stress response in mice. These effects are often associated with sedative and anxiolytic effects.[92] The aerial parts of *Polygala tenuifolia* contain a variety of anxiolytic flavonoids, including isorhamnetin, kaempferol, and quercetin.[93]

7.4.15 POLYGONUM MULTIFLORUM

Polygonum multiflorum is a vine-like herb commonly used in traditional Chinese medicine and officially listed in the *Chinese Pharmacopoeia*. Various parts of the plants have been used for medicinal purposes. The leaves, tubers, and rhizomes have been used as tonic and anti-aging agents. The stems have been used to alleviate insomnia and treat diabetes.[94] The herb is also being evaluated for use in treating Alzheimer's disease.[95] Reports have shown that *Polygonum multiflorum* contains a variety of potentially psychoactive phytochemicals, such as anthraquinones, naphthalenes, stilbenoids, flavonoids, phenylpropanoids, phenolic acids, and dianthrones.[96] Of note, the long-term use of *Polygonum multiflorum* may lead to liver and kidney toxicity.[97]

There are no human clinical studies of anxiolytic effects of *Polygonum multiflorum*. However, it is worth noting that in a study from Taiwan, *Polygonum multiflorum* was found to be the most commonly prescribed single Chinese herb for treatment of insomnia.[98]

There are also no published studies of anxiolytic-like effects of *Polygonum multiflorum* in laboratory animals. However, some of its specific phytochemical constituents, including steroid-like substances such as β-sitosterol; stilbenoids such as resveratrol; and the flavonoids rutin, luteolin, quercetin, kaempferol, apigenin, hyperoside, and vitexin,[99] have been found to possess anxiolytic-like activities. See Chapter 5.

7.4.16 PORIA COCOS

Poria cocos is perhaps the most common ingredient in the herbal combinations used to treat anxiety in traditional Chinese medicine. It has been evaluated in human trials in subjects diagnosed with GAD and was found to be effective in relieving anxiety. It was also found effective in treating distressing symptoms of menopause that included anxiety. It appears to act by a variety of mechanisms, including GABAergic enhancement, buffering of glutamatergic activity, serotonergic effects, anti-inflammatory action, and action as an adaptogen. See Chapter 6.

7.4.17 REHMANNIA GLUTINOSA

Rehmannia glutinosa is a time-honored herb in China. It was described in Shennong's herbal treatise, which is considered one of the oldest texts of Chinese herbal medicine. More than 70 chemical components have been separated and identified from extracts of *Rehmannia glutinosa*. It is especially rich in iridoids and saccharides, along with phenol glycosides and flavonoids.[100]

In a rat model of menopause, 5 weeks of treatment with extract of *Rehmannia glutinosa* showed anxiolytic-like effects in the open field and elevated plus maze tests. These effects were accompanied by normalizations of levels of serotonin, dopamine, glutamate, and GABA throughout the brain.[101] The herb also produced antidepressant-like effects in chronically stressed rats, apparently through elevating diminished levels of monoamines, increasing brain concentrations of BDNF, and dampening levels of the stress hormone corticosterone. These effects have also been associated with anxiolytic effects.[102]

Extracts of *Rehmannia glutinosa* have also been shown to exert anticonvulsant effects. Two of its components, the iridoid catalpol and the sugar alcohol mannitol, were found to produce both anticonvulsant and anxiolytic-like effects in mice. Those effects were attributed to enhancement of GABAergic activity.[103]

7.4.18 SCHISANDRA CHINENSIS

Schisandra chinensis has long been used in traditional Chinese medicine to "calm and quiet the spirit." It is also among the herbs commonly recommended by members of the American Herbalists Guild to treat anxiety. In one study, treatment with a combination of extract of the herb, polyunsaturated fatty acids, and vitamin D3 significantly improved confidence and reduced measurements of anxiety and stress in athletes during training. It contains flavonoids known to enhance GABAergic activity.

Unlike many other phytochemicals, the sedative effects of schisandrins extracted from the herb are apparently not due to enhancement of GABA activity. Rather, the effects are due to increasing serotonin activity in the brain. Extracts of *Schisandra chinensis* have also been reported to have adaptogenic effects. See Chapter 6.

7.4.19 ZIZYPHUS JUJUBA

In traditional Chinese medicine, *Zizyphus jujuba* is one of the most commonly used herbs for treatment of anxiety. When using the seed, it is often referred to as *Zizyphus spinosa*. When using the fruit, it is sometimes referred to as *Zizyphus fructus*. The literature contains only one reference to a controlled clinical study of *Zizyphus jujuba* in patients diagnosed with GAD. See Chapter 6. It significantly reduced anxiety as revealed by use of the Hamilton Anxiety Rating Scale, a standard method of assessment of anxiety. Phytochemicals in *Zizyphus jujuba* enhance activity at GABA-A receptors and dampen glutamatergic activity.

REFERENCES

1. Maciocia G. *The Foundations of Chinese Medicine*. London, UK: Elsevier; 2005. pp. 342–345.
2. Chung YK, Chen J, Ko KM. Spleen function and anxiety in Chinese medicine: A western medicine perspective. *Chin Med*. 2016;7:110–110.
3. Tseng W. The development of psychiatric concepts in traditional Chinese medicine. *Arch Gen Psychiatry*. 1973;29(4):569–575.

4. Aung SKH, Fay H, Hobbs RF. Traditional Chinese medicine as a basis for treating psychiatric disorders: A review of theory with illustrative cases. *Med Acupunct.* 2013;25(6):398–406.

5. Scheid V, Bensky D, Ellis A, Barolet R. *Chinese Herbal Medicine: Formulas & Strategies.* Seattle, WA: Eastland Press; 2009. p. 457.

6. Lao L, Xu L, Xu S. Traditional Chinese Medicine. In: Längler A, Mansky PJ, Seifert G. (Eds), *Integrative Pediatric Oncology.* Berlin, GR: Springer; 2012. pp. 125–135.

7. Zhang E, Shen J, So FK. Chinese traditional medicine and adult neurogenesis in the hippocampus. *J Trad Complement Med.* 2014;4(2):77 81.

8. Chen LSL. Clinical study of *Baizi yangxin* decoction combined with *Shugan ningshen* powder in treating patients with generalized anxiety disorder. *Chin J Exp Tradit Med Formul.* 2014;20(22):200–203.

9. Ping BO. Clinical observations on 46 cases of globus hystericus treated with modified *Banxia Houpu* decoction. *J Tradit Chin Med.* 2010;30(2):103–107.

10. Xiao L, Li Y. Randomized controlled trial of modified *banxia houpo* decoction in treating functional dyspepsia patients with psychological factors. *Chin J Integr Tradit West Med.* 2013;33(3):298–302.

11. Zang H, Zhang H, Wang L. A clinical control study of *baoshen* decoction on treatment of general anxiety disorder. *Liaoning J Tradit Chin Med.* 2007;34(7):951–952.

12. Zhang Y, Cao Y, Wang L. The effects of a new, improved Chinese medicine, *Gengnianchun* formula granules, on hot flushes, depression, anxiety, and sleep in Chinese peri- and postmenopausal women: A randomized placebo-controlled trial. *Menopause.* 2020;27(8):899–905.

13. Scheid V, Bensky D, Ellis A, et al. *Chinese Herbal Medicine: Formulas & Strategies.* Seattle, WA: Eastland Press; 2009. pp. 353–355.

14. Teoh ZY. *Research on Observation and Literature of Gui Pi Tang Treating Insomnia.* Masters Thesis, INTI International University; 2015.

15. Wang S, Zhao L, Qiu X, et al. Efficacy and safety of a formulated herbal granula, *Jiu Wei Zhen Xin,* for generalized anxiety disorder: A meta-analysis. *eCAM.* 2018; Article ID 9090181.

16. Mantani N, Hisanaga A, Kogure T, et al. Four cases of panic disorder successfully treated with *Kampo* (Japanese herbal) medicines: *kami-shoyo-san* and *hange-koboku-to. Psychiat Clin Neurosci.* 2002;56(6):617–620.

17. Tominaga K, Sakata Y, Kusunoki H, et al. *Rikkunshito* simultaneously improves dyspepsia correlated with anxiety in patients with functional dyspepsia: A randomized clinical trial (the DREAM study). *Neurogastroenterol Motil.* 2018;30:e13319.

18. Xiao ZC, Yu XH. Clinical observation on *Shenqi Wuweizi* tablet for anxiety before college entrance examination a report of 113 cases. *J Tradit Chin Med.* 2010;51(2):136–138.

19. Li LB, Sun JG, Shi JF, et al. Clinical analysis of *sensongyangxin* capsule combined with electroacupuncture for anxiety disorder a report of 35 cases. *App J Gen Prac.* 2007;5(12):1073–1074.

20. Song M-F, Hu LL, Liu WJ, et al. Modified *Suanzaorentang* had the treatment effect for generalized anxiety disorder for the first 4 weeks of paroxetine medication: A pragmatic randomized controlled study. *eCAM.* 2017: Article ID 8391637.

21. Hu L-L, Zhang X, Liu WJ, et al. *Suan zao ren tang* in combination with *zhi zi chi tang* as a treatment protocol for insomniacs with anxiety: A randomized parallel-controlled trial. *eCAM.* 2015;2015:7.

22. Yi P-L, Tsai CH, Chen YC, et al. Gamma-aminobutyric acid (GABA) receptor mediates *suanzaorentang,* a traditional Chinese herb remedy, -induced sleep alteration. *J Biomed Sci.* 2007;14(2):285–297.

23. Scheid V, Bensky D, Ellis A, Barolet R. *Chinese Herbal Medicine: Formulas & Strategies.* Seattle, WA: Eastland Press; 2009. pp. 786–789.

24. Li T. Clinical Evaluation of Wendan decoction in the treatment of COPD with anxiety and depression. *Mod Tradit Chin Med.* 2019;06:69–72.
25. Xiao F, Xu B-Y, Li Y, et al. Effect of *Jiawei Xiaoyao San* on anxiety and depression in patients with psychological stress insomnia. *Chin J Tradition Chin Med Pharm.* 2009;27:962–964.
26. Li J, Mu Z, Xie J, et al. Effectiveness and safety of Chinese herbal medicine *Xiaoyao san* for the treatment of insomnia protocol for a systematic review and meta-analysis. *Medicine* (Baltimore). 2019;98(29):e16481.
27. Zhao L, Gan A-P. Clinical and psychological assessment on *Xinwei* decoction for treating functional dyspepsia accompanied with depression and anxiety. *Am J Chin Med.* 2005;33(2):249–257.
28. Qi GF. Clinical observation on anxiety and depression disorder treated with *Yangxin* decoction. *Chin Arch Tradit Chin Med.* 2011;28(5):1181–1183.
29. Mizukami K, Asada T, Kinoshita T, et al. A randomized cross-over study of a traditional Japanese medicine (*kampo*), *yokukansan*, in the treatment of the behavioural and psychological symptoms of dementia. *Int J Neuropsychopharmacol.* 2009;12(2):191–199.
30. Shinno H, Inami Y, Inagaki T, et al. Effect of *Yi-Gan San* on psychiatric symptoms and sleep structure at patients with behavioral and psychological symptoms of dementia. *Prog Neuro-Psychoph.* 2008;32(3):881–885.
31. Miyaoka T, Furuya M, Yasuda H, et al. *Yi-gan san* for the treatment of borderline personality disorder: An open-label study. *Prog Neuro-Psychoph.* 2008;32(1):150–154.
32. Mao LJ, Lu Y, Sun W. The evaluation of effect about generalized anxiety disorder by treatment and syndrome differentiation. *Guangming J Chin Med.* 2012;3:191–193.
33. Meng ZR, Yi XY. Clinical observation to patients with internal phlegm turbidity block in generalized anxiety disorders treated by clear the heart and flush heat decoction. *J Sichuan Trad Chin Med.* 2010;19(1):27–28.
34. Li ZN. A clinic comparison of anxiety disorders healing by traditional Chinese medicine. *J Liaoning Univ Trad Chin Med.* 2011;7:84–85.
35. Wang T, Ding J-Y, Xu G-X, et al. Efficacy of *Yiqiyangxin* Chinese medicine compound combined with cognitive therapy in the treatment of generalized anxiety disorders. *Asian Pac J Trop Med.* 2012;818–822.
36. Park J-S, Kil BH, Kim DW, et al. Two case reports of anxiety disorder patients with gastrointestinal symptoms treated with traditional Korean medicine. *J Int Korean Med.* 2020;41(2):177–185.
37. Hsu HY, Hsu CS. *Commonly Used Chinese Herb Formulas Companion Handbook.* Long Beach, CA: Oriental Healing Arts Institute; 1997.
38. Scheid V, Bensky D, Ellis A, et al. *Chinese Herbal Medicine: Formulas & Strategies.* Seattle, WA: Eastland Press; 2009. pp. 457–482.
39. Kwon C-Y, Choi E-J, Suh H-W, et al. Oriental herbal medicine for generalized anxiety disorder: A stematic review of randomized controlled trials. *Eur J Integr Med.* 2018;20:36–62.
40. Li Y, Zhang X-L, Huang Y-R, et al. Extracts or active components from *Acorus gramineus* Aiton for cognitive function impairment: Preclinical evidence and possible mechanisms. *Oxi Med Cell Longev.* 2020;2020: Article ID 6752876.
41. Ma Y, Tian S, Sun L, et al. The effect of acori graminei rhizoma and extract fractions on spatial memory and hippocampal neurogenesis in amyloid beta 1–42 injected mice. *CNS Neurol Disord Drug Targets.* 2015;14(3):411–420.
42. Chellian R, Pandy V, Mohamed Z. Pharmacology and toxicology of α- and β-Asarone: A review of preclinical evidence. *Phytomedicine.* 2017;32:41–58.
43. Sarris J, McIntyre E, Camfield DA. Plant-based medicines for anxiety disorders, part 1 a review of preclinical studies. *CNS Drugs.* 2013;27(3):207–219.

44. Kim WK, Jung JW, Ahn NY, et al. Anxiolytic-like effects of extracts from *Albizzia julibrissin* bark in the elevated plus-maze in rats. *Life Sci.* 2004;75(23):2787–2795.
45. Jung YH, Ha RR, Kwon SH, et al. Anxiolytic effects of Julibroside C1 isolated from *Albizzia julibrissin* in mice. *Prog Neuropsychopharmacol Biol Psychiatry.* 2013;44:184–192.
46. Wei W-L, Zeng R, Gu C-M, et al. *Angelica sinensis* in China-A review of botanical profile, ethnopharmacology, phytochemistry and chemical analysis. *J Ethnopharmacol.* 2016;190:116–141.
47. Chen SW, Min L, Li WJ, et al. The effects of angelica essential oil in three murine tests of anxiety. *Pharmacol Biochem Behav.* 2004;79:377–382.
48. Matsumoto K, Kohno S, Ojima K, et al. Effects of methylenechloride-soluble fraction of Japanese angelica root extract, ligustilide and butylidenephthalide, on pentobarbital sleep in group-housed and socially isolated mice. *Life Sci.* 1998;62:2073–2082.
49. Zhao KJ, Dong TTX, Tu PF, et al. Molecular genetic and chemical assessment of radix angelica (Danggui) in China. *J Agri Food Chem.* 2003;51(9):2576–2583.
50. Woo JH, Ha T-W, Kang J-S, et al. Potentiation of decursinol angelate on pentobarbital-induced sleeping behaviors via the activation of GABAA-ergic systems in rodents. *Korean J Physiol Pharmacol.* 2017 Jan;21(1):27–36.
51. Lee B-B, Yun H-Y, Shim I-S, et al. *Bupleurum falcatum* prevents depression and anxiety-like behaviors in rats exposed to repeated restraint stress. *J Microbiol Biotech.* 2012;22(3):422–430.
52. Sun N, Ren Y, Wang M, et al. Gallbladder-warming decoction with *Bupleurum* and *Scutellaria* inhibits anxiety and depression of rats. *Earth Environ Sci.* 2020;440:022097.
53. Yang F, Dong X, Yin X, et al. *Radix Bupleuri*: A review of traditional uses, botany, phytochemistry, pharmacology, and toxicology. *BioMed Res Int.* 2017;2017:ID 7597596.
54. Hernandez-Leon A, González-Trujano ME, Fernández-Guasti A. The anxiolytic-like effect of rutin in rats involves GABAA receptors in the basolateral amygdala. *Behav Pharmacol.* 2017;28(4):303–312.
55. Overstreet DH, Kralic JE Morrow AL, et al. NPI-031G (puerarin) reduces anxiogenic effects of alcohol withdrawal or benzodiazepine inverse or 5-HT2C agonists. *Pharmacol Biochem Behav.* 2003;75(3):619–625.
56. Qiu ZK, Zhong DS, He JL, et al. The anxiolytic-like effects of Puerarin are associated with the changes of monoaminergic neurotransmitters and biosynthesis of allopregnanolone in the brain. *Metab Brain Dis.* 2018;33:167–175.
57. Sun X, Li X, Pan R, et al. Total saikosaponins of *Bupleurum yinchowense* reduces depressive, anxiety-like behavior and increases synaptic proteins expression in chronic corticosterone-treated mice. *BMC Complement Altern Med.* 2018;18:117.
58. Lim EY, Kim JG, Lee J, et al. Analgesic effects of *Cnidium officinale* extracts on postoperative, neuropathic, and menopausal pain in rat models. *eCAM.* 2019;9698727:1–8.
59. Ozaki Y, Sekita S, Harada M. Centrally acting muscle relaxant effect of phthalides (ligustilide, cnidilide and senkyunolide) obtained from *Cnidium officinale* Makino. *Yakugaku Zasshi.* 1989;109(6):402–406.
60. Meng F-C, Wu Z-F, Yin Z-Q, et al. *Coptidis rhizoma* and its main bioactive components: Recent advances in chemical investigation, quality evaluation and pharmacological activity. *Chin Med.* 2018;13(1):13.
61. Peng W-H, Wu C-R, Chen C-S, et al. Anxiolytic effect of berberine on exploratory activity of the mouse in two experimental anxiety models: Interaction with drugs acting at 5-HT receptors. *Life Sci.* 2004;75(20):2451–2462.
62. Kong LD, Cheng CHK, Tan RX. Monoamine oxidase inhibitors from Rhizoma of *Coptis chinensis. Planta Med.* 2001;67(1):74–76.
63. Zhou Y, Xie M, Song Y, et al. Two traditional Chinese medicines, *Curcuma Radix* and *Curcuma Rhizoma*: An ethnopharmacology, phytochemistry, and pharmacology review. *eCAM.* 2016;2016:1–30.

64. Hu D, Gao J, Yang X, et al. A comprehensive mini-review of *Curcuma Radix*: Ethnopharmacology, phytochemistry, and pharmacology. *Nat Prod Commun.* 2021;16(5):1–11.

65. Cui ZH, Guo ZQ, Miao JH, et al. The genus *Cynomorium* in China: An ethnopharmacological and phytochemical review. *J Ethnopharmacol.* 2013;147:1–15.

66. Cuia J-L, Gonga Y, Xue X-Z, et al. Phytochemical and pharmacological review of *Cynomorium songaricum. Nat Prod Commun.* 2018;13(4):501–510.

67. Zhao G, Wang J, Qin GW, et al. *Cynomorium songaricum* extracts functionally modulate transporters of gamma-aminobutyric acid and monoamine. *Neurochem Res.* 2010;35:666–676.

68. Wong M. *La Medecine Chinoise par les Plantes.* Le Corps a Vivre: Editions Tchou; 1976.

69. Ambawade SD, Kasture VS, Kasture SB. Anxiolytic activity of *Glycyrrhiza glabra* Linn. *J Nat Remedies.* 2001;2:130–134.

70. Asl MN, Hosseinzadeh H. Review of pharmacological effects of *Glycyrrhiza sp.* And its bioactive compounds. *Phytother Res.* 2008;22:709–724.

71. Parchestani ZN, Rafieirad M. The effect of herniarin on anxiety behaviors and depression following chronic cerebral ischemia hypoperfusion in male rats. *Exp Animal Biol.* 2021;9(3):93–103.

72. Lee B, Yeom M, Shim I, et al. Umbelliferone modulates depression-like symptoms by altering monoamines in a rat post-traumatic stress disorder model. *J Nat Med.* 2020;74:377–386.

73. Wang X, Guan S, Liu A, et al. Anxiolytic effects of Formononetin in an inflammatory pain mouse model. *Mol Brain.* 2019;12:36.

74. Hoffmann KM, Beltrán L, Ziemba PM. Potentiating effect of glabridin from *Glycyrrhiza glabra* on GABAA receptors. *Biochem Biophys Rep.* 2016;6:197–202.

75. Parker S, May B, Zhang C, et al. A pharmacological review of bioactive constituents of *Paeonia lactiflora* Pallas and *Paeonia veitchii* lynch. *Phytother Res.* 2016;30:1445–1473.

76. Wu Y-Q, Wei M-R, Zhao D-Q, et al. Flavonoid content and expression analysis of flavonoid biosynthetic genes in herbaceous peony (*Paeonia lactiflora* Pall.) with double colors. *J Integr Agri.* 2016;15(9):2023–2031.

77. Kamiya K, Yoshioka K, Saiki Y, et al. Triterpenoids and flavonoids from *Paeonia lactiflora. Phytochemistry.* 1997;44:141–144.

78. Wang J, Song C, Gao D, et al. Effects of *Paeonia lactiflora* extract on estrogen receptor β, TPH2, and SERT in rats with PMS. *Anxiety.* 2020;2020: Article ID 4690504.

79. Zhi-Kun Q, Jia-Li H, Xu L, et al. Anxiolytic-like effects of paeoniflorin in an animal model of post traumatic stress disorder. *Metab Brain Dis.* 2018;33:1175–1185.

80. Hu M-Z, Wang A-R, Zhao Z-Y, et al. Antidepressant-like effects of paeoniflorin on post-stroke depression in a rat model. *Neurol Res.* 2019;41(5):446–455.

81. Han M, Yang X, Zhang M, et al. Phytochemical study of the rhizome of *Pinellia ternata* and quantification of phenylpropanoids in commercial *Pinellia* tuber by RP-LC. *Chroma.* 2006;64:647–653.

82. Zhang ZH, Dai Z, Hu XR, et al. Isolation and structure elucidation of chemical constituents from *Pinellia ternata. Zhong Yao Cai.* 2013;36(10):1620–1622.

83. Liu Y, Liu W, Liang Z. Endophytic bacteria from *Pinellia ternata*, a new source of purine alkaloids and bacterial manure. *Pharm Biol.* 2015;53(10):1545–1548.

84. Wu X-Y, Zhao J-L, Zhang M, et al. Sedative, hypnotic and anticonvulsant activities of the ethanol fraction from *Rhizoma Pinelliae Praeparatum. J Ethnopharmacol.* 2011;135(2):325–329.

85. Yoon BH, Choi JW, Jung JW, et al. Anxiolytic-like effects of phenylpropanoid compounds using the elevated plus-maze in mice. *Yakhak Hoeji.* 2005;49(5):437–442.

86. Panayotis N, Freund PA, Marvaldi L, et al. β-sitosterol reduces anxiety and synergizes with established anxiolytic drugs in mice. *Cell Rep.* 2021;2(5):100281.
87. Wagner JA, Katz RJ. Purinergic control of anxiety: Direct behavioral evidence in the rat. *Neurosci Lett.* 1983;43(2–3):333–337.
88. Lacaille-Dubois M-A, Delaude C, Mitaine-Offer A-C, et al. A review on the phytopharmacological studies of the genus *Polygala*. *J Ethnopharmacol.* 2020;249:112417.
89. Lee B, Sur B, Shin S, et al. *Polygala tenuifolia* prevents anxiety-like behaviors in mice exposed to repeated restraint stress. *Anim.* 2015;19(1):1–7.
90. Jung J-W, Yoon B-H, Kim S-Y. Anxiolytic-like effects of *Polygala tenuifolia* Willdenow using the elevated plus maze and hole-board apparatus in mice. *Biomol Ther.* 2005;13(2):84–89.
91. Yao Y, Jia M, Wu J-G, et al. Anxiolytic and sedative-hypnotic activities of polygala saponins from *Polygala tenuifolia* in mice. *Pharm Biol.* 2010;48(7):801–807.
92. Kawashima K, Miyako D, Ishino Y, et al. Anti-stress effects of 3,4,5-trimethoxycinnamic acid, an active constituent of roots of *Polygala tenuifolia* (Onji). *Biol Pharm Bull.* 2004;27:1317–1319.
93. Shi T, Li Y, Jiang Y, et al. Isolation of flavonoids from the aerial parts of *Polygala tenuifolia* Willd. And their antioxidant activities. *Chin Pharm Sci.* 2013;22:36–39.
94. Bound G-A, Feng YU. Review of clinical studies of *Polygonum multiflorum* Thunb. And its isolated bioactive compounds. *Pharmacognosy Res.* 2015;7(3):225–236.
95. Liu LF, Durairajan SS, Lu JH, et al. In vitro screening on amyloid precursor protein modulation of plants used in Ayurvedic and traditional Chinese medicine for memory improvement. *J Ethnopharmacol.* 2012;141(2):754–760.
96. Yang J-B, Sun H, Ma J, et al. New phenolic constituents obtained from *Polygonum multiflorum*. *Chinese Herb Med.* 2020;12(3):342–346.
97. National Toxiclogy Program. NTP technical report. The toxicology and carcinogenesis studies of emodin in F344/N rats and B6C3F1 mice (Report No. 01–3952). *NIH Publication.* 2001:1–278.
98. Chen FP, Jong MS, Chen YC, et al. Prescriptions of Chinese herbal medicines for insomnia in Taiwan during 2002. *eCAM.* 2011;2011:236341.
99. Lin L, Ni B, Lin H, et al. Traditional usages, botany, phytochemistry, pharmacology and toxicology of *Polygonum multiflorum* Thunb.: A review. *J Ethnopharmacol.* 2015;159:158–183.
100. Zhang R-X, Li M-X, Jia Z-P. *Rehmannia glutinosa*: Review of botany, chemistry and pharmacology. *J Ethnopharmacol.* 2008;117:199–214.
101. Zhou X-D, Shi D-D, Zhang Z-J. Ameliorative effects of *Radix rehmanniae* extract on the anxiety- and depression-like symptoms in ovariectomized mice: A behavioral and molecular study. *Phytomedicine.* 2019;63:153012.
102. Wang JM, Pei LX, Zhang YY, et al. Ethanol extract of *Rehmannia glutinosa* exerts antidepressant-like effects on a rat chronic unpredictable mild stress model by involving monoamines and BDNF. *Metab Brain Dis.* 2018;33:885–892.
103. Kim M, Acharya S, Botanas CJ, et al. Catalpol and mannitol, two components of *Rehmannia glutinosa*, exhibit anticonvulsant effects probably via GABAA receptor regulation. *Biomol Ther* (Seoul). 2020;28(2):137–144.

8 Ayurvedic Herbal Treatment of Anxiety

The word *Ayurveda* is derived from the Sanskrit words *ayur*, meaning life, and *veda*, meaning science or knowledge. Thus, Ayurveda is the science of life. It is the ancient health and healing system of India, and it derives from philosophies that can be traced back more than 4,000 years.

Ayurvedic medicine is holistic. It uses not only herbs to treat ill health but also exercise, yoga, breathing techniques, meditation, diet, lifestyle changes, purification, and spiritual exercises. Like traditional Chinese medicine, Ayurveda strives to restore balance. There are, however, some differences in the worldview that produced these two ancient healing systems. Thus, each has its own, unique way of conceptualizing diseases and their treatments.

As in Chinese philosophy, Ayurveda holds that there are five fundamental elements that compose the living body. These are *aakash* (space), *jala* (water), *prithvi* (earth), *teja* (fire), and *vayu* (air). Somewhat in contrast with Chinese medical philosophy, Ayurveda further postulates that these elements combine in each individual to generate three fundamental qualities, or *doshas*, called *vata*, *pitta*, and *kapha*. Although everyone has some of each *dosha*, one *dosha* tends to predominate in each individual. The individual pattern of compositional *doshas* is referred to as one's *prakruti*. Each of the *doshas* is associated with a specific bodily type and certain personality traits. Ayurveda also links each *dosha* with tendencies toward certain health and emotional problems.[1]

Vata is said to consist mostly of the two elements, air and space. It has the qualities of cold, light, dry, rough, flowing, and spacious. Its season is autumn. Those with the *vata dosha* are described as slim, energetic, and creative. However, they are easily distracted. Their mood is easily affected by the weather, people around them, and foods they eat. When stressed they may be forgetful, unstable in mood, and easily overwhelmed. *Kapha* derives from earth and water. It has the qualities of steady, stable, heavy, slow, cold, and soft. Spring is *kapha*'s season. People with this *dosha* are known for keeping things together and being a support system for others. *Kapha*-dominant people rarely get upset. They think before acting and go through life in a slow, deliberate manner. They are empathetic, caring, trusting, patient, calm, wise, happy, and romantic. However, they are also more susceptible than others to depression. *Pitta* is a *dosha* of fire and water. It has the qualities of hot, light, sharp, oily, liquid, and mobile. Its season is summer. People with *pitta dosha* are intelligent and purposeful and make strong leaders. They're highly motivated, goal oriented, and competitive. However, they can become impatient, and their aggressive and tenacious nature can be oppressive to some people. Thus, they are prone to agitation and conflict.

Those that are predominantly *vata* are often seen as most prone to anxiety. However, all three of the *dosha* types can and do experience feelings of anxiety, worry, or feeling overwhelmed. They are simply thought to manifest anxieties in different ways. *Vatas* are likely to experience heart palpitations, tremors, and numbness and tingling of their extremities under stress. *Pittas* may feel overwhelmed with worry often associated with incompletion of tasks or the fear of losing control. *Kaphas* may experience feelings of worry and fear, though often with rumination of melancholic thoughts and disappointments. They are most likely to be driven to inertia and mild depression if faced with anxiety-inducing stressors.[2]

Each *dosha* is also seen as having five sub-*doshas* through which the qualities of the *doshas* affect the various organ systems of the body. This is similar to traditional Chinese medicine. The five sub-*doshas* of *vata* are *prana, udana, vyana, samana,* and *apana*. The sub-doshas of *kapha* are *tarpaka, bodhaka, avalambaka, shleshaka,* and *kledaka*. The sub-*doshas* of pitta are *alochaka, ranjaka, bhrajaka,* and *pachaka*. Each in their own way, the sub-*doshas* affect the balance and function of the brain, heart, lungs, stomach, intestines, skin, joints, and every other system in the body. As in traditional Chinese medicine, there are also thought to be "channels," or *srotas*, 14 in number, that carry various energies through the body. These channels can be blocked with need of release, deficient and in need of supplementation, or excessive in need of calming.

For some sub-*doshas*, imbalances are best addressed by diet, lifestyle changes, or spiritual practices. In other sub-*doshas*, herbs are seen as the most direct route to resolve imbalance. Herbs are chosen, often in combination, to bring the 3 *doshas* and 15 sub-*doshas* back into to the balance that best suits the individual's *prakruti*. Herbs are seen as having properties that are associated with the *doshas* and sub-*doshas*, such as sweet, hot, pungent, oily, heavy, or unstable, and these characteristics lend them advantage for use in certain *prakruti* and their ailments. The choice and effectiveness of Ayurvedic treatment is thus dependent upon thorough examination of the patient and review of all aspects of his or her life. Diagnoses do not simply spring from evaluation of the patient's most prominent symptoms.[3]

Ayurvedic and traditional Chinese medicine share some perspectives, and many of their herbal treatments are similar. A difference is that there is nothing in traditional Chinese medicine leading to categorization of people into types and predispositions for illness, as is the case with Ayurvedic medicine. Yet, despite the ancient concepts and vastly different conceptualization of the nature of illness, the Ayurvedic notion of types is not out of step with modern Western medicine's understanding of genetic predisposition to disease. The Ayurvedic division of people into *vata, pitta,* and *kapha* types with predispositions to certain psychiatric manifestations also calls to mind Sheldon's constitutional psychology from the 1940s, in which individuals were categorized into endomorph, mesomorph, and ectomorph somatotypes.[4] These basic somatotypes, of which each individual was thought to possess certain degrees, were thought to predispose them to personality characteristics. Though long ago abandoned, views such as Sheldon's have influenced the bio-psycho-social model of psychiatric illness.

Before discussing Ayurvedic treatments, it must be noted that India is an advanced society that has embraced modern science and technology. In many ways, Ayurvedic philosophy is at odds with the Western approach to medicine that is increasingly being practiced in India. Ancient Ayurvedic principles, such as the use of astrology, dream interpretations, and relationships of illness to actions of the various gods as bases for diagnosis and treatment, have become anachronisms. The seeming disparities between classical Ayurvedic medicine and Western scientific medical practice have been recognized by many of Ayurveda's own practitioners, and calls have been made for "bridging Ayurveda with evidence-based, scientific approaches in medicine."[5] Perhaps translating and melding Ayurvedic concepts and vocabulary into more modern, scientific perspectives would lessen the apparent dissimilarities. Nonetheless, a growing number of studies have shown that the ancient herbal treatments recommended in Ayurvedic practice provide the same degree of relief as modern pharmaceuticals. Regardless of the philosophical underpinnings that guide the choice of treatments and explain their effects, many herbal treatments have been found effective over thousands of years and deserve consideration.

8.1 HERBAL TREATMENT OF ANXIETY IN AYURVEDIC MEDICINE

Since its ancient beginnings, practitioners of Ayurvedic medicine have used thousands of different herbs to treat human illnesses. Many have been used to treat psychiatric and nervous conditions. Those herbs tend to act as restoratives as well as to calm and improve mood. Among such herbs that have been mentioned in the Ayurvedic literature are: *Acacia nilotica, Aconitum carmichaelii, Achyranthes aspera, Acorus calamus, Adhatoda zeylanica, Albizzia lebbek, Allium cepa, Alphinia galanga, Amanita muscaria, Anacyclus pyrethrum, Andrographis paniculata, Argyreia speciosa, Asparagus racemosus, Azadirachta indica, Bacopa monnieri, Benincasa hispida, Boerhavia diffusa, Bombax ceiba, Boswellia serrata, Brassica nigra, Caesalpinia bonduc, Calotropis procera, Cannabis sativa, Cassia occidentalis, Celastrus paniculatus, Centella asiatica, Citrullus colosynthis, Commiphora wightii, Convolvulus pluricaulis, Coriandrum sativum, Crocus sativus, Curculigo orchioides, Cuscuta reflexa, Cynodon dactylon, Cyperus scariosus, Datura metel, Daucus carota, Eclipta prostrata, Eclipta alba, Ferula foetida, Ficus benghalensis, Glycyrrhiza glabra, Helianthus annuus, Hemidesmus indicus, Hibiscus rosasinensis, Hygrophila spinosa, Hyoscyamus niger, Inula racemosa, Juglans regia, Lawsonia inermis, Moringa oleifera, Mucuna pruriens, Myristica fragrans, Nardostachys jatamansi, Ocimum tenuiflorum, Orchis latifolia, Papaver somniferum, Phoenix dactylifera, Phyllanthus emblica, Picrorbiza kurrooa, Piper cubeba, Piper longum, Piper nigrum, Plumbago zeylanica, Prunus amygdalus, Psidium guajava, Pueraria tuberosa, Punica granatum, Rauwolfia serpentina, Sapindus mukorossi, Saussurea lappa, Semecarpus anacardium, Sesbania grandiflora, Sida cordifolia, Solanum surratense, Sphaeranthus indicus, Strychnos nux vomica, Syzygium aromaticum, Terminalia bellirica, Terminalia chebula, Tinospora cordifolia, Tribulus terrestris, Valeriana jatamansi, Vitex negundo, Vitis vinifera, Withania somnifera, Xeromphis spinosa, Zingiber officinale,* and *Zizyphus mauritiana.*[6-7]

In some cases, there are clinical data establishing the efficacy of specific Ayurvedic herbs that have been used on their own to treat anxiety disorders. These herbs include *Bacopa monnieri, Cannabis sativa, Centella asiatica, Convolvulus pluricaulis, Evolvulus alsinoides, Nardostachys jatamansi, Tinospora cordifolia, Valeriana jatamansi,* and *Withania somnifera.* Each of those herbs has been discussed in Chapter 6 of this book. However, Ayurvedic herbs are often used in well-devised combinations.[8] As in traditional Chinese medicine, Ayurvedic practitioners create combinations for each individual according to what the examination reveals. However, it is not unusual for certain combinations to provide relief in a more general fashion. Some specific combinations were even mentioned in ancient texts. In some cases, the efficacy of such herbal combinations has been established in clinical trials, and these combinations are discussed in the following. Finally, there are a number of herbs that are the mainstays of Ayurvedic herbal treatment of anxiety. The individual herbs among that group that have not been evaluated in clinical studies are discussed using preclinical data to establish the likelihood of efficacy and possible mechanisms of action.

8.1.1 ASHWAGANDHA CHURNA

Ashwagandha (Withania somnifera) is a time-honored herbal treatment in Ayurvedic medicine. As noted in a previous chapter, there are many clinical studies showing that the herb used on its own can relieve anxiety in individuals formally diagnosed with anxiety disorders. One study compared the effects of *ashwagandha* alone with *ashwagandha* combined with two other common Ayurvedic herbs, *shankhapushpi (Evolvulus alsinoides)* and *yastimadhu (Glycyrrhiza glabra),* in the treatment of *chittodvega,* the Ayurvedic term for GAD. The herbal combination was referred to as *ashwagandha churna.*[9]

Patients received either 4g of *ashwagandha churna* or 4g of *ashwagandha* three times a day for a month and were reevaluated for symptoms. None of the patients in either group enjoyed complete resolution of anxiety. However, nearly half of each experienced moderate degree of relief, and almost all of the rest enjoyed at least mild relief. There was found to be a slight advantage to the combination of the herbs over *ashwagandha* alone, though the results were quite similar.

8.1.2 ASHWAGANDHA AND MANDOOKAPARNI

The herbs *ashwagandha (Withania somnifera)* and *mandookaparni (Centella asiatica)* have been found to relieve anxiety by themselves in clinical studies. However, these herbs have been held in high esteem in Ayurvedic medicine for centuries for their ability to resolve anxiety. In one particular study, the combination of *ashwagandha* and *mandookaparni* was used to treat *mandowega,* which is one of several Ayurvedic conceptions of GAD.[10] Subjects in the study had all been diagnosed with GAD. One group was given the combination of *ashwagandha* and *mandookaparni* daily for 3 months. For the first 7 days, half of these subjects also received *shirodhara* using *ksheerabala taila* oil. *Shirodhara* is the slow, persistent pouring of liquid— usually, milk, buttermilk, water, or, in this case, oil—onto the forehead. The authors of that study referred to *shirodhara* as one of the most powerful Ayurvedic techniques "to relieve *Vata* (wind) in the mind preoccupied with swarming thoughts." After 12 weeks, the treatments significantly reduced anxiety in comparison to baseline levels as measured by the Hamilton Anxiety Rating Scale. Those who also received the *shirodhara* treatment appeared to enjoy slightly greater relief.

8.1.3 *ASPARAGUS RACEMOSUS* AND *GLYCYRRHIZA GLABRA*

One herb used in Ayurvedic medicine is held in particularly high regard. This is *Asparagus racemosus*, known in Ayurvedic medicine as *shatavari*. *Shatavari* is the primary Ayurvedic rejuvenating tonic for women, whereas *ashwagandha* is for men. Indeed, the word *shatavari* means "she who possesses a hundred husbands." Accordingly, it is often used for correcting menstrual irregularities, to enhance fertility, to increase female sex drive, and as a general postpartum tonic. It is considered to be among the *medhya*, which are plants thought to enhance intelligence, improve memory, and protect against stress. It is also one of the herbs commonly recommended by members of the American Herbalists Guild to treat both anxiety and depression. However, while there are studies demonstrating anxiolytic and antidepressant-like effects in laboratory animals, there are no published studies of such effects in human patients. There are reports of various herbal combinations containing *Asparagus racemosus* easing anxiety and other disorders in humans. However, the specific contribution *Asparagus racemosus* might have made cannot be known.

There is a study evaluating the effects of *Asparagus racemosus* in combination with only one other herb, *Glycyrrhiza glabra*, more commonly known as licorice root, in the treatment of women suffering symptoms of menopause that included anxiety.[11] It should be noted that licorice root is a common ingredient in Ayurvedic and traditional Chinese herbal combinations to treat anxiety and other psychiatric illnesses. In this study, women suffering symptoms of menopause were given twice daily treatments of 3g of powder of licorice root and *Asparagus racemosus* over 8 weeks. Evaluation of anxiety using the Hamilton Anxiety Rating Scale showed that this combination significantly alleviated symptoms of anxiety in comparison to a placebo of wheat flour.

8.1.4 *BRAHMI GRITHA*

In a well-documented case study, a 57-year-old man presented with complaints of inability to relax, persistent worry, lack of sleep, muscle tension, palpitation, and increased sweating over the previous 3 years. He was diagnosed with GAD according to criteria outlined in the International Statistical Classification of Diseases and Related Health Problems. The treatment he received was *Brahmi gritha*, which consisted of *brahmi*, or *Centella asiatica*; *bach*, or *Acorus calamus*; *kusta*, or *Costus igneus*; and *sankhapuspi*, or *Evolvulus alsinoides*, carried in clarified butter and administered as nasal drops. After 3 weeks of treatment, he enjoyed a significant reduction in anxiety reflected in a drop in his Hamilton Anxiety Rating Scale score from 18 to 13.[12]

8.1.5 GERIFORTE

The herbal treatment Geriforte was designed by Indian psychiatrists based on Ayurvedic herbal traditions. Each Geriforte tablet consists of *chyavanprash* jam (containing *Phyllanthus emblica, Glycyrrhiza glabra, Bacopa monnieri, Agele marmelos, Tribulus terrestris, Pipal longum, Tinospora cordifolia,* and *Terminalia chebula*) *Asparagus adscendens, Withania somnifera, Centella asiatica, Mucuna pruriens, shilajeet* (a mineral supplement), *Asparagus racemosus, Terminalia arjuna, makardhwaj* (a mineral and herbal supplement containing gold, mercury, sulfur, cotton, *Gossypium herbaceum,* and *Aloe vera*), and *Piper longum.* I note that the use of mercury is not uncommon in Ayurvedic formulas but is not here advised.

The Geriforte combination was evaluated in an open study using subjects diagnosed with anxiety disorders. Those subjects were already being treated with standard Western psychiatric medications, but without success. After 6 weeks of three times daily administrations of Geriforte, the patients showed substantial and significant reduction of symptoms as measured by the Hamilton Anxiety Rating Scale.[13] In another study, patients diagnosed with anxiety neurosis were treated with either Geriforte three times a day for 12 weeks or placebo. Those who received Geriforte experienced significant reductions of symptoms of anxiety as per the Presumptive Stressful Life Events Scale.[14]

8.1.6 GUDUCHYADI MEDHYA RASAYANA

Those suffering dementias are prone to anxiety and agitation, as well as depressed mood. Control of agitation, especially if it grows to include disruptive or aggressive behavior, is a major concern in care homes and in families caring for demented elderly relatives. Powerful medications can help control these behaviors, but many come with warnings about stroke and sudden death. Thus, herbal formulas that control anxiety and agitation are much needed.

In a clinical study, an herbal combination called *guduchyadi medhya rasayana* was evaluated for its ability to reduce anxiety, agitation, and depressed mood in patients with evidence of decline in memory and thinking and impairment of personal activities of daily living. Curiously, any patients formally diagnosed with Alzheimer's disease or Parkinson's disease, which can sometimes include dementia, were excluded. The herbal combination consisted of *guduchi* (*Tinospora cordifolia*), *Acarenthus aspera, Embelia ribes, Convolvulus pluricaulis, Acorus calamus, Terminalia chebula, Saussurea lappa,* and *Asparagus racemosus* in ghee and sugar. Subjects were given 5g of the herbal combination three times a day over 3 months.

Hamilton rating scales for anxiety and depression, as well as the Brief Psychiatric Rating Scale, were used to gather data. At the end of the study, there were significant reductions in anxiety, tension, fear, insomnia, inability to relax, and depression.[15] Again, while *Acorus calamus* has been used for centuries in Ayurvedic medicine, it has been banned in the United States for human consumption due to concerns about liver cancer.

8.1.7 KUSHMANDADI GHRITA

Kushmandadi ghrita is an ancient Ayurvedic treatment consisting of *Glycyrrhiza glabra* and *Benincasa hispida* prepared in clarified butter. *Glycyrrhiza glabra,* or licorice root, is an herb quite commonly used in Ayurvedic and traditional Chinese medicine to treat psychiatric disorders. *Benincasa hispida* is known in Ayurvedic tradition as *kushmandadi* and in English as winter melon. This plant, too, has long been used in both Ayurvedic and Chinese medicine. *Kushmandadi* is thought to balance the three *doshas* and has a variety of uses in Ayurvedic medicine. It is thought to improve energy and stamina. However, it is also considered a *medhya*—that is, a brain tonic—and is often used to treat insomnia and normalize sleeping patterns.

Patients diagnosed with *chittodvega*, a disorder comparable to GAD, were treated with *Kushmandadi ghrita*. Treatment with this combination for 4 weeks reduced symptoms of anxiety as shown by significant reductions in Hamilton Anxiety Rating Scale and Brief Psychiatry Rating Scale scores.[16]

8.1.8 *MEDHYARASAYANA GHRITA* AND *VACHADI GHRITA NASYA*

Medhyarasayana ghrita is an herbal combination that contains *sankhapushpi* (*Evolvulus alsinoides*), *mandukaparni* (*Centella asiatica*), *yastimadhu* (*Glycyrrhiza uralensis*), *guduchi* (*Tinospora cordifolia*), *jyotishmati* (*Celastrus paniculatus*), *kushmanda* (*Benincasa hispida*), *ashwagandha* (*Withania somnifera*), *tulsi* (*Ocimum tenuiflorum*), *bhallatak* (*Semecarpus anacardium*), *kapikachchu* (*Mucuna pruriens*), and zinc processed with ghee. *Medhyarasayana ghrita* was given by mouth along with *vachadi ghrita* in the form of nasal drops. *Vachadi ghrita* contained *vacha* (*Acorus calamus*), *kustha* (*Costus igneus*), and *pippali* (*Piper longum*). Subjects were all elderly patients diagnosed with dementia. Subjects were given *medhyarasayana ghrita*, 10g by mouth, and two drops of *vachadi ghrita* nasally twice daily over three months. Data were gathered using the Hamilton Anxiety Rating Scale and Hamilton Depression Rating Scale, as well as the Brief Psychiatry Rating Scale. At the end of the study, the combination of *medhyarasayana ghrita* along with *vachadi ghrita* nasal drops brought statistically significant improvements in fear, insomnia, difficulty with concentration and memory, anxiety, tension, and depressed mood. Interestingly, a significant increase was also noted in scores in the Mini Mental Status Examination.[17]

8.1.9 MENTAT

A now proprietary compound, Mentat, has been studied in regard to effects on anxiety and mental performance. This compound is derived from an Ayurvedic formula containing *brahmi* (*Centella asiatica*), *bach* (*Acorus calamus*), *ashwagandha* (*Withania somnifera*), *giloe* (*Tinospora cordifolia*), *shankhapushpi* (*Evolvulus alsinoides*), and *jatamansi* (*Nardostachys jatamansi*). Each of these herbs has been found in clinical studies to significantly alleviate anxiety on their own, and all are discussed in a previous chapter. Thus, one might expect a synergistic effect when these herbs are combined. I must again caution that *bach*, or *Acorus calamus*, has been banned in the United States as an herbal treatment due to liver cancer being produced in laboratory animals.

Treatment with this Ayurvedic derived formula for 3 months resulted in significant calming and relaxation in executives suffering "burnout" as determined by increased presence of alpha brain waves and decreases in muscle tension in the scalp and forehead muscles.[18] In another study, subjects diagnosed with "anxiety neurosis" exhibited significant improvement in memory and endurance after 3 months of treatment with the Mentat combination.[19]

8.1.10 OCTA

One study evaluated a combination of herbs in a proprietary formula called OCTA.[20] The study was performed in Canada, not India, and the researchers were naturopathic, not Ayurvedic, physicians. The herbs were chosen not out of Ayurvedic diagnosis but due to their adaptogenic qualities. Nonetheless, the three primary herbal ingredients, *Withania somnifera*, *Lagerstroemia speciosa*, and *Bacopa monnieri*, are commonly used herbs in Ayurvedic medicine. *Ashwagandha* is one of the most revered herbs in Ayurvedic medicine. It is seen as a *rasayana*, or tonic, particularly helpful for the mind and brain. The crepe myrtle is often referred to as "the pride of India tree" both for its beauty and medicinal value. Its primary use is for treatment of diabetes. *Bacopa monnieri*, known in Ayurvedic medicine as *brahmi*, is a *rasayana* and favored herb to strengthen the mind. It is seen as a "cooling" agent to calm the mind, reduce anxiety, and promote sleep. It is a constituent of many Ayurvedic treatments of anxiety.

None of the subjects had been formally diagnosed with an anxiety disorder. However, all had some physical or emotional complaint associated with stress, such as reports of anxiety, arthritis, chronic pain, depression, diabetes, eczema, headaches, heart attacks, heart disease, impotence, decreased libido, high blood pressure, or peptic ulceration. Participants were provided with an aqueous-based liquid herbal preparation, OCTA, containing extracts of eight herbs: *Withania somnifera*, *Lagerstroemia speciosa*, *Bacopa monnieri*, *Zizyphus jujuba*, *Morinda citrifolia*, *Punica granatum*, *Schisandra chinensis*, and *Lycium barbarum*. Participants were instructed to consume 2 tablespoons (30ml) of the herbal compound per day each morning for 3 months. Every two weeks, participants were given a battery of psychological tests that included Perceived Stress Scale, State-Trait Anxiety Inventory, and Beck Depression Scale.

By the second week of the study, improvement was noted in each test. Scores continued to improve even further throughout the study. By the end of the study, highly significant improvements continued to be seen in tests of anxiety, as well as in mood.

8.1.11 SARASVATA CHOORNA

Sarasvata choorna is an Ayurvedic herbal formulation mentioned in the classical text *Bhaishajya Ratnavali* for the treatment of various psychiatric illnesses. It contains *Acorus calamus*, *Costus igneus*, *Withania somnifera*, *Apium graveolens*, *Cuminum cyminum*, *Carum carvi*, *Zingiber officinale*, *Piper nigrum*, *Piper longum*, *Convolvulus pluricaulis*, and *Centella asiatica*.

The anxiolytic effects of *sarasvata choorna* combined with *panchagavya ghrita nasya* over 60 days were evaluated in patients suffering *chittodvega*, the Ayurvedic equivalent of GAD. The treatment significantly improved symptoms of anxiety as determined by the Hamilton Anxiety Rating Scale. *Panchagavya ghrita nasya* is a preparation not likely to be seen as having value in modern Western medicine, but it must be explained. This is the use of nose drops prepared from the water of cow dung, milk, cow urine, milk curd, and clarified butter.[21] Whether *sarasvata choorna* alone would have been as successful as the treatment that combined *sarasvata choorna* with *panchagavya ghrita nasya* could not be determined from this study. It must be noted, however, that in another study, *sarasvata choorna* alone was not effective for the treatment of GAD.[22] Aside from how distasteful use of water from cow dung may seem, one wonders if it might not serve a purpose, such as balancing gut bacteria in patients who receive it.

Finally, *sarasvata choorna* was also found to significantly alleviate symptoms of major depression—with diagnoses based on *DSM-IV-TR* criteria—in a group of geriatric patients. The antidepressant effects were similar to those of citalopram. Unfortunately, GAD was an exclusionary diagnosis in that study.[23]

8.1.12 SARPAGANDHA GHANA VATI

Rauwolfia serpentina carries the common English name of Indian snakeroot. In India, the herb is known as *sarpagandha*, and it has been used in Ayurvedic medicine for several thousand years to treat psychiatric conditions such as insomnia, severe anxiety, and psychosis. It is a commonly used and well-regarded herb. Mahatma Gandhi was known to make *Rauwolfia* root tea in the evening to help relax after a hectic day. It has also been used to treat snakebite, which may be the basis for its common name. Because of the effectiveness of the herb in dampening agitation and even psychotic symptoms, the herb was used for a time in mainstream psychiatry. A paper by Gananath Sen and Karthick Chander Bose in 1931 in an Indian medical journal was one of the first scientific reports of the effects of the herb.[24] They reported on the use of an alkaloid extract from the *Rauwolfia serpentina* plant in the successful treatment of hypertension and "insanity with violent maniacal symptoms." The substance extracted from *Rauwolfia serpentina* was reserpine, and it was purified and marketed as a drug for both psychotic agitation and to treat high blood pressure. In a paper from 1955, it was said, "*Rauwolfia serpentina* is an effective sedative for use in mental hospitals although it is not effective in all cases. It reduces anxiety and drive and exerts a calming effect on psychomotor excitement."[25] When the potent, synthetic antipsychotic drug chlorpromazine became available in the early 1950s, it replaced reserpine, as it was more predictable, often more effective, and had fewer (or so it seemed at the time) side effects. Reserpine then fell out of favor as a prescribed psychiatric drug.

Sarpagandha is still used frequently in Ayurvedic medicine, and it is utilized either alone, in what is called *sarpagandha churna*, in the combination *sarpagandha ghana vati*, or in the combination *sarpagandha mishran*. *Sarpagandha ghana vati* contains *Rauwolfia serpentina*, as well as *Hyoscyamus niger*, *Nardostachys jatamansi*, *Cannabis sativa*, and *Piper longum*. *Sarpagandha mishran* contains *Rauwolfia serpentina*, *Nardostachys jatamansi*, *Acorus calamus*, *Boerhaavia diffusa*, *Centella asiatica*, *Tinospora cordifolia*, and *Evolvulus alsinoides*.

Ayurvedic medicine has recognized the syndrome of high blood pressure in the context of anxiety and pressures of life. It is considered to be part of a syndrome of excessive *rakta dhatu*, the primary "fire" of the body. It is said that when *rakta dhatu* is in excess, heat in the body increases, the tissues of the body experience inflammation, the skin may redden, and the mind experiences too great an intensity. There are studies testing the effects of various herbal remedies on blood pressure while at the same time assessing ability of the treatment to reduce anxiety. In one such study, the effects of the combination *sarpagandha ghana vati* were compared against those of *brahmi vati*. *Brahmi vati* contains *Centella asiatica*, *Convolvulus pluricaulis*, *Cyperus rotundus*, *Acorus calamus*, *Piper longum*, *Nardostachys jatamansi*, *swarna makshika* (a combination of copper pyrite and iron pyrite), and *rasa sindoor* (sulfide of mercury that would not be used in Western medicine).[26] Participants suffering both high blood pressure and anxiety were randomly divided into two groups. One group received 500mg of *brahmi vati* and the other group received 500mg of *sarpagandha ghana vati* twice a day for 30 days. Measurements of blood pressure and anxiety, using the Hamilton Anxiety Rating Scale, were performed on days 1, 15, and 30. Both treatments reduced blood pressure but also significantly reduced anxiety scores. Both treatments also significantly improved sleep. I cannot recommend the use of *brahmi vati* due to the inclusion of mercury and *Acorus calamus*, which has been banned from use in the United States due to risk of liver cancer.

Pure reserpine extracted from *Rauwolfia serpentina* has been shown in studies beginning in the 1950s to have significant calming and anxiolytic effects.[27–28] However, the somewhat high doses of reserpine used in severely agitated patients would sometimes cause depression and secondarily worsened anxiety. The drug was long ago abandoned by Western psychiatry.

A special note on dose

When given as a pure drug for psychotic agitation, reserpine extracted from *Rauwolfia serpentina* would often be given in doses of 5 to 15mg by intramuscular injection. In Ayurvedic herbal medicine, when using *sarpagandha* either alone or in an herbal combination, the daily dose of reserpine from the herb amounts to about 0.5 to 1.65mg a day. The typical dose of *sarpagandha* powder supplying that amount of reserpine is about for an adult is 600 to 1,000mg of dried root powder. The German Commission E recommends 600mg a day of dried root. Ayurvedic preparations of *sarpagandha* are available on the internet.

8.1.13 *Shankhapushpi panak* and *Shirodhara* with *Mamsyadi kwatha*

Shankhapushpi, or *Evolvulus alsinoides*, is an herb used often in Ayurvedic formulas for anxiety and other nervous and psychiatric disorders. Such a formula described in an ancient text, *Ayurveda Sara Sangraha*, is called *shankhapushpi panak* and contains *Evolvulus alsinoides*, *Centella asiatica*, and *sharkara*, which is simply cane sugar. In a clinical evaluation of that herbal treatment, patients received *shankhapushpi panak* along with *shirodhara* using the herbal combination *mansyadi kwatha*.[29] *Shirodhara* is the pouring of medicinal liquid, often oil or milk, onto the forehead for long durations of time to relax the mind. It is in part a forehead massage and herbal treatment. The components of the *mansyadi kwatha* administered by *shirodhara* are *Nardostachys jatamansi*, *Withania somnifera*, and *Hyoscyamus niger.* I note that henbane in large doses can cause delirium and death, and use should be left to experts. Patients diagnosed with *chittodvega*, the Ayurvedic equivalent of GAD, received these treatments daily for a month. In this study, the Ayurvedic treatment was compared against treatment with the commonly prescribed antidepressant medication sertraline. Effects of each of those treatments were assessed on the basis of improvement in scores on the Hamilton Anxiety Rating Scale and signs and symptoms of GAD as described in the *DSM-IV*, which is sometimes called the "Bible" of Western psychiatric diagnosis. Statistically significant improvements over baseline were observed in both treatment groups. It is not clear to what degree the herbs delivered by *shirodhara* could have been absorbed to give therapeutic blood levels of the phytochemicals contained in the *mansyadi kwatha* combination.

8.1.14 SHANKHAPUSHPYADI GHANA VATI

It has been noted by Ayurvedic scholars that the term "high blood pressure" was coined only after the invention of the sphygmomanometer. Before that, there was a syndrome identified by Ayurvedic physicians that has more recently included high blood pressure as a symptom. This long-recognized syndrome tended to include headache, palpitations in the chest, a sense of giddiness, and redness of the skin, as well as irritability, anxiety, and agitation. This insight predates what has been referred to as psychosomatic medicine in the West. This syndrome was considered to largely be due to "too much fire," and there have been a number of herbs and combinations of herbs used to treat it. One such herb is *shankhapushpi. Shankhapushpi* was discussed earlier in this text, and, as was noted, there are several anxiolytic herbs that have each been called by the Punjabi-language name *shankpushpi.* Two herbs that carry that name are two species of morning glory, *Evolvulus alsinoides*— which is the species earlier discussed—and *Convolvulus pluricaulis.* The following is a study in which a combination of *Convolvulus pluricaulis*—referred to as *shankpushpi*—is used in an herbal combination to treat high blood pressure in the context of anxiety and agitation.[30] This combination is called *shankhapushpyadi ghana vati*, and it includes *Convolvulus pluricaulis, Centella asiatica, Tinospora cordifolia, Cassia fistula, Azadirachta indica, Costus igneus, Tribulus terrestris*, and *Acorus calamus.* (Again, I note that *Acorus calamus* is banned for internal use in the United States.) In this study, patients suffering high blood pressure in the context of anxiety were treated with 2g *shankhapushpyadi ghana vati* per day in divided doses, along with a restricted diet pattern for 8 weeks. Results at the end of the study were compared against measurements taken at the start for each subject. The herbal treatment resulted in significant reductions in high blood pressure. The treatment also significantly reduced many of the symptoms of anxiety, including headache, insomnia, weakness, fatigue, lack of concentration and decisiveness, mental irritability, forgetfulness, poor appetite, palpitations, uneasiness, and feelings of tension. This study also evaluated the herbal combination *sarpagandha ghana vati*, containing reserpine and already discussed prior. That herbal combination was again found to significantly reduce high blood pressure and symptoms of anxiety.

8.1.15 VACHA BRAHMI GHAN

Acorus calamus, referred to as *vacha* or *bach*, is a common ingredient in Ayurvedic formulas to treat the various presentations of anxiety. *Vacha brahmi ghan* is a combination of *Acorus calamus* and *Centella asiatica*. Administration of 500mg of the combination three times a day over 6 weeks significantly reduced symptoms of anxiety in patients diagnosed with *manodwega*, the Ayurvedic equivalent of anxiety neurosis.[31] Among the symptoms relieved were persistent fear, excessive sweating, indecisiveness, heart palpitations, fatigue, breathlessness, trembling, insomnia, stomach ache, chest pain, and frequent headaches. Authors reported that at the end of the study, about 9% rated improvement as "good" and 70% rated improvement as "fair," whereas about 16% of the patients reported no benefit. No adverse effects were reported.

8.1.16 WORRY FREE

Worry Free is a proprietary product based on an Ayurvedic formula to treat anxiety. It was developed and researched at the Maharishi International University in Fairfield, Iowa. There the university has established a department of Ayurvedic medicine studies. The Worry Free formula contains *Nardostachys jatamansi*, *Withania somnifera*, *Glycyrrhiza uralensis*, *Tinospora cordifolia*, *Centella asiatica*, *Evolvulus alsinoides*, and *Kaempferia galanga*. In a very small but randomly controlled study of individuals diagnosed with GAD, 3 months of treatment significantly reduced symptoms of anxiety. A few subjects experienced full remission of symptoms.[32]

8.2 MAINSTAYS OF AYURVEDIC

Ayurvedic medicine describes a variety of herbs used to treat what would in common Western terms be referred to as anxiety, agitation, hysteria, restlessness, and insomnia. Notable among these herbs are *Acorus calamus*, *Albizzia lebbek*, *Allium cepa*, *Anacyclus pyrethrum*, *Asparagus racemosus*, *Bacopa monnieri*, *Benincasa hispida*, *Cannabis sativa*, *Centella asiatica*, *Convolvulus pluricaulis*, *Cuscuta reflexa*, *Cynodon dactylon*, *Evolvulus alsinoides*, *Ficus religiosa*, *Glycyrrhiza glabra*, *Hyoscyamus niger*, *Juglans regia*, *Lawsonia inermis*, *Moringa oleifera*, *Nardostachys jatamansi*, *Piper nigrum*, *Punica granatum*, *Saussurea lappa*, *Tinospora cordifolia*, *Valeriana jatamansi*, *Vitex negundo*, and *Withania somnifera*.[33] These herbs are among the mainstays of Ayurvedic herbal treatment of various manifestations of anxiety.

8.2.1 ACORUS CALAMUS

As yet another cautionary note, *Acorus calamus* has been banned for use as a medicinal herb in the United States because of well-substantiated reports of causing liver cancer in laboratory animals. This finding has been controversial in herbalist circles, and it must be known that it has been used for perhaps thousands of years by conscientious and observant Ayurvedic physicians without stimulating concern. It is discussed in Chapter 6. Nonetheless, I cannot recommend its use.

8.2.2 ALBIZZIA LEBBEK

Albizzia lebbeck is native to India but also distributed in tropical and subtropical areas of Africa, Asia, and northern Australia. Its leaves, bark, flowers, and seeds are used to treat a range of medicinal purposes including asthma, inflammation, infection, fever, agitation, and heart issues. The whole plant contains a variety of phytochemicals, including saponins, steroid-like triterpenes, flavonoids, phenylpropanoids, and alkaloids. Among those are many that have been shown to possess anxiolytic-like effects, such as β-sitosterol, kaempferol, and quercetin.[34] The closely related herb *Albizzia julibrissin* is widely used in Chinese traditional medicine in the treatment of anxiety and is discussed in Chapter 7.

There are no studies of anxiolytic effects of *Albizzia lebbeck* in humans. While there are some references to anxiolytic and anticonvulsant effects of the herb in animals, these are generally not well documented. However, in one study the saponin-rich, n-butanolic fraction extracted from dried leaves of *Albizzia lebbeck* had an anxiolytic-like effect in mice. Treated mice spent more time in the open arm of the elevated plus maze in a dose-dependent manner. That effect occurred without any significant effect on motor coordination.[35]

8.2.3 ALLIUM CEPA

Allium cepa, the onion bulb, contains a variety of phytochemicals, including ferulic acid, gallic acid, protocatechuic acid, quercetin, myricetin, and kaempferol. It contains phenylpropanoids, anthocyanins, and various sulfur-containing molecules.[36] Animal studies have shown *Allium cepa* to have anxiolytic-like effects. In one such study, 7 days of treatment with a methanolic extract of *Allium cepa* bulbs had an anxiolytic-like effect in mice in the elevated plus maze, open field test, and light and dark transition box. In that study, levels of GABA in the brain were increased with treatment.[37] In another study, 14 days of treatment with powdered *Allium cepa* prevented the typical anxiogenic effects of restraint stress in mice. Significant anxiolytic-like effects were seen in treated animals in the elevated plus maze and light/dark activity tests. Neurochemical analysis further showed potent antioxidant effects in the brain.[38]

8.2.4 ANACYCLUS PYRETHRUM

Anacyclus pyrethrum is an herb native to India, the Middle East, and North Africa. It is widely recognized in Ayurvedic medicine as a tonic and rejuvenator. In Unani and Moroccan folk medicine, it has been used to treat epilepsy. The plant contains flavonoids; polyphenolic compounds, such as chlorogenic acid, that can act on glutamate receptors; sesamin, which can modulate activity of GABA; and eugenol, an aromatic terpene compound that positively modulates GABA-A receptors.[39] An ethanolic extract of roots of *Anacyclus pyrethrum* was found to have anxiolytic-like effects in rats in the hole board and elevated plus maze tests. Unlike rats given diazepam as an active control, the herb did not cause any significant reduction in locomotor activity.[40] Extract of *Anacyclus pyrethrum* also showed an antidepressant-like effect in mice, attributed to enhancement of central catecholaminergic activity.[41]

8.2.5 ASPARAGUS RACEMOSUS

Asparagus racemosus is a common component in Ayurvedic treatments intended to boost immunity and improve longevity, vigor, and mental function. It is also commonly used to treat emotional disorders in women. It is regarded as a *rasayana*—that is, a plant that promotes general well-being by increasing cellular vitality and resistance. Extracts of the root of the plant contain steroidal saponins along with alkaloids, flavonoids, dihydrophenanthrene derivatives, furan derivatives, and volatile constituents.[42]

There is a study described previously in which the combination of *Asparagus racemosus* and *Zingiber officinale* was used successfully to treat anxiety and other symptoms arising in women during menopause. However, there are no published studies of anxiolytic effects of *Asparagus racemosus* alone in humans. There are numerous reports of *Asparagus racemosus* showing anxiolytic-like effects in rodents, including attempts to determine the mechanism of action of the herb.

In one study, 7 days of oral treatment with a methanol extract of *Asparagus racemosus* produced an anxiolytic-like effect in rats in the light/dark box, and this effect was comparable to that of diazepam.[43] In another more comprehensive study, 7 days of treatment with a methanolic extract of *Asparagus racemosus* exerted an anxiolytic-like effect in mice in the open field, hole board, and elevated plus maze tests. These effects were accompanied by increases in levels of serotonin and norepinephrine in the amygdala, as well as increases in the density of 5-HT2A receptors in that area. Perhaps most significant, these effects of *Asparagus racemosus* were reversed with flumazenil, suggesting a GABAergic, benzodiazepine-like mechanism of action.[44] Of note, a study also showed the methanolic extract of *Asparagus racemosus* to have an antidepressant-like effect in rodents. Similar to the study prior, those effects were accompanied by enhancement of serotonergic and noradrenergic activity.[45]

8.2.6 BACOPA MONNIERI

Bacopa monnieri is one of the herbs for which there have been clinical evaluations of anxiolytic effects. No studies have been performed with subjects actually diagnosed with a formal anxiety disorder. Nonetheless, several studies have shown that the herb on its own can relieve complaints of anxiety. See Chapter 6.

8.2.7 BENINCASA HISPIDA

Benincasa hispida, commonly known as wax gourd, is widely used in Ayurvedic medicine as a rejuvenative agent, or *rasayana*, in various nervous disorders including epilepsy, schizophrenia, and mood disorder. The active constituents of *Benincasa hispida* include volatile oils, flavonoids, glycosides, saccharides, proteins, carotenes, vitamins, minerals, β-sitosterin, and ursolic acid.[46]

A methanolic extract of the dried fruit of *Benincasa hispida* produced an anxiolytic-like effect in mice in the open field and elevated plus maze assays.[47] In the marble burying paradigm, thought to be a model of anxiety as well as obsessive compulsive disorder, a methanolic extract of *Benincasa hispida* significantly reduced marble burying behavior of mice.[48] In yet another assessment of effects of *Benincasa hispida* in mice, the herb produced antidepressant-like effects that were accompanied by increases in monoaminergic activities in the brain.[49]

8.2.8 *Cannabis sativa*

Cannabis, also known as marijuana, is a genus of plants in the family *Cannabaceae*. The genus includes three species, *sativa*, *indica*, and the lesser known *ruderalis*. Cannabis is thought to have originally come from central Asia, but it has been spread by humans throughout the temperate and tropical areas of the world. For thousands of years, it has been used for fiber, recreation, and spiritual quests. It has also been used for medicinal purposes. Cannabis has long been thought to reduce anxiety. On the other hand, one of the most common complaints about cannabis is panic attacks and feeling "paranoid." There are clinical and preclinical studies showing that cannabis and some of its constituent phytochemicals can provide anxiolytic effects. It appears the end result may depend upon factors such as the ratio of cannabidiol to tetrahydrocannabinol. See Chapter 6.

8.2.9 *Centella asiatica*

Centella asiatica, also known as gotu kola, is a perennial herbaceous plant of the *Umbellifere* family. Known as *mandukparni* or *jalbrahmi*, it has been used as a medicine in the Ayurvedic tradition of India for thousands of years and was described in the ancient Indian medical text *Sushruta Samhita*. The herb was also known to the ancient Chinese herbalists and was referred to as a "miracle elixir of life." It is one of the herbs that has been found to offer anxiolytic effects in human subjects suffering GAD. See Chapter 6.

8.2.10 *Convolvulus pluricaulis*

Convolvulus pluricaulis, a species of morning glory, is one of several Ayurvedic herbs referred to as *shankhapushpi*. Another such herb, *Evolvulus alsinoides*—the dwarf morning glory—has been found to have anxiolytic effects in human trials and is discussed in Chapter 6. *Convolvulus pluricaulis* is a common ingredient in herbal combinations to treat a variety of mental illnesses. It has been shown to have anxiolytic effects in humans suffering GAD.

8.2.11 *Cuscuta rflexa*

Cuscuta reflexa, known in Ayurvedic literature as *akashvalli* or *aftimooni*, has for centuries been used in treatments for relief of anxiety and insomnia. Many phytochemicals have been isolated from *Cuscuta reflexa*, including cuscutin, amarbelin, β-sitosterol, stigmasterol, myricetin, qurecetin, cuscutamine, luteolin, and bergenin.[50] There are no human trials of the herb for such use. However, several animal studies have revealed anxiolytic-like effects of the herb. In one such study, a methanol extract of the whole plant produced an anxiolytic-like effect in mice in the elevated plus maze and light and dark chamber.[51] In a similar study, treatment with *Cuscuta reflexa* produced anxiolytic-like effects in those tests that compared well with those of the benzodiazepine diazepam.[52] In a study of the closely related herb *Cuscuta epithymum*, the enhancement of pentobarbital-induced sleep was attenuated with flumazenil, suggesting benzodiazepine receptor involvement.[53]

8.2.12 *CYNODON DACTYLON*

Cynodon dactylon, also known as *doob* in India and Bermuda grass in English, is a perennial grass native to East Africa, Asia, Australia, and southern Europe. It has been used in Ayurveda and other regional traditional medicines to treat varied ailments such as cough, headache, diarrhea, cramps, epilepsy, dropsy, dysentery, hemorrhage, hypertension, hysteria, measles, snakebite, sores, stones, urogenital disorders, tumors, and warts.[54] Phytochemicals contained in *Cynodon dactylon* include apigenin, orientein, gallic acid, morin, rutin, C-glycosides, β-sitosterol, luteolin, citronellol, phytol, truxillic acid, docosanoic acid, linolenic acid, docosanoic acid, syringol, hexadecanoic acid, eicosanoic acid, and other steroids, flavonoids, alkaloids, and saponins.[55]

Cynodon dactylon has not been evaluated for anxiolytic effects in human trials. However, several studies have found anxiolytic-like effects of the herb in laboratory animals. An alcohol extract exhibited anxiolytic-like effects of mice in the elevated plus maze and open field tests, and did so without affecting motor coordination.[56] In another study, treatment with aqueous extract of *Cynodon dactylon* in mice produced anxiolytic-like effects in the elevated plus maze and open field that were comparable to those of diazepam. The treatment also produced significant antidepressant effects in the forced swim and tail suspension tests.[57] Treatment with a hydroalcoholic extract of *Cynodon dactylon* also ameliorated irradiation-induced anxiety-like behaviors of mice in the open field. In that study, potent antioxidant effects were noted.[58]

8.2.13 *EVOLVULUS ALSINOIDES*

Evolvulus alsinoides, also known as dwarf morning glory, is an herb whose anxiolytic effects have been studied in clinical trials. The herb on its own has shown significant relief from anxiety in human subjects. See Chapter 6.

8.2.14 *FICUS RELIGIOSA*

Ficus religiosa is a food and medicinal plant whose bark, fruit, leaves, and seeds are widely used in indigenous systems of medicine. The plant has a wide spectrum of pharmacological activities including anticonvulsant, anthelmintic, anti-amnesic, anti-anxiety, anti-asthmatic, antibacterial, antioxidant, anti-inflammatory, and anti-ulcer effects.[59] The stem, bark, root, bark, and fruit of the plant have medicinal properties and contain a variety of phenols, tannins, steroids, alkaloids, and flavonoids. Among these are stigmasterol, β-sitosterol, kaempferol, quercetin, myricetin, bergapten, and begaptol.[60]

There are no human studies of anxiolytic effects of *Ficus religiosa*. However, several animal studies have shown such anxiolytic-like effects. In one such study, an aqueous extract of trunk bark showed an anxiolytic-like effect in rats in the Vogel conflict test. Additional testing in the hole board apparatus showed no reduction in motor activity or coordination.[61] Another study showed that an aqueous extract of the root attenuated anxiety-like behavior in the open field, potentiated pentobarbital-induced sleep, and ameliorated pentylenetetrazol-induced seizures.[62]

8.2.15 GLYCYRRHIZA GLABRA

Glycyrrhiza glabra, one of several species referred to as licorice, is a common ingredient in Ayurvedic treatments of anxiety and mood disorder. The closely related herb *Glycyrrhiza uralensis* is also used in Ayurvedic medicine as well as in traditional Chinese herbal treatments. Indeed, the dried rhizome and root of *Glycyrrhiza glabra* and related species have been used by the Egyptian, Chinese, Greek, Indian, and Roman civilizations. Licorice was known in Chinese medicine as early as 2800 BCE. Phytochemical screening of the *Glycyrrhiza glabra* root has revealed the presence of alkaloids, glycosides, carbohydrates, starches, phenolic compounds, flavonoids, proteins, pectin, mucilage, saponins, lipids, tannins, sterols, and steroids. Prominent among them are liquiritic acid, glycyrretol, glabrolide, iso-glaborlide, liquiritin, isoliquiritin, isoliquiritigenin, neoisoliquiritin, licuraside, glabridin, shinptcrocarpin, linalool, prasterone, anethole, eugenol, pinene, lavandulol, α-terpineol, β-caryophyllene, and carvacrol.[63] Many among those phytochemicals have been found to exert their own anxiolytic effects.

Despite its widespread use, there are no clinical studies of anxiolytic effects of *Glycyrrhiza glabra*. Nonetheless, there are animal studies demonstrating such effects. In a study of mice, hydroalcoholic extract of roots and rhizomes of *Glycyrrhiza glabra* produced anxiolytic effects in the elevated plus maze and foot shock-induced aggression paradigms.[64] Treatment with a hydroalcoholic extract of *Glycyrrhiza glabra* also ameliorated stress-induced anxiety-like behavior in mice in the mirror chamber paradigm. In that study, the extract was administered daily prior to forced swimming over 15 days. The herbal extract did not cause any motor impairment. Indeed, treated animals exhibited more locomotor activity than stressed control animals.[65] In a voltage clamp electrophysiological study, glabridin, a flavonoid found in *Glycyrrhiza glabra*, enhanced the effects of GABA in *Xenopus laevis* oocytes expressing recombinant GABA-A receptors. This effect of glabridin was insensitive to flumazenil. Thus, some anxiolytic effects of *Glycyrrhiza glabra* may be mediated by increases in GABAergic activity.[66]

8.2.16 HYOSCYAMUS NIGER

Hyoscyamus niger, known as *parasika yavani* in Ayurvedic medicine, is a potent yet potentially perilous treatment. It seeds are seen as useful in the treatment of various *unmada*, or psychological disorders; *anidra*, or insomnia; and *pralapa*, or restlessness. It is a common ingredient in combinations of herbs used to treat *chittod-vega*, or anxiety. It is perilous in that it contains potent anticholinergic substances, in particular the alkaloids scopolamine and atropine. Several case studies report severe adverse effects.[67]

There are no accessible, formal studies of anxiolytic effects of *Hyoscyamus niger* in human subjects. Interestingly, there are several reports (albeit from a single set of researchers) about clinical anxiolytic effects of scopolamine, a primary active component of *Hyoscyamus niger*. This treatment is the combination of scopolamine and the beta-blocker atenolol.[68] This treatment would essentially disable large components of the autonomic nervous system.

8.2.17 JUGLANS REGIA

Juglans regia, the walnut, is most commonly seen as a food plant. However, the nut, bark, leaf, and seed husks have long been used as natural remedies in folk medicines throughout Asia, Europe, and the Indian subcontinent. Its uses have been as varied as a mosquito repellant and lice killer; for the treatment of itching, chronic dysentery, frostbite, constipation, rheumatism, dandruff, muscular pain, and poor eye sight; and as a brain tonic and aphrodisiac.[69] The phytochemical analysis of the bark of *Juglans regia* showed that it contained alkaloids, tannins, phenols, and saponins. The leaves contain alkaloids, cardiac glycosides, flavonoids, saponins, steroids, and tannins. The nuts contain saturated, monounsaturated, and polyunsaturated fats.[70]

There are no evaluations of anxiolytic effects of *Juglans regia* in humans. However, a hydroalcoholic extract of *Juglans regia* kernels in mice significantly increased exploration and time spent in open areas of the elevated plus maze, as well as time spent in the light areas in the light and dark model. These are recognized as anxiolytic-like effects. Increases were also noted in head twitching, an indicator of enhancement of activity at 5-HT2 receptors.[71] Extract of *Juglans regia* has also produced antidepressant-like effects in the forced swimming and tail suspension tests.[72] Of note, extract of the nut kernel exhibited an anticonvulsant effect in rats, an effect that is common among anxiolytic medications, particularly those that affect GABA activity. However, the anticonvulsant effects of the plant were not attenuated by flumazenil. On the other hand, it enhanced the anticonvulsant effect of diazepam.[73]

8.2.18 LAWSONIA INERMIS

Lawsonia inermis, commonly known as henna, is a perennial herbaceous plant belonging to the family *Lythraceae*. Traditionally it has been used to treat skin diseases, dysentery, bronchitis, anemia, and inflammation. The plant contains a variety of phenolic compounds, flavonoids, saponins, proteins, alkaloids, terpenoids, quinones, coumarins, and xanthones.[74]

In one study, a methanolic extract of the leaves of *Lawsonia inermis* produced an anxiolytic-like effect in mice in the elevated plus maze.[75] In a similar study, treatment of mice with a hydroalcoholic extract of *Lawsonia inermis* increased both open arm exploration in the elevated plus maze and nose poking in the hole board test. Interestingly, no antidepressant-like effects were noted.[76]

8.2.19 MORINGA OLEIFERA

Moringa oleifera is commonly known as the drumstick tree or shevga. Different parts of these plants—the leaves, pods, seeds, gums, bark, and flowers—are used for the treatment of various ailments in Ayurvedic medicine. Among the conditions treated with the herb is anxiety. Several bioactive compounds have been purified from the leaves of Moringa oleifera, including carotenoids, polyphenols, phenolic acids, flavonoids, alkaloids, glucosinolates, isothiocyanates, tannins, saponins, oxalates, and phytates.[77]

There are no dependable human trials of Moringa oleifera for anxiety. However, several studies have shown anxiolytic-like effects of the herb in rodents. In one study, an aqueous but not ethanolic extract of Moringa oleifera produced an anxiolytic-like effect in mice in the open field and light/dark box.[78] In another study, treatment of mice with an aqueous extract of Moringa oleifera produced significant anxiolytic effects in the elevated plus maze, open field test, and hole board apparatus. In that study, the herb also had significant antiepileptic effects. It was suggested, though not proved, that those effects were mediated by GABAergic activity.[79] A study of mice found that the anxiolytic effects of Moringa oleifera were blocked by flumazenil, suggesting an enhancement of GABAergic activity through agonist effects at the benzodiazepine binding site.[80]

8.2.20 NARDOSTACHYS JATAMANSI

Nardostachys jatamansi is one of the few herbs in this discussion that has been evaluated in a human trial and found to be an effective anxiolytic. Several of its constituent phytochemicals, including ursolic acid, aristolen-9 β-ol, and β-sitosterol, have themselves been found to have anxiolytic effects in animals. See Chapter 6.

8.2.21 PIPER NIGRUM

Piper nigrum is one of the most popular spice products in Asia. The fruits of Piper nigrum have been widely used for thousands of years in household spices as the condiment, black pepper. However, it has also traditionally been used for the treatment of malaria in India and epilepsy in China. It is a component of many herbal combinations used to treat anxiety. Piper nigrum contains many bioactive compounds, including betaine, achyranthine, 10-tricosanone, 10-octacosanone, 4-tritriacontanone, piperolactam D, pellitorine, piperidine, piperine, sylvamide, cepharadione A, and paprazine.[81]

There are several studies of anxiolytic effects of Piper nigrum in rodents. A methanolic extract of Piper nigrum produced an anxiolytic-like effect in mice in the elevated plus maze, and this effect was comparable to that of diazepam.[82] A methanolic extract of Piper nigrum also produced anxiolytic- and antidepressant-like effects in a rat model of Alzheimer's disease.[83] In another study, the anxiolytic-like effect of the essential oil of Piper nigrum on mice in the elevated plus maze was blocked by the 5-HT1A antagonist WAY-100635 but not by the benzodiazepine antagonist flumazenil. Of note, the essential oil also produced an antidepressant-like effect in the mice in the tail suspension test.[84]

8.2.22 PUNICA GRANATUM

Punica granatum, the common pomegranate, is one of the first domesticated fruits. It is indigenous to the Middle East, the Mediterranean, Anatolia, Central Asia, and regions of India up into the Himalayas. Many parts of the plant have been used for medicinal purposes. Pomegranate fruit has anti-inflammatory and antibacterial activities. The seed oil has been thought to have inhibitory effects on skin and breast cancers. The pomegranate seed oil has phytoestrogenic compounds, and the fruit is rich in phenolic compounds with strong antioxidant activity. The fruit and bark of *Punica granatum* are used against intestinal parasites, dysentery, and diarrhea. The leaves have been used in traditional medicines for epilepsy and anxiety. Phytochemicals in *Punica granatum* include ellagic acid, gallic acid, chlorogenic acid, cinnamic acid, hydroxy protocatechuic acid, hydroxy benzoic acid, caffeic acid, ferulic acid, coumaric acid, p-coumaric acid, o-coumaric acid, pelletierine, isopelletierine, methylpelletierine, pseudopelletierine, punicalagin, punicalin, phloridzin, quercetin, luteolin, kaempferol, and narigenin.[85] Many of these substances have been found to possess anxiolytic effects.

There are no published studies of anxiolytic effects of *Punica granatum* in humans. However, there are numerous such studies in laboratory animals. Administration of the juice of *Punica granatum* for 15 days produced modest anxiolytic-like effects in rats in the open field and elevated plus maze. Antidepressant-like effects were also noted in the forced swimming test.[86] Single doses of the juice of *Punica granatum* produced similar anxiolytic-like effects in mice in the elevated plus maze and hole board apparatus.[87] In another study, an ethanolic extract of leaves of *Punica granatum* exerted an anxiolytic-like effect in mice in the elevated plus maze that was similar to that produced by diazepam. The extract also produced a potent anticonvulsant effect in rats.[88]

8.2.23 SAUSSUREA LAPPA

Saussurea lappa is a plant native to the mountainous regions of India. In Ayurvedic tradition, the root of this plant is used for skin conditions, vomiting, headache, epilepsy, hysteria, and as a tonic to balance the three *doshas*. Its active principles are costunolide, germacrene, lappadilactone, isodihydrocostunolide, cynaropicrin, linoleic acid, cyclocostunolide, alantolactone, isoalantolactone, and various sesquiterpene-saussureamines.[89] It is also used in traditional Chinese medicine and was discussed in Shen Nong's ancient text on herbal treatments.[90]

There are no human trials of *Saussurea lappa*. However, animal studies reveal anxiolytic effects and possible mechanisms. Administration of extract of *Saussurea lappa* to mice had anxiolytic effects in the open field and elevated plus maze.[91] Anticonvulsant effects of the plant in mice were attributed to enhancement of GABA activity.[92]

8.2.24 TINOSPORA CORDIFOLIA

Tinospora cordifolia is known in Ayurvedic medicine as *guduchi*. The herb is native to India and is an ancient Ayurvedic herbal remedy for anxiety and other nervous disorders. It is considered as a *rasayana*, with the ability to rejuvenate and build resiliency. It is an herb that has been shown in clinical study to have anxiolytic effects in patients diagnosed with GAD. It also has antidepressant effects in human subjects. See Chapter 6.

8.2.25 VALERIANA JATAMANSI

Valeriana jatamansi has long been used in both Ayurvedic and traditional Chinese medicine as a sedative and anxiolytic. It is one of the few herbs that has been evaluated in a clinical study, although none of the subjects had been diagnosed with a formal anxiety disorder. Its ability to relieve presurgical anxiety was comparable to that of the benzodiazepine diazepam. See Chapter 6.

8.2.26 VITEX NEGUNDO

Vitex negundo is an ancient medicinal plant. Its Sanskrit name is nirgundi. However, it is sometimes referred to as the Chinese chaste tree. As with Vitex agnus-castus, it has found use in treating disorders of the female reproductive system and increasing sexual desire. As discussed in Chapter 6, Vitex agnus-castus has been used to treat the emotional disturbances of menopause. Leaves, seeds, and roots have medicinal properties. Among the many flavonoids, alkaloids, saponins, and iridoid glycosides identified in Vitex negundo are β-sitosterol, stigmasterol, vitexin, isovitexin, luteolin, orientin, wogonin, pinene, 3-carene, limonene, linalool, geraniol, β-caryophyllene, and ursolic acid.[93] Many of those phytochemicals have been found to exhibit anxiolytic properties on their own.

In a study in mice, acute administration of an ethanolic extract of the roots of Vitex negundo showed an anxiolytic-like effect in the elevated plus maze and light/dark exploration test. The effect was seen as comparable to that of the benzodiazepine diazepam. These effects occurred without any overt motor dysfunction.[94] An ethanolic extract of the leaves of this plant produced a similar anxiolytic effect.[95]

8.2.27 WITHANIA SOMNIFERA

Withania somnifera, known in India as ashwagandha, is a medicinal herb from the Solanaceae, or nightshade, family. It is native to India, China, and Nepal and is commonly used in Ayurvedic medicine to calm the mind, relieve weakness and nervous exhaustion, build sexual energy, and promote healthy sleep. The herb is considered to be a rasayana, meaning it bestows longevity and vitality. It has been shown in clinical studies to be effective in relieving anxiety in patients diagnosed with GAD, mixed anxiety and depression, adjustment disorder with anxiety, and panic disorder. See Chapter 6.

REFERENCES

1. Chopra A, Doiphode VV. Ayurvedic medicine. Core concept, therapeutic principles, and current relevance. *Med Clin North Am.* 2002;86(1):75–89.

2. Amin H, Vyas M. Evaluation of *Pradhana sharira* and *Manas prakriti* (bodily and mental constitution) on disease manifestations in generalized anxiety disorder. *Int J Clin.* 2016;3(4):171–179.

3. Pole S. *Ayurvedic Medicine: The Principles of Traditional Practice.* London: Jessica Kingsley Publishers; 2013.

4. Sheldon WH. *The Varieties of Human Physique.* New York: Harper; 1940.

5. Patwardhan B. Bridging Ayurveda with evidence-based scientific approaches in medicine. *EPMA.* 2014;5(1):1–7.

6. Meena AK, Bansal P, Kumar S. Plants-herbal wealth as a potential source of Ayurvedic drugs. *Asian J Tradit Med.* 2009;4(4):152–170.

7. Balkrishna A, Misra LN. Ayurvedic plants in brain disorders: The herbal hope. *J Tradit Med Clin Natur.* 2017;6:221–230.

8. Parasuraman S, Thing GS, Dhanaraj SA. Polyherbal formulation: Concept of ayurveda. *Pharmacog Rev.* 2014;8(16):73–80.

9. Vishal G, Narayan Prakash B, Suhas KS, et al. Comparative study on the efficacy of *ashvagandha churna* and *ashvagandha* compound in the management of generalized anxiety disorder (*chittodvega*). *Int J Pharm Thera.* 2014;5(3):220–226.

10. Ramana GV. Clinical evaluation of *Ashwagandha* and *Mandookaparni* in the management of *Manodwega* (generalized anxiety disorder). *J Res Ayurvedic Sci.* 2018;2(2):70–79.

11. Farzana M, Sultana A. *Clinical Study of Glycyrrhiza Glabra Linn and Asparagus Racemosus Linn on Menopausal Symptoms.* Proceedings in Medicine, 8th International Research Conference—KDU, Sri Lanka; 2015. pp. 27–29.

12. Pillai CC, Chacko J, Soman D, et al. Ayurvedic management of generalized anxiety disorder—a case report. *J Ayu Herb Med.* 2018;4(3):111–113.

13. Boral GC, Bandopadyaya G, Boral A, et al. Geriforte in anxiety neurosis. *Indian J Psychiat.* 1989;31(3):258–260.

14. Upadhyaya L, Tiwari AK, Agrawal A, et al. Role of an indigenous drug geriforte on blood levels of biogenic amines and its significance in the treatment of anxiety neurosis. *Activ Nerv Super.* (Czechoslovakia). 1990;32:1.

15. Kulatunga RDH. A clinical study on the effect of *Medhya Rasayana* therapy on anxiety and depression in senile dementia. *IAMY.* 2018;6(4):752–758.

16. Ahir Y, Tanna I, Ravishankar B, et al. Evaluation of clinical effect of *Kushmandadi Ghrita* in generalized anxiety disorder. *Indian J Tradit Know.* 2011;10(2):239–246.

17. Chaudhuri K, Samarakoon SM, Chandola HM, et al. Clinical evaluation of *Medhyarasayana Ghrita* along with *Vachadi Ghrita Nasya* (*Pratimarsha*) on senile dementia. *Indian J Ancient Med Yoga.* 2010;3(3):113–120.

18. Dixit SP, Agrawal U, Dubey G. Executive fatigue and its management with 'mentat.' *Pharmacopsychoecologia.* 1993;6:7–9.

19. Sharma AK, Agrawal A, Agrawal U, et al. Influence of mentat on memory and mental fatigue in cases of anxiety neurosis and depression. *Ind J Cancer Bio Res.* 1990;3(1):27–30.

20. Seely D, Singh R. Adaptogenic potential of a polyherbal natural health product: Report on a longitudinal clinical trial. *eCAM.* 2007;4(3):375–380.

21. Divya Z, Kalpana P. *A Comparative Clinical Study of Panchagavya Ghrita Nasya and Sarsvata Choorna in the Management of Chittodvega w.s.r. to Generalized Anxiety Disorder.* Jamnagar: Department of Panchakarma, PG Dissertation Submitted to Gujrat Ayurved University; 2017.

22. Gupta K, Mamidi P, Thakar A. Randomized placebo controlled study on *Sarasvata choorna* in generalized anxiety disorder. *Int J Green Pharm.* 2014;231–236.

23. Radheyshyam T, Tripathi JS, Sanjay G, et al. Pharmaceutical and clinical studies on compounds Ayurvedic formulations, *Saraswatha churna. Int Res J Pharm.* 2011;2:77–84.

24. Sen G, Bose K. Rauwolfia serpentina, a new Indian drug for insanity and high blood pressure. *Indian Med World*. 1931;2:194–201.

25. Glynn JD. Rauwolfia serpentina (Serpasil) in psychiatry. *J Neurol Neurosurg Psychiat*. 1955;18:225–227.

26. Mishra D, Tubaki BR. Effect of *Brahmi vati* and *Sarpagandha Ghana vati* in management of essential hypertension—a randomized, double blind, clinical study. *J Ayurveda Integr Med*. 2019;10(4):269–276.

27. Ferguson RS. A clinical trial of reserpine in the treatment of anxiety. *J Ment Sci*. 1956;102(426):30–42.

28. Muller JC, Pryor WW, Gibbons JE, et al. Depression and anxiety occurring during *Rauwolfia* therapy. *JAMA*. 1955;159(9):836–839.

29. Rao P, Saroj UR, Joshi RK. Clinical evaluation of the efficacy of *shankhapushpi panak* and *shirodhara* with *mansyadi kwatha* in the management of *chittodvega* w.S.R. To generalized anxiety disorder. *World J Pharm Res*. 2016;5(1):1312–1328.

30. Mishra J, Joshi NP, Pandya DM. A comparative study of *Shankhapushpyadi Ghana Vati* and *Sarpagandhadi Ghana Vati* in the management of "essential hypertension." *Ayu*. 2012;33(1):54–61.

31. Mangal A, Jadhav AD. Evaluation of the efficacy and safety of Ayurvedic drug (*vacha brahmi ghan*) in the management of *manodwega* (anxiety neurosis). *J Res Educ Indian Med*. 2012;18(3–4):143–148.

32. Mills PJ, Farag NH, Newton RP, et al. Effects of a traditional herbal supplement on anxiety in patients with generalized anxiety disorder. *J Clin Psychopharmacol*. 2002;22:443–444.

33. Balkrishna A, Misra LN. Ayurvedic plants in brain disorders: The herbal hope. *J Tradit Med Clin Natur*. 2017;6:2.

34. Verma SC, Vashishth E, Singh R, et al. A review on parts of *Albizia lebbeck* (L.) Benth. Used as Ayurvedic drugs. *Res J Pharm Tech*. 2013;6(11):1235–1241.

35. Une HD, Kasture V. Nootropic and anxiolytic activity of saponins of *Albizzia lebbeck* leaves. *Pharmacol Biochem Behav*. 2001;69(3–4):439–444.

36. Teshika JD, Zakariyyah AM, Zaynab T, et al. Traditional and modern uses of onion bulb (*Allium cepa* L.): A systematic review. *Crit Rev Food Sci Nutr*. 2019;59(Supp 1):S39–70.

37. Pitchaiah G, Anusha VL, Hemalatha CH, et al. Anxiolytic and anticonvulsant activity of methanolic extract of *allium cepa* Linn (Onion) bulbs in Swiss albino mice. *J Pharmacog Phytochem*. 2015;4(3):131–135.

38. Samad N, Saleem A. Administration of *Allium cepa* L. bulb attenuates stress-produced anxiety and depression and improves memory in male mice. *Metab Brain Dis*. 2018;33:271–281.

39. Usmani A, Khushtar M, Arif M, et al. Pharmacognostic and phytopharmacology study of *Anacyclus pyrethrum*: An insight. *J Appl Pharm Sci*. 2016;6(3):144–150.

40. Sujith K, Suba V, Darwin CR. Neuropharmacological profile of ethanolic extract of *Anacyclus pyrethrum* in Albino wister rats. *IJPSR*. 2011;2(8):2109–2114.

41. Badhe SR, Badhe RV, Ghaisas MM, et al. Evaluation of antidepressant activity of *Anacyclus pyrethrum* root extract. *Int J Green Pharm*. 2010;4:79–82.

42. Singla R, Jaitak V. *Shatavari* (*Asparagus racemosus* wild): A review on its cultivation, morphology, phytochemistry and pharmacological importance. *IJPSR*. 2014;5(3):742–757.

43. Yadav R, Maheshwari KK, Gupta A, et al. Evaluation of anti-anxiety activity of *Asparagus racemosus* (*satavari*) in rats by using light and dark model. *Int J Rec Res Pharm*. 2020;1(1A):119–125.

44. Garabadu D, Krishnamurthy S. *Asparagus racemosus* attenuates anxiety-like behavior in experimental animal models. *Cell Mol Neurobiol*. 2014;34:511–521.

45. Singh GK, Garabadu D, Muruganandam AV, et al. Antidepressant activity of *Asparagus racemosus* in rodent models. *Pharmacol Biochem Behav.* 2009;91(3):283–290.

46. Al-Snafi AE. The pharmacological importance of *Benincasa hispida.* A review. *Int J Pham Sci Res.* 2013;4(12):165–170.

47. Rachchh MA, Aghera RR, Gokani RH, et al. Evaluation of anxiolytic and anticonvulsant effect of *Benincasa hispida. Res J Pharmacog Phytochem.* 2010;2(6):464–466.

48. Girdhar S, Wanjari M, Prajapati S K, et al. Evaluation of anti-compulsive effect of methanolic extract of *Benincasa hispida* Cogn. fruit in mice. *Acta Pol Pharm.* 2010;67(4):417–421.

49. Dhingra D, Joshi P. Antidepressant-like activity of *Benincasa hispida* fruits in mice: Possible involvement of monoaminergic and GABAergic systems. *J Pharmacol Pharmacother.* 2012;3(1):60–61.

50. Patel S, Sharma V, Chauhan NS, et al. An updated review on the parasitic herb of *Cuscuta reflexa* Roxb. *J Chinese Integr Med.* 2012;10:249–255.

51. Thomas S, Shrikumar S, Velmurugan C, et al. Evaluation of anxiolytic effect of whole plant of *Cuscuta reflexa. World J Pharm Sci.* 2015;4:1245–1253.

52. Ara I, Kalam MA, Maqbool M, et al. Phytochemical standardization and anti-anxiety (*Izterab-e-Nafsani*) study of *Aftimoon Hindi* (*Cuscuta reflexa* Roxb.) on an animal model. *Cell Med.* 2021;11(3):e14, 1–9.

53. Forouzanfar F, Vahedi MM, Aghaei A, et al. Hydroalcoholic extract of *Cuscuta Epithymum* enhances pentobarbital-induced sleep: Possible involvement of GABAergic system. *Curr Drug Dis Tech.* 2020;17(3):332–337.

54. Ashokkumar K, Selvaraj K, Muthukrishnan SD. *Cynodon dactylon* (L.) Pers.: An updated review of its phytochemistry and pharmacology. *J Med Plant Res.* 2013;7(48):3477–3483.

55. Annapurna HV, Apoorva B, Ravichandran N, et al. Isolation and in silico evaluation of antidiabetic molecules of *Cynodon dactylon* (L.). *J Molec Graph Mod.* 2013;39:87–97.

56. Sherief SH, Sindhura S, Anusha S, et al. Evaluation of anti-anxiety activity of alcoholic extract of *Cyndon dactylon* Linn. In experimental animal models. *Res J Sci Tech.* 2012;4(5):197–202.

57. Kothari S, Sahu M. Evaluation of antianxiety and antidepressant activity of aqueous extract of *Cynodon dactylon* (Doob grass) in Swiss albino mice. *Int J Green Pharm.* 2021;15(2):182.

58. Poojary R, Kumar NA, Kumarchandra M, et al. *Cynodon dactylon* alleviates radiation-induced behavioral and biochemical changes in the cerebral cortex of mice. *Res J Pharm Tech.* 2021;14(5):2569–2575.

59. Kaur A, Rana AC, Tiwari V, et al. Review on ethnomedicinal and pharmacological properties of *Ficus religiosa. J Appl Pharm Sci.* 2011;1(08):6–11.

60. Chandrasekar SB, Bhanumathy M, Pawar AT, et al. Phytopharmacology of *Ficus religiosa. Pharmacogn Rev.* 2010;4(8):195–199.

61. Ratnasooriya WD, Jayakody JRAC, Dharmasiri MG. An aqueous extract of trunk bark of *Ficus religiosa* has anxiolytic activity. *Med Sci Res.* 1998;26:817–819.

62. Panday DR, Rauniar GP. Effect of root-extracts of *Ficus benghalensis* (Banyan) in memory, anxiety, muscle co-ordination and seizure in animal models. *BMC Complement Altern Med.* 2016;16:429.

63. Al-Snafi AE. *Glycyrrhiza glabra*: A phytochemical and pharmacological review. *IOSR J Pharm.* 2018;8(6):1–17.

64. Ambawade SD, Kasture VS, Kasture SB. Anxiolytic activity of *Glycyrrhiza glabra* Linn. *J Nat Remedies.* 2001;2:130–134.

65. Trivedi R, Sharma KJ. Hydroalcoholic extract of *Glycyrrhiza glabra* Linn. Attenuates chronic fatigue stress induced behavioral alterations in mice. *Int J Pharm.* 2011;2(3):996–1001.

66. Hoffmann KM, Beltrán L, Ziemba PM, et al. Potentiating effect of glabridin from *Glycyrrhiza glabra* on GABAA receptors. *Biochem Biophys*. 2016;6:197–202.
67. Aparna K, Joshi AJ, Vyas M. Adverse reaction of *Parasika Yavani* (*Hyoscyamus niger* Linn): Two case study reports. *Ayu*. 2015;36(2):174–176.
68. Dooley TP, Benjamin AB, Thomas T. Treating anxiety with a beta blocker—antimuscarinic combination a review of compounded atenolol—scopolamine. *Clin Psychiat*. 2019;5(3):63.
69. Hassan GA, Tali Bilal A, Ahmad BT, eta al. Economic and ethnomedicinal uses of *Juglans regia* in Kashmir Himalaya. *UJAHM*. 2013;1(3):64–67.
70. Al-Snafi AE. Chemical constituents, nutritional, pharmacological and therapeutic importance of *Juglans regia*-a review. *IOSR J Pharm*. 2018;8:1–21.
71. Chandel HS, Singh S, Pawar A. Neuropharmacological investigation of *Juglans regia* fruit extract with special reference to anxiety. *Int J Drug Res Tech*. 2012;2(7):461–471.
72. Rath BP, Pradhan D. Antidepressant activity of *Juglans regia* L. fruit extract. *Int J Toxicol Pharmacol Res*. 2009;1:24–26.
73. Asadi-Shekaari M, Eslami A, Kalantaripour T. Potential mechanisms involved in the anticonvulsant effect of walnut extract on pentylenetetrazole-induced seizure. *Med Princ Pract*. 2014;23:538–542.
74. Al-Snafi AE. A review on *Lawsonia inermis*: A potential medicinal plant. *Int J Curr Pharm Res*. 2019;11(5):1–13.
75. Mandloi P, Pandey R. Evaluation of anti-anxiety activity of *Lawsonia inermis* Linn. *Int J Pharm Life Sci*. 2019;10(1):6016–6019.
76. Roy P, Thahimon PA, Carla B, et al. CNS activities of hydroalcoholic extract of *Lawsonia inermis* Linn. Root. *Asian J Pharmacol Toxicol*. 2020;3(7):7–13.
77. Mishra G, Singh P, Verma R, et al. Traditional uses, phytochemistry and pharmacological properties of *Moringa oleifera* plant: An overview. *Der Pharmacia Lettre*. 2011;3:141–164.
78. Islam MT, Martins N, Imran M, et al. Anxiolytic-like effects of *Moringa oleifera* in Swiss mice. *Cell Mol Biol*. 2020;66(4):73–77.
79. Ingale SP, Gandhi FP. Effect of aqueous extract of moringa oleifera leaves on pharmacological models of epilepsy and anxiety in mice. *Int J Epilepsy*. 2016;03(01):12–19.
80. Aburawi S, Shushni M, Alkateb M. Effect of *Moringa Oleifera* extract on behavior using male albino mice. *Alq J Med App Sci*. 2021;4(1):1–12.
81. Ee G, Lim C, Lim C, et al. Alkaloids from *Piper sarmentosum* and *Piper nigrum*. *Nat Prod Res*. 2009;23(15):1416–1423.
82. Emon NU, Kaiser M, Islam M, et al. Anxiolytic and thrombolytic investigation of methanol extract of *Piper nigrum* L. Fruits and *Sesamum indicum* L. seeds. *J Adv Biotechnol Exp Ther*. 2020;3(3):158–164.
83. Hritcu L, Noumedem JA, Cioanca O, et al. Anxiolytic and antidepressant profile of the methanolic extract of *Piper nigrum* fruits in beta-amyloid (1–42) rat model of Alzheimer's disease. *Behav Brain Funct*. 2015;11(13):1–13.
84. Ghosh S, Kumar A, Sachan N, et al. Anxiolytic and antidepressant-like effects of essential oil from the fruits of *Piper nigrum* Linn. (Black pepper) in mice: Involvement of serotonergic but not GABAergic transmission system. *Heliyon*. 2021;7(4):e06884.
85. Shaygannia E, Bahmani M, Zamanzad B, et al. A review study on *Punica granatum* L. *J Evid Based Complementary Altern Med*. 2016;21(3):221–227.
86. Riaz A, Khan RA. Effect of *Punica granatum* on behavior in rats. *Afr J Pharmacy Pharmacol*. 2014;8(44):1118–1126.
87. Kulkarni S, Bathe R, Javalgikar A. Evaluation of *Punica granatum* fruit juice for anti-anxiety activity. *Int J Biomed Adv Res*. 2016;7(9):452–455.
88. Das S, Sarma P. A study on the anticonvulsant and anti-anxiety activity of ethanolic extract of *Punica granatum* Linn. *Int J Pharm Sci*. 2014;6:389–392.

89. Madhuri K, Elango K, Ponnusankar S. *Saussurea lappa* (Kuth root): Review of its traditional uses, phytochemistry and pharmacology. *Orient Pharm Exp Med*. 2012;12:1–9.
90. Wei H, Yan LH, Feng WH, et al. Research progress on active ingredients and pharmacologic properties of *Saussurea lappa*. *Curr Opin Complement Alternat Med*. 2014;1(1):16–22.
91. Ambavade SD, Mhetre NA, Patil KM. Anxiolytic activity of root extract of *Saussurea lappa* Clark. in mice. *J Nat Remedies*. 2006;6:103–108.
92. Ambavade SD, Mhetre NA, Muthal AP, et al. Pharmacological evaluation of anticonvulsant activity of root extract of *Saussurea lappa* in mice. *Eur J Integr Med*. 2009;1(3):131–137.
93. Vimal A, LoharVikram SS, Anil B. *Vitexnegundo*: A Chinese chaste tree. *IJPI*. 2011;1(5):9–20.
94. Adnaik RS, Pai PT, Sapakal VD, et al. Anxiolytic activity of *Vitex Negundo* Linn. In experimental models of anxiety in mice. *Int J Green Pharm*. 2009;3:243–247.
95. Aswar MK, Bidkar AA, Gujar KN, et al. Anxiolytic like effects of leaves extract of *Vitex negundo* (L) -(Fam:Verbaceae) in elevated plus maze test. *J Nat Remedies*. 2012;72(2):141–150.

9 Adaptogens

Some herbs can act rapidly to provide relief from occasional, acute anxiety. However, for many individuals, anxiety is a severe and ongoing problem. In those cases, a different form of treatment is required. A concern in the management of chronic anxiety is building resistance to stress and maintaining the body's ability to remain resilient against the damage chronic stress can produce. Such damage in the body and central nervous system has been referred to as allostatic load.

An important manifestation of allostatic load is dysregulation of the hypothalamic-pituitary-adrenal axis. Chronic stress can result in decreased activity of corticotrophin-releasing hormone in the hypothalamus but increased activity in the amygdala. These effects diminish the ability of the hypothalamic-pituitary-adrenal axis to mount a stress response and at the same time amplify the amygdala's response during states of fear and anxiety.[1] Individuals with PTSD may suffer states of hypocortisolemia that can produce persistent states of inflammation in the body and central nervous system.[2] Inflammation then contributes to the underlying pathophysiology of chronic anxiety.[3] It has long been known that individuals suffering severe major depression can have a diminished response to cortisol, as if a state of cortisol resistance has evolved. This is revealed in failures to reduce cortisol levels in the dexamethasone suppression test. However, individuals suffering GAD can have the paradoxical combination of basal hypocortisolemia as well as failure to respond to dexamethasone suppression of cortisol release.[4] Persistent stress also contributes to metabolic syndrome, with insulin resistance and increased release of inflammatory cytokines from visceral fat. Those conditions then further exacerbate anxiety and depression.[5] All in all, it may be said that ongoing anxiety and stress perpetuate further anxiety and stress.

There is a class of herbs, referred to as adaptogens, that may help build resiliency against stress as well as maintain the ability of the brain to respond to new physiological challenges, which can be compromised during chronic stress.[6] This would lessen the reactivity of the brain under anxiety-provoking conditions, as well as allow the nervous system to re-equilibrate between episodes of stress. The term *adaptogen* was coined by the Russian researcher Israel Brekhman and was initially used to describe the ability of the herb *Eleutherococcus senticosus* to improve stamina and optimize utilization of oxygen during extreme physical exertion.[7] In subsequent years, research has led to the compilation of a long list of herbs that act as adaptogens. Many have been used since antiquity in Chinese, Ayurvedic, and Western traditions to build strength and resiliency against stress and disease. These herbs can be used to address the variety of cumulative pathological changes that chronic stress and illness can cause.

Clinical studies suggest that adaptogenic herbs act, at least in part, by buffering and bolstering the hypothalamic-pituitary-adrenal axis. Daily treatment with *Withania somnifera* over 60 days significantly decreased serum cortisol and C-reactive protein,

DOI: 10.1201/9781003300281-9

a protein positively associated with inflammation.[8] Acute administration of *Bacopa monnieri* lowered cortisol levels in saliva.[9] A single treatment with *Ginkgo biloba* extract similarly lowered levels of cortisol in the saliva of stressed human subjects.[10] Human subjects suffering from stress-related fatigue, or burnout, treated for 28 days with extract of *Rhodiola rosea* had lower morning levels of cortisol and lower degrees of burnout.[11] The same effect was seen in human subjects who, during extreme physical exertion, had lower levels of cortisol after treatment with *Schizandra chinensis* or *Bryonia alba*.[12]

Many adaptogen plant species, for example, *Panax ginseng*, *Scutellaria baicalensis*, *Schizandra chinensis*, *Withania somnifera*, *Poria cocos*, and *Eleutherococcus senticosus*, contain tetra- or pentacyclic triterpenoids that structurally resemble glucocorticoids.[13–16] Thus, adaptogens may act in part at glucocorticoid receptors to buffer extremes of glucocorticoid effects in the brain and body. They may normalize stress-induced cortisol release and cortisol resistance, which prolong the stress response and exacerbate anxiety and mood instability.

Ginsenoside Rg1, a steroid-like tetracyclic triterpene glycoside found in *Panax ginseng*, acts as a glucorticoid agonist and anti-inflammatory agent.[17] Bacopaside I, a tetracyclic saponin extracted from *Bacopa monneri*, is also steroid-like in structure. It has antidepressant-like effects in chronically stressed rodents. This effect appeared to be due, at least in part, to buffering of the hypothalamic-pituitary-adrenal axis. It also activates the brain-derived neurotrophic factor signaling pathway.[18] Steroid-like triterpenes from *Ganoderma lucida*, *Poria cocos*, and other mushrooms have been found to act at glucocorticoid receptors.[19]

Some phytochemicals in adaptogens may act upon the hypothalamic-pituitary-adrenal axis, but without having steroid-like structures. Schisandrin A is one of several tricyclic lignans contained in *Schisandra chinensis*. Although not a steroid in structure, it was found to reverse dexamethasone-induced muscle atrophy in rodents.[20] Salidroside is one of the primary active components in *Rhodiola rosea*. It is a small, phenylethanoid glucoside molecule and not even remotely steroid-like in structure. Nonetheless, it acts as a buffer of glucocorticoid activity. For example, it was found to block steroid-induced avascular necrosis of the femoral head in rodents.[21] Curcumin, from *Curcuma longa*, is not a steroid-like molecule, but rather a diarylheptanoid. Still, it was found to alleviate glucocorticoid-induced osteoporosis in rodents, perhaps indirectly, through the regulation of the Wnt signaling pathway.[22]

In a recent in-depth review of adaptogens, Alexander Panossian, one of the leading figures in the area, suggested mechanisms of action other than modulating the hypothalamic-pituitary-adrenal axis. He noted that some herbs contain phenylpropanoids and lignan dimers that might instead buffer the autonomic nervous system, an important arm of the stress response. He also noted the ability of adaptogens to influence the activities of BDNF, CREB, mTOR, FOXO3 SIRT, NRF2, Nf-kB, and other cell signaling participants to reduce inflammation and enhance cell repair and maintenance.[23] In this regard, it should be noted that adaptogens, and virtually all other herbs, contain flavonoids that have the capacity to interact with the MAPK cascades within neurons. This biochemical cascade mediates many of the cell signaling systems involved in inflammation, stress, and cell maintenance.[24] Those systems, in turn, modulate mood and resiliency. Thus, it must be appreciated that there are various systems deep in the chemical machinery of neurons that mediate stress, inflammation, oxidative damage, and other challenges that can destabilize the brain and prevent it from functioning properly. Buffering these chronic weaknesses and imbalances can enhance brain function and general well-being and can help break the cycles of recurring episodes of debilitating anxiety.

In his review, Panossian lists a large number of such adaptogen herbs, albeit identified not from clinical studies but rather from traditional use or animal studies. Among those herbs are: *Ajuga turkestanica, Alstonia scholaris, Anacyclus pyrethrum, Andrographis paniculate, Argyreia nervosa, Argyreia speciosa, Bergenia crassifolia, Bryonia alba, Caesalpinia bonduc, Centella asiatica, Chlorophytum borivilianum, Chrysactinia mexicana, Convolvulus prostrates, Curculigo orchioides, Curcuma longa, Dioscorea deltoidei, Drypetes roxburghii, Evolvulus alsinoides, Firmiana simplex, Gentiana pedicellate, Heteropterys aphrodisiaca, Hippophae rhamnoides, Holoptelea integrifolia, Hoppea dichotoma, Hypericum perforatum, Lepidium peruvianum, Ligusticum striatum, Melilotus officinalis, Morus alba, Mucuna pruriens, Nelumbo nucifera, Oplopanax elatus, Pandanus odoratissimus, Paullinia cupana, Pfaffia paniculate, Potentilla alba, Ptychopetalum olacoides, Rhaponticum carthamoides, Rhodiola heterodonta, Rostellularia diffusa, Salvia miltiorrhiza, Serratula inermis, Sida cordifolia, Silene italica, Sinomenium acutum, Solanum torvum, Sutherlandia frutescens, Trichilia catigua, Trichopus zeylanicus, Turnera diffusa,* and *Vitis vinifera.*

In older, primarily herb-based medical traditions, the use of adaptogens is well accepted. In traditional Chinese medicine, there are tonic herbs that have long been used to improve low body resistance and weak constitution or to add support when the body is finding it difficult to fight severe diseases.[25] These various herbs have been categorized as those that strengthen *Qi,* blood, *yin,* or *yang* in the body. Among these tonic herbs are *Panax ginseng, Rhodiola crenulata, Astragalus membranaceus, Glycyrrhiza uralensis, Eleutherococcus senticosus, Atractylodes macrocephala, Angelica sinensis, Epimedium brevicornu, Psoralea corylifolia, Stachys geobombycis, Asparagus cochinchinensis,* and *Polygonatum odoratum.* Many of these herbs are found on various lists of adaptogenic herbs as well as in traditional Chinese combinations used for the treatment of depression-like syndromes. In Ayurveda, the ancient traditional medicine of India, adaptogenic herbs are referred to as *rasayana* and have included *Tinospora cordifolia, Asparagus racemosus, Emblica officinalis, Withania somnifera, Piper longum, Terminalia chebula,* and others.[26]

In traditional Western herbalism, there has never been a specific category of herbs defined as "antidepressants." Rather, there have been herbs known as nervines that act upon the nervous system as tonics, relaxants, or stimulants. Marisa Marciano, a naturopath, herbalist, and author, has noted similarities between nervines and adaptogens. "Nervine tonics are perhaps the most important contribution herbal medicine can make in the area of stress and anxiety, as they will strengthen and feed the nervous system in cases of nervous debility and exhaustion. Adaptogens may also be considered in this group due to their ability to aid the whole body and mind to cope with demands made upon it."[27] David Hoffmann, also a Western herbalist and member of the American Herbalists Guild, provided a list of adaptogens in his book, *Medical Herbalism.*[28] This list includes: *Acanthopanax sessiliflorum, Albizzia julibrissin*, *Aralia alata*, *Aralia manchuria*, *Aralia schmidtii*, *Cicer arietinum*, *Codonoposis pilosula*, *Echinopanax elatus*, *Eleutherococcus senticosus*, *Eucommia ulmoides*, *Ganoderma lucidum*, *Hoppea dicotoma*, *Leuzea carthamoides*, *Ocimum sanctum*, *Panax ginseng*, *Panax quinquefolius*, *Rhodiola rosea*, *Schisandra chinensis*, *Tinospora cordifolia*, *Trichopus zeylanicus*, and *Withania somnifera*. This list overlaps with other such lists, both modern and traditional. Some of these herbs have not been clinically evaluated in human subjects. However, some have been found to have significant anxiolytic and antidepressant effects in clinical studies, whereas others are ingredients of clinically studied Chinese and Ayurvedic herbal combinations.

Many herbs categorized as adaptogens have been found to alleviate anxiety on their own, and they are discussed in Chapter 6. Among those herbs are *Bacopa monnieri*, *Centella asiatica*, *Convolvulus pluricaulis*, *Curcuma longa*, *Eleutherococcus senticosus*, *Evolvulus alsinoides*, *Ganoderma lucidum*, *Ginkgo biloba*, *Hypericum perforatum*, *Lepidium peruvianum*, *Ocimum sanctum*, *Panax ginseng*, *Poria cocos*, *Rhodiola rosea*, *Schisandra chinensis*, *Scutellaria baicalensis*, *Tinospora cordifolia*, and *Withania somnifera*. These herbs, and many other adaptogenic herbs, are also common ingredients in combinations of herbs used in traditional Chinese medicine and Ayurvedic medicine to treat anxiety. Although these herbs can useful for treatment of acute anxiety, one should certainly consider the addition of such adaptogenic herbs in cases of chronic, persisting anxiety disorders.

REFERENCES

1. McEwen BS. Allostasis and allostatic load: Implications for neuropsychopharmacology. *Neuropsychopharmacol.* 2000;22:108–124.
2. Sriram K, Rodriguez-Fernandez M, Doyle FJ. Modeling cortisol dynamics in the neuro-endocrine axis distinguishes normal, depression, and post-traumatic stress disorder (PTSD) in humans. *PLoS Comput Biol.* 2012;8:e1002379.
3. Michopoulos V, Powers A, Gillespie CF, et al. Inflammation in fear- and anxiety-based disorders: PTSD, GAD, and beyond. *Neuropsychopharmacol.* 2017;42:254–270.
4. Hacimusalar Y, Esel E. Evaluation of hypothalamo-pituitary-adrenal axis activity by using dexamethasone suppression test in patients with panic disorder and generalized anxiety disorder. *Dusunen Adam J Psychiatry Neurol Sci.* 2017;30:15–24.
5. Mendelson SD. *Metabolic Syndrome and Psychiatric Illness: Interactions, Pathophysiology, Assessment and Treatment.* London, UK: Academic Press; 2008.
6. Panossian A, Wikman G. Evidence-based efficacy of adaptogens in fatigue, and molecular mechanisms related to their stress-protective activity. *Curr Clin Pharmacol.* 2009;4:198–219.
7. Brekhman II. A new medicinal plant of the family *Araliceae* the spiny *Eleutherococcus.* *Iz Sibir Otdel Akad Nauk USSR.* 1960;9:113–120.
8. Auddy B, Hazra J, Mitra A, et al. A standardized *Withania somnifera* extract significantly reduces stress-related parameters in chronically stressed humans: A double blind, randomized, placebo-controlled trial. *J Am Nutraceut Assoc.* 2008;11(1):50–56.
9. Benson S, Downey LA, Stough C, et al. An acute, double-blind, placebo-controlled cross-over study of 320 mg and 640 mg doses of *Bacopa monnieri* (CDRI 08) on multitasking stress reactivity and mood. *Phytother Res.* 2014;28(4):551–559.
10. Jezova D, Duncko R, Lassanova M, et al. Reduction of rise in blood pressure and cortisol release during stress by *Ginkgo biloba* extract (EGb 761) in healthy volunteers. *J Physiol Pharmacol.* 2002;53(3):337–348.

11. Olsson EM, von Schéele B, Panossian AG. A randomized, double-blind, placebo-controlled, parallel-group study of the standardized extract shr-5 of the roots of *Rhodiola rosea* in the treatment of subjects with stress-related fatigue. *Planta Med.* 2009;75(2):105–112.

12. Panossian AG, Oganessian AS, Ambartsumian M, et al. Effects of heavy physical exercise and adaptogens on nitric oxide content in human saliva. *Phytomedicine.* 1999 Mar;6(1):17–26.

13. Pawar VS, Shivakumar H. A current status of adaptogens: Natural remedy to stress. *Asian Pac J Trop Dis.* 2012;2(Suppl 1):S480–S490.

14. Song QY, Jiang K, Zhao QQ, et al. Eleven new highly oxygenated triterpenoids from the leaves and stems of *Schisandra chinensis. Org Biomol Chem.* 2013;11:1251–1258.

15. Jin-Wook S, Jae-Hun J, Cha-Gyun S, et al. Overexpression of squalene synthase in *Eleutherococcus senticosus* increases phytosterol and triterpene accumulation. *Phytochem.* 2005;66(8):869–877.

16. Tong X-G, Liu J-L, Cheng Y-X, et al. A new pregnane steroid from *Poria cum Radix Pini. J Asian Nat Prod Res.* 2010;12(5):419–423.

17. Du J, Cheng B, Zhu X, et al. Ginsenoside Rg1, a novel glucocorticoid receptor agonist of plant origin, maintains glucocorticoid efficacy with reduced side effects. *J Immunol.* 2011;187(2):942–950.

18. Zu X, Zhang M, Li W, et al. Antidepressant-like effect of Bacopaside I in mice exposed to chronic unpredictable mild stress by modulating the hypothalamic—pituitary—adrenal axis function and activating BDNF signaling pathway. *Neurochem Res.* 2017;42(11):3233–3244.

19. de la Soledad Lagunes-Castro M, Aguila S, Herrera-Covarrubias D, et al. Structure-based virtual screening of sterols and triterpenoids isolated from *Ganoderma* (*Agaricomycetes*) medicinal mushrooms shows differences in their affinity for human glucocorticoid and mineralocorticoid receptors. *Int J Med Mushrooms.* 2021;23(9):1–13.

20. Yeon M, Choi H, Jun HS. Preventive effects of schisandrin a, a bioactive component of *Schisandra chinensis*, on dexamethasone-induced muscle atrophy. *Nutrients.* 2020;12(5):1255.

21. Xue XH, Feng ZH, Li ZX, et al. Salidroside inhibits steroid-induced avascular necrosis of the femoral head via the PI3K/Akt signaling pathway: In vitro and in vivo studies. *Mol Med Rep.* 2018;17(3):3751–3757.

22. Chen Z, Xue J, Shen T, et al. Curcumin alleviates glucocorticoid-induced osteoporosis through the regulation of the Wnt signaling pathway. *Int J Mol Med.* 2016;37(2):329–338.

23. Panossian A. Understanding adaptogenic activity: Specificity of the pharmacological action of adaptogens and other phytochemicals. *Ann NY Acad Sci.* 2017;1401:49–64.

24. Spencer JPE. The interactions of flavonoids within neuronal signaling pathways. *Genes Nutr.* 2007;2(3):257–273.

25. Liao L-Y, He Y-F, Li L. A preliminary review of studies on adaptogens: Comparison of their bioactivity in TCM with that of ginseng-like herbs used worldwide. *Chinese Med.* 2018;13:57.

26. Rege NN, Thatte UM, Dahanukar SA. Adaptogenic properties of six *rasayana* herbs used in Ayurvedic medicine. *Phytother Res.* 1999;13(4):275–291.

27. Marciano M, Vizniak NA. *Botanical Medicine.* Toronto: Prohealth; 2016. p. 52.

28. Hoffmann D. *Medical Herbalism: The Science and Practice of Herbal Medicine.* Rochester, VT: Healing Arts Press; 2003. p. 483.

10 Aromatherapy

Aromatherapy is a technique of using essential oils extracted from herbs to treat diseases. The use of aromatic plant fragrances and oils is ancient. It is mentioned in the Judeo-Christian Bible and in medical texts from ancient Egypt and India. Although the practice is ancient, the word *aromatherapy* is modern. The term was coined in 1937 by French chemist Rene-Maurice Gattefossé in his famous book on the subject.[1] He had some fanciful notions about aromatic oils. He thought that particles of oil may absorb certain frequencies of light or affect magnetic fields in the body. He was a man of his times, but he was wise enough to state in his book, "The chemical action is beyond us, as is the chemical action of most of the remedies already in use. But chemistry is gradually moving toward physics, and physics provides us with some interesting hypotheses." Despite some errors in thinking, his methods were methodical, and he can be said to be the father of modern aromatherapy.

There are two primary methods used in aromatherapy to expose a person to essential oils. One is to inhale the vapors of the oil from the air, either by using some type of vaporizer or placing an oil-infused cloth close to the nose. The other most common technique is to apply the essential oils during massage. Of course, during massage the patient will also be exposed to the aroma of the essential oil. The ancient Ayurvedic technique of *shirodhara* might be considered a special form of aromatherapy. *Shirodhara* comes from the two Sanskrit words, *shiro* (head) and *dhara* (flow). It's a healing technique that involves pouring warm liquid—usually oil, milk, buttermilk, or water containing the essences of herbs—onto the forehead. *Shirodhara* is often combined with a body, scalp, or head massage.

Many physicians and other mainstream health providers discount the effectiveness of aromatherapy. But blanket dismissal is unwarranted. When trying to distinguish between genuine, physiological effects of aromatherapy and merely effects of belief and wishful thinking, i.e., placebo effects, there is a very useful body of scientific literature to rely upon. This is the literature concerning effects of aromatherapy on animals. One might think this means only laboratory rats and mice. Certainly there are many studies showing effects of inhalation of essential oils on laboratory rodents. However, there are also well-documented effects of aromatherapy in sheep,[2] cats,[3] and dogs.[4] One of the most interesting studies—performed at a college of veterinary medicine and published in a well-respected journal of veterinary medicine—concerns calming effects of aromatherapy in horses.[5] This study measured effects of several different essential oils on "Equine Facial Expression, Heart Rate, Respiratory Tidal Volume and Spontaneous Muscle Contractures in M. Temporalis and M. Cleidomastoideus." Most of us are oblivious as to whether horses have facial expression, yet apparently they do. In any case, the far more objective measurements, including muscle tension in the head and neck muscles, clearly show significant effects. Vaporized essential oils of *Chrysopogon zizanioides*, *Nardostachys jatamansi*, *Chamaemelum nobile*, and *Lavandula angustifolia* were evaluated for

DOI: 10.1201/9781003300281-10

effects. The results revealed that all the essential oils significantly lowered heart rate and respiratory tidal volume, a sign of relaxation. Oil of *Nardostachys jatamansi* was best at inducing a relaxed facial expression, whereas *Chamaemelum nobile* oil was most successful at reducing spontaneous muscle twitches. Such clear results in subjects unable to be swayed by placebo effects lend credence to the technique.

Due to a growing number of clinical studies showing successful use of aroma-therapy, and the aforementioned reports of effects in animals, there can no longer be doubt about the effectiveness of this technique. The most compelling question is thus, "What is the mechanism of action?" The most satisfying explanation—especially for doctors trained in Western medicine—is that the active components of the essential oils actually enter the body to produce their effects like any other medication. Phytochemicals in the oil would be absorbed through the skin during vigorous massage. When essential oils are inhaled, some of the volatile components of the oil would enter the nose, get absorbed through mucous membranes of the nasal cavity, and then travel on into the bloodstream to take effect in the body. There is a study in which mice were placed in cages filled with essential oil of lavender that they were forced to inhale. These animals showed evidence of the well-known sedating effect of lavender. Blood samples taken from the mice later showed that linalool, an active phytochemical in lavender, had been absorbed into their bodies from the air they inhaled.[6] Thus, aromatherapy may simply be an unorthodox way to get phytochemicals into the bloodstream and the body, where they then act like any other medicine. Indeed, one study evaluated the effects of inhalation of 1,8-cineol, extracted from *Rosmarinus officinalis*, on cerebral blood flow in human subjects. Significant effects were observed that seemed consistent with previous reports of aromatherapeutic effects of 1,8-cineol. However, one of the so-affected subjects in this study was anosmic, which led to the conclusion that pharmacological effects of absorbed 1,8-cineol, rather than the aroma of the substance, were responsible for the observations.[7]

Although aromatherapy may be just another way to introduce therapeutic phyto-chemicals into the body and bloodstream, a more interesting possibility is that simply smelling the essential oil—without phytochemicals entering the bloodstream—might have its own special effect. Stimulation of the primary olfactory neurons in the nasal epithelium is first processed in the olfactory bulb of the brain. This information is relayed to the main secondary olfactory structure, the piriform cortex. The informa-tion moves on into the tertiary olfactory structures, the thalamus, hypothalamus, amygdala, hippocampus, and orbitofrontal and insular cortices, where the process-ing of olfaction and emotion might become intertwined. Indeed, these structures are deeply embedded in the limbic system. Thus, it would not be at all surprising that odors would have a significant effect on emotional state.[8]

However, the olfactory system of the mammalian brain is complex. It is one of the last frontiers of neuroscience, and much of its workings remains a mystery. We do not yet understand how the nose and brain can analyze, recognize, and respond to an almost endless variety of odors and combinations of odors. Nonetheless, it is common knowledge that foul smells, such as the odor of rotten food or body odor, are repellant and make us feel bad. We do what we can to avoid such smells. Other smells are pleasant and rewarding. We have all at one time or another gone out of our way to walk over and smell the sweet fragrance of a flower. Thus, it is possible that part of the beneficial effects of aromatherapy is simply being distracted by a pleasant experience. You might gain similar relief from anxiety by listening to a piece of music by Bach or being distracted by a pleasant conversation with a friend. Also, as Marcel Proust so elegantly described in his novel *Remembrance of Things Past*, pleasant aromas are perhaps the most powerful gateway to memories. If the odor of lavender brings to mind a past walk in a spring garden, then so much the better.

One study has indeed suggested that simply being distracted by any pleasant smell can relieve anxiety.[9] Women waiting in a clinic to receive abortions—obviously a stressful situation—were told to sniff either a container of a mixture of essential oils of *Chrysopogon zizanioides*, *Citrus bergamia*, and *Pelargonium graveolens* or a container of a pleasant-smelling hair conditioner. Both the herbal and control treatments resulted in very slight, non-significant reductions in anxiety in women waiting to receive an abortion. Of course, they did not try to rule out the possibility that some ingredient of the hair conditioner offered aromatherapeutic effects. In any case, other studies provide evidence that the responses to aromatherapy are deeply psychological and may change according to expectations. That is, they are highly susceptible to placebo effects. A study showed that if subjects were told the lavender oil they were given to inhale might prevent them from relaxing, they tended not to relax. If, on the other hand, they were told the oil would help them relax, those subjects tended to relax even more than they would have without that advice. Thus, expectancy played a major role.[10]

Whereas some effects of aromatherapy may jog memories and stimulate unique and personal responses, other responses to smells may be triggered by extremely sensitive and specific mechanisms with hard-wired connections to the brain. In many animal species, there is a special organ of smell, sometimes in the hard palate and sometimes on the nasal septum, called the vomeronasal organ.[11] The vomeronasal organ is filled with nerve endings, and, like nerves in the nose that sense regular odors, it sends signals to the odor-processing area of the brain called the olfactory bulb. The vomeronasal organ is extremely sensitive to molecules called pheromones. Pheromones are in many respects hormones released by animals to affect the behavior of others around them. When pheromones land on special receptors in the vomeronasal organ, they almost immediately cause changes in behavior. This is quite obvious in male animals responding to the pheromones produced by females in heat. Another example is that the exposure of young female mice to airborne pheromones from the urine of male mice accelerates the onset of puberty in those females, ostensibly mediated by the vomeronasal organ.[12]

The main olfactory systems and the vomeronasal system have long been thought to process mutually exclusive aromatic stimuli. However, recent studies have shown that the two systems can influence each other.[13] Thus, subtle interactions between the main and accessory olfactory systems could subserve the effects of aromatherapy.

There is a vomeronasal organ in humans, but there has long been controversy about what role it serves. The common understanding is that during development of the human embryo, the organ regresses and the neural connections disappear. The vomeronasal cavities can still be observed by endoscopy in some adults, but they lack sensory neurons and nerve fibers. Nonetheless, a scientific report as recent as 2018 acknowledges that the existence of a human vomeronasal organ is "still the subject of heated controversy."[14]

Although the existence of the vomeronasal organ is controversial, there is strong evidence that humans can release substances into the air that affect the physiology and behavior of other humans. For example, it has been shown that the scent of ovulating women causes testosterone levels to increase in men.[15] Consistent with those findings, men sniffing an estrogen-like molecule swabbed from the armpits of women show changes in the activity of neurons in the hypothalamus of the brain. Women sniffing secretions swabbed from the armpits of men show similar changes in the brain. Those changes in activity of the brain occurred too rapidly for them to have been due to substances being absorbed and brought to the brain by the bloodstream.[16] The most obvious way that humans picked up those chemical signals in the air was by some aspect of the sense of smell alone. If the vomeronasal organ is not active in humans, then perhaps other components of the human nose have adapted to take over the role that organ plays in lower mammals. Is it possible that essential oils could mimic human pheromones? Some human pheromones appear to be derivatives of steroids humans have in their bodies. When one considers that many essential oils contain steroid-like triterpenes, it is reasonable to suspect that these substances could generate such effects. There are studies showing that substances in essential oils of plants mimic pheromones of various insects, possibly serving to attract pollinators or warn away potential pests.[17] Nonetheless, there is no evidence to make the leap to humans.

Is there anything in between the extremes of an aroma simply being generically pleasant and an aroma causing a specific, hardwired response such as a pheromone might produce? That is, can certain aromas reliably be expected to cause specific responses, such as relaxation, joy, concentration, alertness, joy, or sexual attraction? Might certain types of olfactory stimulation evoke specific emotional tones in the same inexplicable ways that minor keys elicit feelings of melancholy[18] and bright yellow and green hues give rise to cheerfulness?[19]

Studies have shown that the effects of aromas are not necessarily generic. The aromas of different herbs can generate different effects on brain activity. In one study, aromas of *Lavandula angustifolia* and *Rosmarinus officinalis* produced different effects on cognitive performance. Oil of *Lavandula angustifolia* mildly diminished performance of working memory, whereas oil of *Rosmarinus officinalis* enhanced working memory. Both herbs reportedly improved mood.[20] Although the essential oils of both *Lavandula angustifolia* and *Rosmarinus officinalis* have been found to reduce anxiety when used as aromatherapy, the prior study makes it difficult to conclude that they both act in the same way as mere pleasant, distracting fragrances. In several cases, differences were observed in electroencephalographic data, which arguably are objective and real. One group recorded the brain waves of subjects exposed to the aromas of *Eucalyptus*, *Lavandula angustifolia*, spiced apple, and odorless solvent as control. The results showed that each aroma produced a distinct pattern of alpha wave and theta wave distributions. Spiced apple odor was the most effective in increasing alpha activity as well as producing subjective feelings of relaxation.[21] In Japanese studies, electroencephalography was used to evaluate the effects of the aromas of *Lavandula angustifolia*, 1,8-cineol, *Jasminum officinale*,

Santalum album, and alpha-pinene. Inhalation of the odors of *Lavandula angustifolia*, 1,8-cineol, *Santalum album*, and alpha-pinene all increased alpha waves, suggesting relaxation. However, inhalation of *Jasminum officinale* increased beta wave activity, suggesting an arousing, stimulant effect.[22-23] For a thorough discussion of differential effects of olfactory stimulation on EEG, see the excellent review by Sowndhararajan and Kim.[24]

In this chapter, examples are given of essential oils of herbs that can be used to reduce anxiety when used as aromatherapy through massage, inhalation, or the Ayurvedic practice of *shirodhara*. While many herbs have been used for this purpose, discussion is limited to herbs and combinations for which there is at least one clinical study demonstrating anxiolytic effects. The studies almost invariably involve not persisting anxiety disorders, such as GAD, but rather subjects experiencing anxiety-provoking situations. Also among these studies are several reports concerning the use of aromatherapy for the treatment of agitation in elderly patients suffering dementia. Whereas agitation arising from degenerative processes in the brain is not the same as anxiety, anxiety is certainly a component of the phenomenon. Moreover, since many medical treatments include heavily sedating medications, all non-pharmacological treatment of such behavior is worth introducing. A recent review by the well-regarded Cochrane Database of Systemic Reviews stated that most studies of the use of aromatherapy for reduction of agitation in dementia are either negative in results or of poor quality.[25] In general, the rigor in research on aromatherapy tends not to be high. There is also likely to be publication bias. That is, while positive reports can be found in the literature, negative results often never see the light of day. Yet, in a few cases, the fragrances of oils used in aromatherapy have been reported to make people feel worse rather than better. In one study, patients about to receive radiation treatment for cancer were given to inhale either a combination of essential oils of lavender, bergamot, and cedarwood or simply a neutral, odorless oil. Anxiety was significantly lower in the group that inhaled only the odorless oil.[26] Of course, the observation of any significant effect suggests that these treatments are in some way psychoactive.

Of final note, the current focus is anxiolytic effects of herbal aromatherapy. However, aromatherapy has also been utilized in the management of psychiatric concerns including insomnia, depression, pain, attention deficit hyperactivity disorder, addiction, sexual dysfunction, autism, dementia, schizophrenia, and psychiatric disorders associated with Parkinson's disease. For an enlightening review, including discussion of possible mechanisms, see Perry and Perry.[27]

10.1 HERBS UTILIZED IN AROMATHERAPY

In the following are discussions of 17 individual herbs whose essential oils have been found to successfully relieve anxiety when utilized in aromatherapy.

10.1.1 *Boswellia carterii*

Frankincense is the aromatic resin of the *Boswellia carterii* tree. Most frankincense comes from Somalia and India but also Oman, Yemen, and western Africa. It was used and traded throughout the ancient world, including in China, where it has been used as a medicinal herb often in combination with myrrh. In the Bible, the ancient Hebrews burned frankincense as a sacrament. The rare and expensive resin has long been a highly esteemed gift. The "three wise men" were said to have brought gold, frankincense, and myrrh as gifts to the Christ child. Such was the esteem in which the herb was held. Frankincense has been used to treat a variety of respiratory and inflammatory illnesses such as asthma, rheumatoid arthritis, irritable bowel diseases, osteoarthritis, and most recently relapsing-remitting multiple sclerosis. However, it has also long been used to relieve pain and anxiety. The main chemical components of *Boswellia carterii* include α-ursolic, α-thujene, myrcene, limonene, and alpha-boswellic acid, a steroid-like terpene.[28]

One study of the anxiolytic effects of frankincense included 126 women undergoing labor for the first time, arguably a very anxiety-provoking condition. Women received either gauze infused with essential oil of frankincense or saline, with gauze exchanged every 30 minutes to maintain the strength of treatment. Data was collected using the Spielberger State-Trait Anxiety Inventory and then statistically analyzed. Inhaling frankincense significantly reduced anxiety.[29] In a similar subsequent study, frankincense was found also to reduce level of pain during labor.[30]

10.1.2 CITRUS AURANTIUM

Citrus aurantium, or bitter orange, is a common ingredient in Chinese herbal treatments. It is one of the herbs that has been found to have anxiolytic effects when ingested. It is discussed in a previous chapter. *Citrus aurantium* has also been found to be effective as aromatherapy.

Inhaling the essential oil of *Citrus aurantium* placed by the nose was found to significantly reduce levels of anxiety in women during the first stages of labor.[31] Similar reductions in anxiety after smelling the essential oil have been seen in women recovering from cesarean birth[32] and in hospitalized patients recovering from heart attacks.[33]

10.1.3 CITRUS SINENSIS

Citrus sinensis is sometimes referred to as sweet orange. The essential oil of this type of orange is particularly rich in d-limonene.[34] Effects of ambient aroma of the essential oil were evaluated in patients waiting for a dental procedure. The nebulizing device was hidden from view, and the subjects were not informed that the study involved aromatherapy. Data were collected using the State-Trait Anxiety Inventory. The aroma was found to have a significant relaxing effect in female but not male patients when compared to the control group, who experienced no odor in the air of the waiting room.[35]

10.1.4 CYMBOPOGON CITRATUS

Cymbopogon citratus is commonly known as lemongrass or citronella grass. It is a tall, fragrant member of the grass family that grows in many tropical and subtropical areas of the world. Many cultures, on virtually every continent, use *Cymbopogon citratus* both for flavoring of food and as medicine. It is the source of citronella oil, which has been used in perfume and as mosquito repellant. The phytochemicals citronellal, citronellol, geraniol, and linalool are largely responsible for the spicy aroma and may offer some medicinal effects as well. However, it also contains a wide variety of flavonoids, such as apigenin, luteolin, kaempferol, and quercetin; phenolics; terpenes; and other compounds that might add to its benefits for health.[36]

Cymbopogon citratus has been used in traditional Chinese medicine and Ayurvedic medicine to soothe stress and in the folk medicine of Brazil to relieve anxiety. It is also one of the herbs more commonly recommended by American herbalists for the treatment of anxiety. Unfortunately, there are few studies demonstrating that the herb is actually effective. In one such study, healthy volunteers who inhaled the aroma of six drops of oil of *Cymbopogon citratus* experienced an acute relief of tension. They also recovered more quickly than control subjects after a stressful cognitive challenge.[37] Curiously, although *Cymbopogon citratus* is often recommended by herbalists as a tea or other ingestible form for anxiety, another study found a single dose of strong tea made of *Cymbopogon citratus* had no anxiolytic effects at all in healthy adults subjected to a similar stressful cognitive test.[38]

10.1.5 *EUGENIA AROMATICUM*

Cloves are the aromatic flower buds of a tree in the family *Myrtaceae* scientifically referred to as *Eugenia aromaticum* or *Syzygium aromaticum*. The trees are native to Indonesia but are now grown in subtropical areas throughout the world. It is most often used as spice, and it has an unmistakable spicy, sweet aroma. In Indonesia, buds of *Eugenia aromaticum* are also used to make a kind of cigarette called kreteks. No formal research has been done to determine what, if any, pleasurable effects smoking kreteks may offer. Nonetheless, since this form of cigarette is by far the preferred form of cigarette in Indonesia, it must offer some pleasure for those who smoke them. The essential oil of *Eugenia aromaticum* contains a variety of phytochemicals. Perhaps most important is eugenol, which is known to act as a local anesthetic as well as an enhancer of activity at GABA-A receptors. The oil also contains the terpene linalool, which on its own is known to exert anxiolytic and pain-relieving effects.[39]

In a study from Iran, the effects of the essential oils of *Eugenia aromaticum* and *Mentha piperita* were compared in abilities to reduce anxiety and pain experienced by women in labor.[40] In this study, large for its kind, women about to give birth for the first time were divided into two groups of 63 each and given either *Eugenia aromaticum* oil or *Mentha piperita* oil to inhale from oil-infused gauze attached to the collars of their gowns. The gauze was replaced every 30 minutes. Data were gathered using the Spielberger State-Trait Anxiety Inventory and McGill Pain Questionnaire and later statistically analyzed by standard methods. Pain and anxiety were reduced in both groups. Indeed, at least one other study mentioned in this text found *Mentha piperita* to have such effects. However, the essential oil of *Eugenia aromaticum* was significantly better than oil of *Mentha piperita* in reducing anxiety and pain.

10.1.6 *JASMINUM OFFICINALE*

Jasminum officinale, known as the common jasmine, is a species of flowering plant in the olive family *Oleaceae*. It is native to the Caucasus, northern Iran, Afghanistan, Pakistan, the Himalayas, Tajikistan, India, Nepal, and western China. It has a long history of use in traditional Chinese medicine. The Chinese call it *mo li hua* and believe that it regulates *Qi* and calms the spirit. *Jasminum officinale* has also long been used in India as an Ayurvedic remedy for anxiety. It is there referred to as *jatipushpa* and is considered to have the quality of *saumanasya janaka*, or pleasure giving, due to its pleasant aroma.[41]

In a study published in an Ayurvedic medical journal, patients were given essential oil of *Jasminum officinale* to inhale for 5 minutes a day over 10 days. The subjects' levels of anxiety were determined before the treatment and after the 10-day course. Data was collected using the Hamilton Anxiety Rating Scale and statistically analyzed using a paired samples t-test. The analysis showed that anxiety scores were significantly lower after the 10 days of treatment than before.[42]

In a rather poorly documented study, the anxiolytic effect of massage with oil of *Jasminum officinale* was compared with that of simple aromatherapy by inhalation of the same essential oil as well as an oil-free control treatment in women in active labor.[43] Data were collected using the Spielberger State-Trait Anxiety Inventory. Both the massage with *Jasminum officinale* oil and inhalation of the oil offered anxiolytic effects in comparison to no extra treatment. However, the combination of massage and the essential oil was the most effective.

In one study subjects who received an abdominal massage with essential oil of *Jasminum officinale* reported feeling more alert and vigorous but also less relaxed after treatment.[44] Stimulation rather than relaxation is consistent with a subsequent report that inhalation of essential oil of *Jasminum officinale* shifted EEG activity to beta waves.[45] Beta waves are observed in subjects in alert states whereas relaxed states are associated with increased alpha wave activity.

10.1.7 *LAVANDULA SPP*

Species of *Lavandula*, collectively known as lavender, have been shown to exert anxiolytic effects either by ingestion or by aromatherapy. General discussion of *Lavandula officinalis*—the representative and most commonly used species—as well as descriptions of its anxiolytic effects after ingestion (see *Lavandula angustifolia*, Chapter 6).

Some studies have shown that the aroma of *Lavandula* can reduce anxiety and stress. One example is a study showing that the scent of a candle laced with its essential oil substantially reduced the level of anxiety in patients awaiting their dental appointments.[46] In some cases, those appointments entailed anxiety-provoking procedures such as drilling and tooth extraction. The scent of *Lavandula* has been reported to reduce anxiety in women postpartum.[47] It is important to state that not all studies have found lavender oil aromatherapy effective in reducing anxiety prior to medical procedures.[48]

One study found that inhalation of essential oil of lavender over 3 weeks was significantly more effective than inhalation of odorless sunflower oil in reducing agitation in elderly Chinese patients suffering dementia.[49] Data was gathered using the standard Cohen-Mansfield Agitation Inventory and Neuropsychiatric Inventory. However, at least one other group found no benefits of using inhalation of essential oil of lavender for reducing levels of agitation in patients with dementia.[50]

Another study involved patients in an intensive care unit given massage, exposure to lavender oil, or simply periods of rest. There were no statistically significant differences in the physiological stress indicators or observed ability of patients to cope following any of the three interventions. However, those patients who received aromatherapy reported significantly greater, albeit temporary, improvement in their mood and perceived levels of anxiety immediately following the therapy.[51]

10.1.8 *MATRICARIA RECUTITA*

Matricaria recutita is known commonly as German chamomile. Ingestion of extract of *Matricaria recutita* or consumption as tea has been found to significantly reduce anxiety in patients diagnosed with GAD. Information about chamomile and discussion of the relevant studies appear in Chapter 6. The essential oil of this sweet-smelling herb is commonly used as an anxiolytic agent in aromatherapy. In one study, the anxiety of eight cancer patients was measured using the Rotterdam Symptom Checklist and State-Trait Anxiety Inventory. After three weekly sessions of massage with essential oil of *Chamaemelum nobile* or Roman chamomile, the levels of anxiety significantly dropped in those patients. The weakness of this study was that there were no control groups to help determine what effect massage alone or exposure to aroma of the essential without massage may have contributed.[52]

10.1.9 *MELISSA OFFICINALIS*

Melissa officinalis, or lemon balm, is an herb whose extract has been found to significantly reduce anxiety, though there is no data from patients formally diagnosed with an anxiety disorder. For further discussion, see Chapter 6. The fragrant essential oil has also been found to reduce agitation when applied as aromatherapy.

In a study, 72 patients with severe dementia were treated with massages of faces and arms using lotion containing essential oil of *Melissa officinalis*. After 4 weeks of twice daily treatment, those patients showed significant reductions in agitation along with significant improvement in social interaction as measured by the Cohen-Mansfield Agitation Inventory and Quality of Life Index. In total, 60% of those treated with *Melissa officinalis* but only 14% of those treated with only lotion experienced at least a 30% reduction of agitation scores.[53]

10.1.10 *MENTHA PIPERITA*

Mentha piperita, or simple peppermint, is one of the herbs that has been found to reduce anxiety when ingested as tea. A complete discussion of *Mentha piperita* can be found in Chapter 6. However, there have been at least two published studies of the effects of aromatherapy using the essential oil of *Mentha piperita* for relief from anxiety. None of the subjects carried diagnoses of GAD or any other formal diagnosis of anxiety. Rather, the anxiety was situational, in the context of women's first experience of labor. Women in labor were given gauze infused with essential oil of *Mentha piperita* that was attached to the collar of their hospital gown and refreshed every 30 minutes. Data was collected using the Spielberger State-Trait Anxiety Inventory and then statistically analyzed. Results demonstrated that inhaling the essential oil significantly reduced both anxiety and pain throughout the process of labor.[54]

In another study, the aroma of essential oil of *Mentha piperita* infused into the air inside cars significantly reduced frustration and anxiety in individuals undergoing driving tests. It also reduced subjective sense of anxiety and fatigue. Interestingly, infusion of aroma of essential oil of *Cinnamomum* similarly increased alertness and lowered impatience and frustration but did not lead to reports of less anxiety.[55]

10.1.11 *NARDOSTACHYS JATAMANSI*

Nardostachys jatamansi, with the common name of spikenard, is able to provide anxiolytic effects either by ingestion or through aromatherapy. Details about *Nardostachys jatamansi* can be found in Chapter 6. Significant anxiolytic effects of *Nardostachys jatamansi* were observed in patients diagnosed with anxiety neurosis after 14 days of daily administration by the classical Ayurvedic practice of *shirodhara*.[56] In this case, sesame oil carried the herbal extracts onto the forehead of the patients. Unlike its cousin, *Valeriana officinalis*, *Nardostachys jatamansi* is sweet smelling and may in that way give comfort and distraction to subjects. It is not known how or to what degree the active phytochemicals may have been absorbed into the bodies of the patients.

10.1.12 NEROLI OIL

Neroli oil is an essential oil produced from the blossom rather than the peel of *Citrus aurantium*, the bitter orange tree. It was the favorite fragrance of Louis XIV of France and is a common essential oil used in aromatherapy. Neroli oil is extracted by steam distillation. Among the phytochemicals in contains are linalool, limonene, farnesol, geraniol, citral, nerolidol, α-terpinyl acetate, and farnesol. It has many of the same constituent phytochemicals as in the oil extracted from the peel of bitter orange. However, neroli oil is sweeter and more floral, likely due to its higher content of linalool and somewhat lower content of spicier limonene.[57]

Neroli oil was studied for its ability to relieve stress, anxiety, depression, and autonomic nervous system activity in high-risk hospitalized pregnant women entering labor. These women received neroli oil for inhalation three times a day over 5 days. The only statistically significant finding was a lowered subjective sense of stress.[58]

10.1.13 *PELARGONIUM GRAVEOLENS*

Pelargonium graveolens, with the common name Rose geranium, is a species of geranium native to South Africa, Zimbabwe, and Mozambique. The main components of the essential oil are eugenol, geranic, citronellol, geraniol, linalool, citronellyl formate, citral, myrtenol, terpineol, methone, and sabinene.[59]

The effects of the essential oil of *Pelargonium graveolens* used as aromatherapy were evaluated in women in labor for the first time. Anxiety levels were measured using the Spielberger State-Trait Anxiety Inventory before and after treatment. Physiological measurements, including blood pressure, respiratory rate, and heart rate, were also measured. The data that were collected were statistically analyzed by standard methods. The anxiety levels of the women inhaling the essential oil of *Pelargonium graveolens* decreased in comparison to the anxiety of women in the placebo group. There was also a significant decrease in diastolic blood pressure.[60] In a study of women experiencing menstrual pain and anxiety, self-massage of the abdomen with essential oil of *Pelargonium graveolens* helped relieve both the pain and anxiety. The data were statistically analyzed, and the self-massage with the oil was significantly more effective than either massage without *Pelargonium graveolens* or no treatment at all.[61]

There was also an uncontrolled clinical trial carried out in a psychiatric ward of a general hospital in São Paulo, Brazil. In this study massage of the neck and back using the essential oil of *Pelargonium graveolens* significantly reduced levels of anxiety of the patients. However, there was no comparison group to help determine how much the oil may have contributed the anxiolytic effect beyond the effects of the massage alone.[62]

10.1.14 ROSA DAMASCENA

Rosa damascena, the rose bush, is native to Asia. In Chinese herbology, dried buds, or *mei gui hua*, have been used to promote the movement of *Qi* to relieve feelings of constraint. The ancient Persians cultivated *Rosa damascena* to obtain perfume as rose water. They also believed the petals cooked in sugar or honey could cool the mind and body as well as cleanse the blood. The much-loved flower is now cultivated throughout the world for its fragrance and beauty. Rose oil is extracted from the petals of various types of roses by steam distillation. The essential oil is full of phytochemicals, including citronellol, geraniol, nerol, linalool, phenyl ethyl alcohol, farnesol, stearoptene, α-pinene, β-pinene, α-terpinene, limonene, p-cymene, camphene, β-caryophyllene, neral, citronellyl acetate, geranyl acetate, neryl acetate, eugenol, methyl eugenol, rose oxide, α-damascenone, β-damascenone, benzaldehyde, benzyl alcohol, rhodinyl acetate, and phenyl ethyl formate.[63] Many of those substances are shared in common with other herbal essential oils, and the mechanisms of action of those herbs are likely due to many of the same molecules.

Many people fear the dentist's office, and dental anxiety is a common focus of study for anxiolytic effects. In one study, patients were given essential oil of *Lavandula* or *Rosa damascena* or a mere placebo. The aroma of the oils or placebo was maintained with a candle warmer, and the patients were made to wait in their respective rooms for 15 minutes before seeing the orthodontist. During that time, heart rate and blood pressure, physiological indicators of anxiety, were measured. A questionnaire containing the Dental Anxiety Scale was also given. The data were then statistically analyzed by paired t-test, analysis of variance, and the Wilcoxon signed-rank tests. Analyses showed that both essential oils in the room air significantly reduced dental anxiety. However, *Lavandula* oil more effectively reduced anxiety when compared to oil of *Rosa damascena*.[64] Depression, anxiety, and stress are also very common among patients undergoing hemodialysis, a treatment to cleanse the blood in patients suffering kidney failure. A study showed that inhalation of oil of *Rosa damascena* for 1 hour prior to treatments over 4 weeks significantly reduced anxiety in those patients.[65]

Anxiety in women during labor is a common emotional reaction, especially in women giving birth for the first time. There are many studies of anxiolytic effects of aromatherapy in these women. In one such study, women inhaled essential oil of *Rosa damascena* and received foot baths in warm water containing the oil for 10 minutes, once at the beginning of the active phase of labor and a second time at the beginning of the transition phase. One control group was given a warm foot bath, whereas another received no extra treatment. Anxiety was assessed during labor using the Visual Analogue Scale for Anxiety at baseline for all participants and again before and after each treatment. Although the baseline levels of anxiety were the same among all groups of women, the treatments with essential oil of *Rosa damascena* significantly lowered anxiety in comparison with both control groups.[66]

In yet another study, aromatherapy with rose oil was evaluated in patients facing a quite anxiety-provoking situation of rhinoplasty.[67] Patients received aromatherapy by ultrasonic nebulizer for 15 minutes before being taken to the operating room for surgery. Treatments included *Rosa damascena* oil, a mixture of distilled water and ethyl alcohol, or no nebulizer treatment. The data were collected by the Spielberger State-Trait Anxiety Inventory on the morning of the surgical procedure and a second test soon after the aromatherapy treatments. Aromatherapy with oil of *Rosa damascena* was significantly more effective in reducing anxiety than the alcohol or no treatment conditions.

Whereas *Rosa damascena* has been one of the most studied and apparently successful herbs used in aromatherapy treatment of anxiety, not all studies of the herb have been successful. In one study, inhalation of the oil for 10 minutes the night prior to surgery and then 1 hour before surgery was not sufficient to quell the anxiety of patients awaiting coronary artery bypass graft surgery.[68] The results, collected with the Spielberger State-Trait Anxiety Inventory, showed no difference in levels of anxiety between those who inhaled rose oil and those who did not.

10.1.15 *ROSMARINUS OFFICINALIS*

Rosmarinus officinalis, or common rosemary, is yet another herb that has been found to offer anxiolytic effects either ingested or used in aromatherapy. Details about *Rosmarinus officinalis* are provided in Chapter 6. Sachets of essential oils of *Rosmarinus officinalis* and *Lavandula officinalis* reduced levels of stress and anxiety in student nurses during stressful midterm examinations. Those subjects were otherwise healthy and did not carry diagnoses of any type of anxiety disorder.[69]

10.1.16 *SALVIA OFFICINALIS*

Salvia officinalis, with the common name of sage, is also one of several herbs that has been found to have benefits when used either by ingestion or in aromatherapy.

Details about *Salvia officinalis* can be found in Chapter 6. In one study performed in an Iranian hospital, drops of essence of sage significantly relieved pain and anxiety in women who had undergone cesarean section surgery.[70] Essential oil of *Salvia officinalis* dropped onto a cotton that hung around the neck as a pendant was similarly found to shorten latency to sleep and improve sleep quality in postmenopausal women.[71] In neither of those studies had subjects been diagnosed with an anxiety disorder.

10.1.17 SANTALLUM SPP

Sandalwood is a fragrant tree native mostly to Asia. However, species of sandalwood are also found in Australia, Indonesia, Hawaii, and other Pacific Islands. There are several true sandalwood species, with *Santallum album* and *Santalum spicatum* perhaps being the most valued. There are also many so-called false sandalwood species from around the world that are fragrant but quite different from true sandalwood. *Santallum* trees have been cultivated since antiquity for their yellowish heartwood, which plays a major role in many Asian funeral ceremonies and religious rites. However, for centuries, East Indian *Santallum* oil has also been a popular ingredient in Indian Ayurvedic and traditional Chinese medicine. Steam distillation is the most common method used to obtain the essential oil. The essential oil contains some phytochemicals somewhat unique to *Santallum*, including cis-α-santalol and cis-β-santalol. It also contains molecules shared by other medicinal herbs, including β-curcumen-12-ol, -nuciferol and α-bisablol, bergamatol, and lanceol.[72]

Essential oil of *Santallum* is commonly used in aromatherapy, alone or in combination with other oils, to calm and relax individuals. However, there are few studies that substantiate the anxiolytic effects of *Santallum spp*. In a study of healthy women under non-stressful conditions, it was found that application of essential oil of sandalwood as perfume significantly increased subjective sense of well-being, calmness, and ability to manage.[73] In one of the more unusual studies, a group evaluated the ability of sandalwood, bossa nova music, or the combination of the two to reduce anxiety in pediatric patients undergoing a non-painful dental procedure. Measurements were taken of blood pressures and heart rate—both being objective physiological reflections of anxiety and stress—before and after treatments. Both *Santallum* aromatherapy and bossa nova music significantly reduced blood pressure and heart rate in comparison to no treatment. However, the strongest effect was when the two treatments were combined.[74] *Santallum* aromatherapy has also been reported to improve sleep in adolescents.[75]

10.2 HERBAL COMBINATIONS IN AROMATHERAPY

In some cases, essential oils of two or more herbs were used in combination in aromatherapy. Because the exact mechanism by which any one essential oil acts to relieve anxiety through aromatherapy is unknown, it is difficult to say how a combination of essential oils might work better or in a different way than a single one. Moreover, many combinations that are employed include essential oil of lavender, which alone has been found effective in reducing anxiety. Nonetheless, it is not uncommon for combinations of essential oils to be used as aromatherapy to relieve anxiety and agitation. Some are noted in the following.

10.2.1 CYMBOPOGON CITRATUS AND EUCALYPTUS MASSAGE WITH LAVANDULA OFFICINALIS INHALATION

Among studies of effects of aromatherapy on agitation in patients with dementia is one study that combined techniques of aromatherapy by using massage with oil containing essential oils of *Cymbopogon citratus* and *Eucalyptus* along with inhalations of essential oil of *Lavandula officinalis*. The subjects in the study had significant illness, with some subjects in both the treatment group and the control group requiring antipsychotic medications to maintain safety. Massages were given 3 days a week for 1 hour, and inhalation of *Lavandula officinalis* took place for 1 hour daily by placing a sponge infused with six drops of the essential oil at the outlet of a cool mist air humidifier. Data were collected using the Neuropsychiatric Inventory and the Cohen-Mansfield Agitation Inventory. After 4 weeks of treatment, patients who received the combined massage and inhalation therapies showed significantly less agitation than those who received no forms of aromatherapy.[76]

10.2.2 LAVANDULA OFFICINALIS, CANANGA ODORATA, AND CITRUS BERGAMIA

A study was performed to determine the effect of aromatherapy in women scheduled to undergo hysterectomy. None of the women had been diagnosed with an anxiety disorder, but one can assume that anticipation of major surgery was anxiety provoking. Women received either the combination of essential oils of *Lavandula officinalis*, *Cananga odorata* (common name ylang ylang), and bergamot oil inhaled in aromatherapy or the usual preoperative care. Bergamot oil is extracted from the inner rind of *Citrus bergamia*. Anxiety was rated using the Visual Analogue Scale after inhaling the essential oils on the previous day and just before surgery. The data were analyzed by the chi-square test and the independent t-test comparing the treatment group and a control group. The study found that inhalation of the combination of the essential oils of *Lavandula officinalis*, *Cananga odorata*, and *Citrus bergamia* significantly reduced anxiety.[77]

10.2.3 LAVANDULA OFFICINALIS, CHAMAEMELUM NOBILE, AND CITRUS AURANTIUM

A study found that the combination of essential oils of *Lavandula officinalis*, *Chamaemelum nobile*, and *Citrus aurantium* blossoms applied to warm "aroma stones" significantly improved anxiety and sleep quality in patients in an ICU. None of the patients were formally diagnosed with any anxiety disorder. However, all were being hospitalized for serious and anxiety-provoking cardiac procedures classified as percutaneous coronary intervention. Results were obtained using the Spielberger State-Trait Anxiety Inventory and the Verran and Snyder-Halpern (VSH) Sleep Scale. Effects of aromatherapy were compared against measurements from patients receiving standard nursing care.[78]

10.2.4 LAVANDULA OFFICINALIS, PELARGONIUM GRAVEOLENS, AND CITRUS RETICULATA

In a study of severely demented patients, daily skin application of the combination of *Lavandula officinalis, Pelargonium graveolens*, and *Citrus reticulata* essential oils carried in almond oil significantly reduced agitation and social isolation, increased alertness and contentment, and improved sleep.[79]

10.2.5 LAVANDULA OFFICINALIS AND ROSA DAMASCENA

Anxiety is common in women during pregnancy and in the postpartum period. About 5% of women who had not previously experienced major depression can develop major depression in the weeks following giving birth. In women that have previously suffered depression, relapse can be quite common. Thus, any treatments to help prevent those symptoms are worth pursuing. This study evaluated the effects of aromatherapy using a combination of the essential oils of *Lavandula officinalis* and *Rosa damascena* in postpartum women.[80] Groups receiving either inhalation of oils or hand massage with oils were compared against a control group that was simply instructed to avoid any form of aromatherapy for 4 weeks. All subjects completed the Edinburgh Postnatal Depression Scale and Generalized Anxiety Disorder scale at the beginning of the study. The scales were then repeated after 2 weeks and at the end of all treatments at 4 weeks. The midpoint and final scores indicated that aromatherapy had significant improvements greater than the control group on both the depression and anxiety scores. No adverse effects were reported.

10.2.6 LAVANDULA OFFICINALIS AND SANTALUM ALBUM

The combination of the essential oils of *Lavandula officinalis* and *Santalum album* were evaluated for anxiolytic effects in women about to undergo breast biopsy to potentially diagnose breast cancer. Women received either the *Lavandula officinalis* and *Santalum album*, a combination of neroli and essential oil of *Mentha piperita*, or a placebo aromatherapy with no active essential oil. Anxiety was self-reported before and after undergoing a breast biopsy using the Spielberger State-Trait Anxiety Inventory. There was a statistically significant reduction in self-reported anxiety with the use of the combination of *Lavandula officinalis* and *Santalum album* aromatherapy compared with the placebo group. Curiously, the neroli oil and *Mentha piperita* aromatherapy combination also evaluated in this study offered no benefits.[81]

10.3 AROMATHERAPY AND SLEEP

Another important consideration of aromatherapy is that it may be useful in treating insomnia. Sleep disorders are common among those suffering anxiety disorders. Indeed, up to 75% of patients diagnosed with GAD also report symptoms of insomnia.[82] It is likely that one condition exacerbates the other. Several essential oils administered in aromatherapy to treat anxiety are also reported to be effective in relieving insomnia. Aromatherapy utilizing essential oil of *Lavandula officinalis* is perhaps the most thoroughly studied and demonstratively effective such treatment for insomnia.[83] Other essential oils that have been used to help resolve insomnia when administered as aromatherapy include *Rosa damascena*,[84] *Jasminum spp*,[85] *Citrus aurantium*,[86] and *Chamaemelum nobile*.[87]

As in aromatherapy treatment of anxiety, combinations of oils are often used for treatment of insomnia. In one study, a blend of essential oils of *Ocimum basilicum, Juniperus communis, Lavandula angustifolia*, and *Origanum majorana* was applied by hand massage; satisfactory sleep increased from 73% to 97% of patient nights, while the use of sedatives was reduced from 90% to 36% of patient nights.[88] In perhaps the most sophisticated study of effects of combined herbal aromatherapy on sleep, two commercially available spray-on combinations of essential oils were evaluated. One combination consisted of essential oils of *Lavandula angustifolia, Pogostemon cablin, Cinnamomum camphora, Vetiveria zizanoides*, and *Ormenis multicaulis*. The other combination included *Pogostemon cablin, Cananga odorata*, and *Boswellia carterii*. In an initial fMRI evaluation of effects on the olfactory system, the first combination specifically activated the superior temporal gyrus, whereas the second activated the caudate. In the sleep component of the study, participants sprayed one of the two herbal combinations or an odor-neutral control substance on their pillowcase before retiring. Both treatments significantly improved components of sleep, though the second combination was more effective.[89]

10.4   SOME FINAL THOUGHTS ABOUT AROMATHERAPY

There are many reports about the ability of aromatherapy to reduce anxiety and stress. Unfortunately, the scientific view of aromatherapy is not terribly supportive. Several reviews on the subject by well-regarded medical organizations, e.g., the Cochrane Library, tend to dismiss aromatherapy by saying there is simply not enough solid, scientific evidence of meaningful, clinical benefits.[90] Indeed, many if not most studies lack the rigor that most large, scientific studies of medical treatments are required to follow.[91] In the present context, it must also be emphasized that studies of effects of aromatherapy on anxiety rarely include individuals actually diagnosed with anxiety disorders. Rather, subjects are most often healthy individuals under stressful situations. Thus, one could argue that there is little if any compelling evidence that aromatherapy helps people who suffer significant, ongoing anxiety disorders. Nonetheless, the fact remains that studies have shown significant calming effects in patients, including some in quite trying clinical situations.

Aside from the question of efficacy, the exact mechanisms by which aromatherapy might act remain unclear. This is in part because aromatherapy is applied in at least two different ways. One method is simply to allow the person to inhale the aroma of essential oil. Even by this method, it is unclear if the sense of smell alone mediates the effect or if some of the essential oil must also be absorbed into the body through the mucous membranes to add a genuine pharmacological component to the overall effect. The other method is to add essential oils to massage oil, which is then applied to the skin. Through this method, the patient may benefit from the aroma of the essential oils as well as from the medicinal effects of any phytochemicals that may be absorbed through the skin. Because massage is comforting, as is any kind of human touch, one might wonder if massage itself is the actual active principle when the techniques are combined. Thankfully, several studies have shown that addition of essential oil to massage adds anxiolytic benefits beyond those obtained from massage alone.

Practitioners of aromatherapy often claim that each essential oil has specific effects and can be chosen for specific conditions. There are data showing differences among various essential oils in how they affect objective measurements, including EEG and fMRI. However, there is little basis to suggest that one essential oil fragrance is more effective than another in dampening anxiety. Moreover, as alluded to in Chapter 5, many of the highly aromatic herbs favored by aromatherapists have phytochemicals in common and duplicate some of the medicinal effects of each other. One consideration in choosing one versus another aromatherapeutic treatment arises from the fact that our sense of smell habituates to odors fairly quickly.[92] If, for example, the aroma of the essential oil of lavender was always in the air, then its usefulness would likely begin to wane with time. Thus, if purely olfactory stimulation contributes to the overall effect of aromatherapy, it might be prudent at least to rotate essential oils to help maintain the benefits of fragrances.

Perhaps the best conclusion is the compelling evidence that aromatherapy is safe and, by whatever mechanism, can help people feel better. As is often the case with anxiolytic agents, many essential oils employed in aromatherapy can also aid sleep, which is often disturbed in those suffering anxiety. Aromatherapy is compatible with other therapies with stronger track records and better elucidations of mechanism of action. Thus, while other herbal or even prescription treatments should probably be relied upon for severe symptoms, aromatherapy may be a safe, helpful, and pleasant addition.

REFERENCES

1. Gattefossé R-M. *Gattefosse's Aromatherapy*, 2nd edition. Saffron Walden: CW Daniels UK; 1996.
2. Hawken PAR, Fiol C, Blache D. Genetic differences in temperament determine whether lavender oil alleviates or exacerbates anxiety in sheep. *Physiol Behav*. 2012;105(5):1117–1123.
3. Goodwin S, Reynolds H. Can aromatherapy be used to reduce anxiety in hospitalized felines. *Vet Nurse*. 2018;9(3):167–171.
4. Wells DL. Aromatherapy for travel-induced excitement in dogs. *J Am Vet Med Assoc*. 2006;229(6):964–967.
5. Kosiara S, Harrison AP. The effect of aromatherapy on equine facial expression, heart rate, respiratory tidal volume and spontaneous muscle contractures in m. temporalis and m. cleidomastoideus. *Open J Vet Med*. 2021;11:87–103.
6. Buchbauer G, Jirovetz L, Jäger W. Aromatherapy: Evidence for sedative effects of the essential oil of lavender after inhalation. *Z Naturforschung*. 1991;46:1067–1072.
7. Našel C, Našel B, Samec P, et al. Functional imaging of effects of fragrances on the human brain after prolonged inhalation. *Chemical Senses*. 1994;19(4):359–364.
8. Soudry Y, Lemogne C, Malinvaud D, et al. Olfactory system and emotion: Common substrates. *Eur Ann. Otorhinolaryngol Head Neck Dis*. 2011;128(1):18–23.
9. Wiebe E. A randomized trial of aromatherapy to reduce anxiety before abortion. *ECP*. 2000;3(4):166–169.

10. Howard S, Hughes BM. Expectancies, not aroma, explain impact of lavender aromatherapy on psychophysiological indices of relaxation in young healthy women. *Br J Health Psych.* 2008;13(4):603–617.

11. Keverne EB. The vomeronasal organ. *Science.* 1999;286(5440):716–720.

12. Novotny MV, Jemiolo B, Wiesler D, et al. A unique urinary constituent, 6-hydroxy-6-methyl-3-heptanone, is a pheromone that accelerates puberty in female mice. *Chem Biol.* 1999;6:377–383.

13. Suárez R, García-González D, De Castro F. Mutual influences between the main olfactory and vomeronasal systems in development and evolution. *Front Neuroanat.* 2012;6:50.

14. Stoyanov GS, Matev BK, Valchanov P, et al. The human vomeronasal (Jacobson's) organ: A short review of current conceptions, with an English translation of Potiquet's original text. *Cureus.* 2018;10(5):e2643.

15. Miller SL, Maner JK. Scent of a woman: Men's testosterone responses to olfactory ovulation cues. *Psychol Sci.* 2010;21:276–283.

16. Savic I, Berglund H, Gulyas B, et al. Smelling of odorous sex hormone-like compounds causes sex-differentiated hypothalamic activations in humans. *Neuron.* 2001;31:661–668.

17. Müller M, Buchbauer G. Essential oil components as pheromones. A review. *Flavour Fragr J.* 2011;26(6):357–377.

18. Cook ND, Hayashi T. The psychoacoustics of harmony perception: Centuries after three-part harmony entered Western music, research in starting to clarify why different chords sound tense or resolved, cheerful or melancholy. *Am Sci.* 2008;96(4):311–319.

19. Valdez P, Mehrabian A. Effects of color on emotions. *J Exp Psychol Gen.* 1994;123(4);394–409.

20. Moss M, Cook J, Wesnes K, et al. Aromas of rosemary and lavender essential oils differentially affect cognition and mood in healthy adults. *Int J Neurosci.* 2003;113(1):15–38.

21. Lorig TS, Schwartz GE. Brain and odor I. Alteration of human EEG by odor administration. *Psychobiol.* 1988;16:281–289.

22. Sugano H. Psychophysiological studies of fragrances. In: *Perfumery: The Psychology and Biology of Fragrance.* New York: Chapman & Hill; 1988. pp. 221–228.

23. Sugano H. Effects of odors on mental function. *Chem Senses.* 1989;14:303.

24. Sowndhararajan K, Kim S. Influence of fragrances on human psychophysiological activity: With special reference to human electroencephalographic response. *Sci Pharm.* 2016;84(4):724–751.

25. Ball EL, Owen-Booth B, Gray A, et al. Aromatherapy for dementia. *Cochrane Database Syst Rev.* 2020;(8):CD003150.

26. Graham PH, Browne L, Cox H, et al. Inhalation aromatherapy during radiotherapy: Results of a placebo-controlled double-blind randomized trial. *J Clin Oncol.* 2003;21(12):2372–2376.

27. Perry N, Perry E. Aromatherapy in the management of psychiatric disorders. *CNS Drugs.* 2006;20(4):257–280.

28. Mertens M, Buettner A, Kirchhoff E. The volatile constituents of frankincense—a review. *Flavour Fragr J.* 2009 Nov;24(6):279–300.

29. Esmaelzadeh-Saeieh S, Torkashvand S, Rahimzadeh KM, et al. Effect of aromatherapy with *Boswellia carterii* on anxiety in first stage of labor in nulliparous women. *Compl Med J Fac Nur Midwifery.* 2016;5(4):1314–1323.

30. Esmaelzadeh-Saeieh S, Rahimzadeh M, Khosravi-Dehaghi N, et al. The effects of inhalation aromatherapy with *Boswellia carterii* essential oil on the intensity of labor pain among nulliparous women. *Nurs Midwifery Stud.* 2018;7(2):45–49.

31. Namazi M, Akbari SA, Mojab F, et al. Aromatherapy with *Citrus Aurantium* oil and anxiety during the first stage of labor. *Iran Red Crescent Med J.* 2014;16(6):e18371.

32. Sharifipour F, Bakhteh A, Mirmohammad Ali M. Effects of *Citrus aurantium* aroma on post-cesarean anxiety. *Iran J Obstet Gynecol Infert.* 2015;18:12–20.

33. Moslemi F, Alijaniha F, Naseri M, et al. *Citrus aurantium* aroma for anxiety in patients with acute coronary syndrome: A double-blind placebo-controlled trial. *J Alt Compl Med*. 2019;25(8):833–839.

34. Bauer K, Garbe D, Surburg H. *Common Fragrance and Flavor Materials*, 4th edition. Weinheim: Wiley VCH; 2001. p. 189.

35. Lehrner J, Eckersberger C, Walla P, et al. Ambient odor of orange in a dental office reduces anxiety and improves mood in female patients. *Physiol Behav*. 2000;71(1–2):83–86.

36. Magotra S, Singh AP, Singh AP. A review on pharmacological activities of *Cymbopogon citratus*. *Int J Pharm Drug Anal*. 2021;6:151–157.

37. Goes TC, Ursulino FR, Almeida-Souza TH, et al. Effect of lemongrass aroma on experimental anxiety in humans. *J Alt Compl Med*. 2015;21(12):766–773.

38. Leite JR, Maria De Lourdes VS, Maluf E, et al. Pharmacology of lemongrass (*Cymbopogon citratus* Stapf). III. Assessment of eventual toxic, hypnotic and anxiolytic effects on humans. *J Ethnopharmacol*. 1986;17(1):75–83.

39. Kaur K, Kaushal S. Phytochemistry and pharmacological aspects of *Syzygium aromaticum*: A review. *J Pharmacogn Phytochem*. 2019;8(1):398–406.

40. Ozgoli G, Torkashvand S, Moghaddam FS, et al. Comparison of peppermint and clove essential oil aroma on pain intensity and anxiety at first stage of labor. *Iran J Obstet Gynecol Infert*. 2016;19(21):1–11.

41. Arun M, Satish S, Anima P. Phytopharmacological profile of *Jasminum grandiflorum* Linn. (*Oleaceae*). *Chinese J Integr Med*. 2016;22(4):311–320.

42. Arhanthkumar A. Effect of jasmine essential oil in generalized anxiety disorder: A pilot clinical study. *J Ayur Holistic Med*. 2013;1(7). http://jahm.co.in/index.php/jahm/article/view/124.

43. Alavi A. Study the effect of massage with jasmine oil in comparison to aromatherapy with jasmine oil on childbirth process in hospitals of Abadan city in 2013. *Ann Trop Med Pub Health*. 2017;10(4):904–909.

44. Hongratanaworakit T. Stimulating effect of aromatherapy massage with jasmine oil. *NPC*. 2010;5(1):157–162.

45. Sayowan W, Siripornpanich V, Hongratanaworakit T, et al. The effects of jasmine oil inhalation on brain wave activities and emotions. *J Health Res*. 2013;27(2):73–77.

46. Kritsidima M, Newton T, Asimakopoulou K, et al. The effects of lavender scent on dental patient anxiety levels: A cluster randomized-controlled trial. *Community Dent Oral Epidemiol*. 2010;38:83–87.

47. Kianpour M, Mansouri A, Mehrabi T, et al. Effect of lavender scent inhalation on prevention of stress, anxiety and depression in the postpartum period. *Iran J Nurs Midwifery Res*. 2016;21(2):197–201.

48. Muzzarelli L, Force M, Sebold M. Aromatherapy and reducing pre-procedural anxiety a controlled prospective study. *Gastroenterol Nurs*. 2006;29(6):466–471.

49. Lin PW-K, Chan WC, Ng BF, et al. Efficacy of aromatherapy (*Lavandula angustifolia*) as an intervention for agitated behaviours in Chinese older persons with dementia: A cross-over randomized trial. *Int J Geriatr Psych*. 2007;22(5):405–410.

50. Snow AL, Hovanec L, Brandt J. A controlled trial of aromatherapy for agitation in nursing home patients with dementia. *J Alt Compl Med*. 2004;10(3):431–437.

51. Dunn C, Sleep J, Collett D. Sensing an improvement: An experimental study to evaluate the use of aromatherapy, massage and periods of rest in an intensive care unit. *J Adv Nurs*. 1995;21(1):34–40.

52. Wilkinson S. Aromatherapy and massage in palliative care. *Int J Palliative Nursing*. 1995;1:21–30.

53. Ballard CG, O'Brien JT, Perry EK. Aromatherapy as a safe and effective treatment for the management of agitation in severe dementia: The results of a double-blind, placebo-controlled trial with Melissa. *J Clin Psychiatry*. 2002;63:553–558.

54. Ozgoli G, Zeinab A, Faraz M, et al. A study of inhalation of peppermint aroma on the pain and anxiety of the first stage of labor in nulliparous women: A randomized clinical trial. *Qom Univ Med Sci J.* 2013;7(3):21–27.

55. Raudenbush B, Grayhem R, Sears T, et al. Effects of peppermint and cinnamon odor administration on simulated driving alertness, mood and workload. *N Am J Psych.* 2009;11(2):245–256.

56. Jain A. Clinical evaluation of *Jatamansi siddha taila shirodhara* on anxiety-neurosis. *JAHM.* 2013;4(2):16–25.

57. Boussaada O, Chemli R. Chemical composition of essential oils from flowers, leaves and peel of *Citrus aurantium* L. var. *amara* from Tunisia. *J Essent Oil-Bear Plants.* 2006;9(2):133–139.

58. Go GY, Park H. Effects of aroma inhalation therapy on stress, anxiety, depression, and the autonomic nervous system in high-risk pregnant women. *Korean J Women Health Nurs.* 2017;23(1):33–41.

59. Ćavar S, Maksimović M. Antioxidant activity of essential oil and aqueous extract of *Pelargonium graveolens* L'Her. *Food Control.* 2012;23(1):263–267.

60. Fakari FR, Tabatabaeichehr M, Kamali H, et al. Effect of inhalation of aroma of geranium essence on anxiety and physiological parameters during first stage of labor in nulliparous women: A randomized clinical trial. *J Caring Sci.* 2015;4(2):135–141.

61. Kim Y-J, Lee MS, Yang YS, et al. Self-aromatherapy massage of the abdomen for the reduction of menstrual pain and anxiety during menstruation in nurses: A placebo-controlled clinical trial. *Eur J Integr Med.* 2011;3(3):e165–e168.

62. Domingos TS, Braga EM. Massage with aromatherapy: Effectiveness on anxiety of users with personality disorders in psychiatric hospitalization. *Rev Esc Enferm USP.* 2015;49(3):453–459.

63. Nayebi N, Khalili N, Kamalinejad M, et al. A systematic review of the efficacy and safety of *Rosa damascena* Mill. with an overview on its phytopharmacological properties. *Complement Ther Med.* 2017;34:129–140.

64. Muacevic A, Syed Aafaque J, Sumalatha S, et al. Effect of aromatherapy on dental anxiety among orthodontic patients: A randomized controlled trial. *Cureus.* 2019;11(8):e5306.

65. Dehkordi AK, Tayebi A, Ebadi A, et al. Effects of aromatherapy using the damask rose essential oil on depression, anxiety, and stress in hemodialysis patients: A clinical trial. *Nephrourol Mon.* 2017;9(6):e60280.

66. Kheirkhah M, Haghani H. Effect of aromatherapy with essential oil of damask rose oil on anxiety of the active phase of labor in nulliparous women. *J Urmia Nurs Midwifery Facult.* 2013;11(6):428–433.

67. Daglia R, Avcu M, Metin M, et al. The effects of aromatherapy using rose oil (*Rosa damascena* Mill.) on preoperative anxiety: A prospective randomized clinical trial. *Eur J Integr Med.* 2019;26:37–42.

68. Fazlollahpour-Rokni F, Shorofi SA, Mousavinasab N, et al. The effect of inhalation aromatherapy with rose essential oil on the anxiety of patients undergoing coronary artery bypass graft surgery. *Complement Ther Clin.* 2019;34:201–207.

69. McCaffrey R, Thomas DJ, Kinzelman AO. The effects of lavender and rosemary essential oils on test-taking anxiety among graduate nursing students. *Holist Nurs Pract.* 2009;23(2):88–93.

70. Sharifipour F, Sohailbaigi S, Dastmozd L. Comparison of the *Citrus arantium* and *Salvia officinalis* aroma impacts on post cesarean anxiety. *Acta Medica Mediterranea.* 2016;32(Special):977–981.

71. Heydarpour S, Sharifipour F, Salari N. Effect of aromatherapy using *Salvia officinalis* on sleep quality of postmenopausal women. *Iran J Obstet Gynecol Infert.* 2020;23(3):50–57.

72. Sindhu RK, Upma KA, Arora S. *Santalum album* linn: A review on morphology, phytochemistry and pharmacological aspects. *Int J PharmTech Res.* 2010 Jan;2(1):914–919.
73. Sheen J Stevens J. Self-perceived effects of Sandalwood. *Int J Aromather.* 2001;11(4):213–219.
74. Gradiyanto V, Dewi AM, Tedjosasongko U, et al. The effects of sandalwood aromatherapy (*Santalum album*) and bossa nova music on anxiety levels of pediatric patients undergoing topical fluoride treatment. *Eur J Mol Clin Med.* 2020;7(5):860–865.
75. Ariani NWN. Effect of sandalwood aromatherapy in sleep quality of adolescents at dharma jati orphanage ii in the year 2012. *Coping: Community of Publishing in Nursing.* 2013;1(1):1–7.
76. Kaymaz TT, Ozdemir L. Effects of aromatherapy on agitation and related caregiver burden in patients with moderate to severe dementia: A pilot study. *Geriatr Nurs.* 2017;38:231–237.
77. Oh Y-H, Jung HM. The effects of inhalation method using essential oils on the preoperative anxiety of hysterectomy patients. *Korean J Rehab Nurs.* 2002;5(1):18–26.
78. Cho MY, Min ES, Hur MH, et al. Effects of aromatherapy on the anxiety, vital signs, and sleep quality of percutaneous coronary intervention patients in intensive care units. *eCAM.* 2013;2013:381381.
79. Kilstoff K, Chenoweth L. New approaches to health and well-being for dementia day-care clients, family careers and day-care staff. *Int J Nurs Pract.* 1998;4:70–83.
80. Conrad P, Adams C. The effects of clinical aromatherapy for anxiety and depression in the high-risk postpartum woman—a pilot study. *Compl Ther Clinl Pract.* 2012;18(3):164–168.
81. Trambert R, Kowalski MO, Wu B, et al. A randomized controlled trial provides evidence to support aromatherapy to minimize anxiety in women undergoing breast biopsy. *Worldviews Evid Based Nurs.* 2017;14:394–402.
82. Bélanger L, Morin CM, Langlois F, et al. Insomnia and generalized anxiety disorder: Effects of cognitive behavior therapy for gad on insomnia symptoms. *J Anxiety Disord.* 2004;18(4):561–571.
83. Karadag E, Samancioglu S, Ozden D, et al. Effects of aromatherapy on sleep quality and anxiety of patients. *Nurs Crit Care.* 2017;22(2):105–112.
84. Babaii A, Adib-Hajbaghery M, Hajibagheri A. The effect of aromatherapy with damask rose and blindfold on sleep quality of patients admitted to cardiac critical care units. *Iran J Nurs.* 2015;28(93):96–105.
85. Widayati H, Indarwati R, Wahyuni E. The influence of jasmine essential oil through foot submersion and inhalation method in elderly sleep quality and quantity. In: *Proceedings of the 9th International Nursing Conference.* Setúbal, PT: INC; 2018. pp. 215–219.
86. Asgari MR, Vafaei-Moghadam A, Babamohamadi H, et al. Comparing acupressure with aromatherapy using citrus aurantium in terms of their effectiveness in sleep quality in patients undergoing percutaneous coronary interventions: A randomized clinical trial. *Complement Ther Clin Pract.* 2020;38:101066.
87. Connell FEA, Tan G, Gupta I, et al. Can aromatherapy promote sleep in elderly hospitalized patients? *J Can Geriatr Soc.* 2001;4(4):191–195.
88. Cannard G. The effect of aromatherapy in promoting relaxation and stress reduction in a general hospital. *Complement Ther Nurs Midwifery.* 1996;2:38–40.
89. Ackerley R, Croy I, Olausson H, et al. Investigating the putative impact of odors purported to have beneficial effects on sleep: Neural and perceptual processes. *Chem Percept.* 2020;13:93–105.
90. Lee MS, Choi J, Posadzki P, et al. Aromatherapy for health care: An overview of systematic reviews. *Maturitas.* 2012;71(3):257–260.
91. Janca A, van der Watt G. Aromatherapy in nursing and mental health care. *Contemp Nurse.* 2008;30(1):69–75.
92. Pellegrino R, Sinding C, De Wijk RA, et al. Habituation and adaptation to odors in humans. *Physiol Behav.* 2017;177:13–19.

11 Choosing an Herbal Treatment for Anxiety

There are a number of factors to consider when choosing an herb or combination of herbs to treat an individual's anxiety. Perhaps the first consideration is efficacy of the treatment. Many herbs and herbal combinations discussed in this text have been found to be effective in relieving anxiety. One must certainly consider the type of anxiety being treated. That includes whether the anxiety is acute and temporary or a persistent problem that may require ongoing treatment. It may be possible to relieve symptoms with a single herb, or it may be prudent to use herbs in combination. An important factor that may direct the decision-making process is if the person suffers significant comorbidities. Many herbs can help anxiety as well as other psychiatric and somatic ailments, and those extra benefits should be taken advantage of. Last, but not least, the herbal treatment must be safe.

11.1 EFFICACY

Herbs have been used for thousands of years to treat human illnesses and relieve human suffering. Certain herbs have gained reputations for efficacy, and these herbs are repeatedly mentioned in the literature and prescribed by experienced practitioners of Western, Chinese, and Ayurvedic schools of herbal medicine. Nonetheless, very few of those herbs have been shown to be both effective and safe in clinical studies. Because mainstream medicine has tended to dismiss herbal treatments due to lack of evidence—and to shun those that employ them—little effort has been made to initiate the very research that might prove their efficacy. It is distressing and unfair that mainstream medicine would on one hand dismiss the value of research into the efficacy of herbal treatment while on the other hand decrying the lack of evidence. One might resort to the old canard, "Lack of evidence is not evidence of lack." However, that would smack of avoidance.

There are many studies demonstrating efficacy of herbs in treating anxiety. However, the quality of those studies varies. In the doctrine of evidence-based medicine,[1] the highest form of evidence is from randomized, double-blinded controlled studies. That is, subjects are randomly divided into active treatment and placebo groups, and neither the subjects of the study nor the doctors giving the treatment know who is getting which treatment. The resulting data are then analyzed by statistical methods, and if significant differences between the treatment and placebo groups are found, it is assumed the differences are real and not just the result of chance, bias, or self-fulfilling prophecy. There have been such rigorous evaluations of herbs, and they have provided conclusive evidence that some herbal treatments can relieve anxiety. In some studies, the anxiety levels of a single

DOI: 10.1201/9781003300281-11

group were compared before and after a treatment, but without a placebo group to compare it against. Those results are considered less robust and must be carefully weighed. Still, they have provided evidence of efficacy. In some instances, authors have reported unusually good responses of individual patients to a treatment. Such "case reports" are considered to be weak evidence. Of course, those motivated to fight the current and swim against the mainstream may also be more vulnerable to bias than is the case with more accepted areas of research. That possibility must be taken into consideration. Admittedly, not all the evidence for the efficacy of herbs in treating anxiety is strong by the established tenets of evidence-based medicine. Nonetheless, evidence-based medicine recognizes that all these types of reports have validity and provide useful information. All in all, the existence of clinical evidence, along with expert opinion, bolstered by elucidation of plausible, scientifically sound mechanisms of action, makes the use of herbal treatments a reasonable path to take.

All the herbs and herbal combination discussed in this book have had some kind of study, or at least a published case report, to point to their efficacy. Any of the individual herbs discussed in this book should be considered as reasonable choices to use for treatment of anxiety, albeit with due caution and diligence and in accordance with the type of anxiety being treated. The herbs that have on their own been clinically found to relieve anxiety include:

Acorus calamus (not recommended for safety reasons), *Avena sativa, Bacopa monnieri, Camellia sinensis, Cannabis sativa, Centella asiatica, Cinnamomum spp, Citrus aurantium, Convolvulus pluricaulis, Crocus sativus, Curcuma longa, Echinacea angustifolia, Echium amoenum, Eleutherococcus senticosus, Eschscholzia californica, Evolvulus alsinoides, Foeniculum vulgare, Galphimia glauca, Ganoderma lucidum, Ginkgo biloba, Humulus lupulus, Hypericum perforatum, Lavandula angustifolia, Leonurus cardiaca, Lepidium meyenii, Lilium brownii, Lippia citriodora, Magnolia officinalis, Matricaria recutita, Melissa officinalis, Mentha piperita, Nardostachys jatamansi, Ocimum sanctum, Panax ginseng, Passiflora incarnata, Piper methysticum, Poria cocos, Psilocybe spp, Rhodiola rosea, Rosmarinus officinalis, Salvia officinalis, Schisandra chinensis, Scutellaria baicalensis, Silybum marianum, Tinospora cordifolia, Trifolium pratense, Valeriana jatamansi, Valeriana officinalis, Vitex agnus-castus, Withania somnifera,* and *Zizyphus jujuba.*

Although expert opinion alone is seen as weak by the standards of evidence-based medicine, when choosing from a list of already proven remedies, such opinion strengthens existing evidence. In his excellent doctoral dissertation, Luke Einerson, Ph.D., sought the opinions of master herbalist members of the American Herbalists Guild in regard to their most favored herbs to treat anxiety.[2] The experts named some herbs that are not among those listed prior. However, from among the list of proven herbs prior, expert opinion chose, in order of preference: *Lavandula spp, Leonurus cardiaca, Passiflora spp, Scutellaria lateriflora, Matricaria recutita, Avena sativa, Ganoderma lucidum, Schisandra chinensis, Melissa officinalis, Escholzchia californica, Humulus lupulus,* and *Piper methysticum.* This smaller list may be relied upon with use of others noted prior for personal preferences, comorbidities, or enhancement through combinations.

11.2   WHAT TYPE OF ANXIETY IS BEING TREATED?

A salient point in choosing an herbal treatment is the type of anxiety being treated. For the most part, the herbal treatments described in this book have been evaluated either in patients diagnosed with GAD or in otherwise healthy individuals who are simply suffering anxiety-provoking circumstances. In some cases, the efficacies of herbs were established under unique circumstances, such as treating the anxiety of menopause or premenstrual dysphoria. The herbs discussed in this book have not been tried across the full range of anxiety disorders, which would include phobias, social anxiety disorder, panic disorder, agoraphobia, substance- or medication-induced anxiety disorder, and anxiety disorder due to a medical condition. It may not be wise to generalize from existing data to make conclusions about other patient populations. However, one might also ask if the various types of anxiety disorders are different enough from one another to warrant specific forms of treatment for each. Some treatments might very well be helpful across the different categories. Clearly, some forms of anxiety disorder, such as phobias, have unique characteristics that define them. The most efficacious approach to treating phobias is to specifically address the trigger of symptoms through psychotherapeutic techniques such as exposure and desensitization. Similarly, there are components of social anxiety disorder that are known to respond to psychotherapies that address the root psychic causes and persisting misconceptions that perpetuate unnecessary feelings of anxiety. Nonetheless, many of the psychic and somatic symptoms that are shared among the various anxiety disorders are responsive to pharmacological and, in turn, herbal treatment. Moreover, many individuals do not sufficiently benefit from non-pharmacological treatment, and addition of an herbal treatment may contribute to relief from symptoms. Thus, it is both reasonable and compassionate to consider phytochemicals, or even anxiolytic medications, to help relieve the suffering of any patient suffering any type of anxiety disorder.

Another important consideration might thus be whether the anxiety is temporary and occasional or chronic and persistent. In most of the human trials of herbs discussed in this book, the anxiolytic effects of individual herbs or combinations of herbs were evaluated after weeks or more of administration. Such protocols do not allow testing of one of the most sought after effects of anxiolytic medication: rapid relief from sudden symptoms of anxiety with a single, acute dose. However, in almost every case, the individual herbs discussed in this book as having anxiolytic effects in humans after chronic administration have also been shown to have rapid anxiolytic effects after acute administration in animal studies. Common use of these herbs suggests this to be the general case in humans.

11.3   SINGLE HERBS OR COMBINATIONS?

In Western herbalism, herbs are often used on their own. If a single herb is effective, then there is no compelling reason to pursue others in addition. As in mainstream psychiatry, it is prudent to avoid two medications if one is sufficient. Of course, the question of using a single herb versus a combination of herbs might be tempered by the fact that each individual herb contains many phytochemicals that may contribute to the overall effect of the herb. Thus, the use of any one herb, by its nature, is an example of the much-maligned polypharmacy. In any case, if more than one herb is required, strategies can be employed to produce the most efficacious combinations.

Some herbs produce their anxiolytic effects, at least in part, through action at benzodiazepine receptors. These herbs would include *Centella asiatica*,[3] *Crocus sativus*,[4] *Curcuma longa*,[5] *Eleutherococcus senticosus*,[6] *Hypericum perforatum*,[7] and *Passiflora incarnata*,[8] as the anxiolytic effects of all of them can be reversed by flumazenil. On the other hand, the anxiolytic effects of *Ginkgo biloba*,[9] *Glycyrrhiza uralensis*,[10] *Leonurus cardiaca*,[11] *Rhodiola rosea*,[12] and *Withania somnifera*[13] are not fully reversed by flumazenil. Rosmanol, cirsimaritin, and salvigenin from *Rosmarinus officinalis* have all been found to have anxiolytic effects in rodents on their own. Those effects also were not reversed by flumazenil.[14] Combining from those two somewhat distinct groups, that is, flumazenil sensitive and flumazenil resistant, might be expected to have synergistic effects.

There are also individual herbs containing anxiolytic phytochemicals that are blocked by flumazenil and some that are not. For example, the anxiolytic effects of bisabolol in *Matricaria recutita* are blocked by flumazenil,[15] whereas the anxiolytic effects of the borneol[16] the herb contains are not. The anticonvulsant effects of wogonin, a flavonoid contained in *Scutellaria baicalensis*, are blocked by flumazenil,[17] whereas the anxiolytic effects of baicalein from the herb are not. Interestingly, those effects of baicalein can be reversed by the neurosteroid DHEAS.[18] Thus, the anxiolytic effects of those two flavonoids in *Scutellaria baicalensis* may have synergistic effects that, in turn, might augment the anxiolytic effects of other herbs. *Nardostachys jatamansi* also contains phytochemicals, some of whose effects are blocked by flumazenil as well as some that are not.[19] Whereas *Piper methysticum* may enhance GABAergic activity, studies have found that the anxiolytic effects of extract of the root are resistant to flumazenil.[20]

Some herbs exhibit the ability to dampen glutamatergic activity, which physiologically tends to enhance GABAergic effects. For example, some of the triterpenes in *Poria cocos* reduce glutamatergic activity in the brain.[21] Tinosporicide, from *Tinospora cordifolia*, does also.[22] Some effects of *Zizyphus jujuba* are reversed by flumazenil.[23] Jujuboside A extracted from the herb is known to enhance GABAergic activity and increase GABA receptor density in the hippocampus with repeated treatment. However, this substance also dampens activity of glutamate.[24]

Non-GABAergic mechanisms are apparent in other herbs that can be exploited to augment the effects of herbs that do act through GABAergic mechanisms. For example, some of the effects of *Echium amoenum*[25] and *Trifolium pratense*[26] may be due to stimulation of opiate receptors. *Eschscholzia californica* can displace binding at both opiate and cannabinoid receptors.[27] *Galphimia glauca* has antinociceptive effects that are mediated by opiate receptors,[28] while its constituent triterpene, galphimine-B, may contribute antagonism of the NMDA receptor.[29]

Of course, most of the effects of *Cannabis sativa* are mediated by cannabinoid receptors. However, there are many non-cannabis cannabinoids. A recent study has shown the combination of L-theanine extracted from *Camellia sinensis*, *Melissa officinalis*, and bark of *Magnolia officinalis* has potent anxiolytic-like effects in rats. These effects were not blocked by flumazenil, showing it was not mediated by benzodiazepine receptors. However, it was blocked by AM251, a cannabinoid receptor type 1 (CB1) antagonist.[30] Recent research shows the *Piper methysticum* constituent yangonin to be a novel cannabinoid.[31] Linalool, a monoterpenoid and a major constituent of *Lavandula angustifolia* and other fragrant medicinal herbs, may stimulate cannabinoid receptors as well as acting at opioid and NMDA receptors.[32-33] Addition of such herbs and constituent substances to those acting primarily at benzodiazepine or other GABA receptor complex sites may result in more efficacious treatment.

While combining herbs is not the rule in Western herbalism, as it is in Chinese and Ayurvedic herbalism, it is certainly not uncommon. Browsing both the formal literature and anecdotal reports shows that combinations of herbs are often recommended by Western herbalists. The combination Euphytose, a European concoction containing *Passiflora incarnata*, *Valeriana officinalis*, *Crataegus oxyacantha*, *Ballota nigra*, *Paullinia cupana*, and *Cola acuminata*, was shown to be effective in a clinical trial. It is discussed in Chapter 6. The relatively conservative German Commission E also discusses several "fixed combinations" of herbs for nervousness, unrest, or insomnia.[34] The combinations they discuss are *Valeriana officinalis* and *Melissa officinalis*; one pairing *Valeriana officinalis* and *Humulus lupulus*; another combining *Valeriana officinalis*, *Humulus lupulus*, and *Passiflora incarnata*; and yet another utilizing *Valeriana officinalis*, *Humulus lupulus*, and *Melissa officinalis*. Certainly, while the Chinese and Ayurvedic combinations discussed in this text were tested in chronic or sub-chronic regimens, they contain herbs with relatively rapid action and can be helpful in relieving anxiety acutely. Finally, while the data is not as compelling as one might like, it may also be worthwhile to consider aromatherapy, using single essential oils or combinations of oils, to help relieve acute anxiety. If administered with massage as part of the treatment, one can expect positive results.

11.4 TREATMENT OF CHRONIC ANXIETY DISORDERS

Most of the herbs and combinations discussed in this book were evaluated after weeks or more of administration and thus have proved themselves as useful for treating chronic anxiety disorders. However, there are at least two ways through which this approach can be helpful. One way is that chronic, scheduled treatment can, over time, help dampen persisting anxiety and make escalation into more severe bouts of anxiety less likely. Such a technique is not uncommon in mainstream psychiatry in which, rather than offering high, "as needed" doses of rapidly acting benzodiazepine, low doses of a long-acting benzodiazepine (such as clonazepam) might be used in a scheduled regimen to diminish the severity of persistent anxiety. It is helpful to explain to patients with histories of frequent panic attacks or other paroxysmal forms of anxiety that it is better to prevent bouts of anxiety than chase them.

The other way in which chronic, scheduled herbal treatments can be successful is by, over time, building resiliency and improved function of the nervous system. This occurs when adaptogens are among the herbs used for such treatment. In traditional Chinese and Ayurvedic medicine, herbs are almost always used in combination to treat anxiety, and in most cases, those combinations include herbs with adaptogenic effects. Among the herbs categorized as adaptogens that have been found on their own to alleviate anxiety are *Bacopa monnieri, Centella asiatica, Convolvulus pluricaulis, Curcuma longa, Eleutherococcus senticosus, Evolvulus alsinoides, Ganoderma lucidum, Ginkgo biloba, Hypericum perforatum, Lepidium peruvianum, Ocimum sanctum, Panax ginseng, Poria cocos, Rhodiola rosea, Schisandra chinensis, Scutellaria baicalensis, Tinospora cordifolia,* and *Withania somnifera.* It may be useful to include one or more of these anxiolytic adaptogens in any herbal combination used to treat chronic anxiety disorders.

11.5 COMORBIDITIES

Another reason to pick one herb over another is comorbidity—that is, the presence of an illness or condition along with the anxiety one may suffer. This could be a comorbid mental health condition, such as depression, or insomnia, menopausal symptoms, dysmenorrhea, pain, irritable bowel syndrome, diabetes, or dementia. Many herbs have been clinically shown to relieve anxiety as well as the symptoms of one or more comorbidities. It is wise to take advantage of such plural activities.

11.5.1 MAJOR DEPRESSION

Anxiety and depression are often comorbid. It has been reported that up to 40% of patients receiving treatment for an anxiety disorder also suffer from major depression.[35] As discussed in Chapter 4, antidepressants are considered a first-line treatment of anxiety. This may be because of the frequent comorbidity with anxiety or due to shared underlying pathology. In any case, the two conditions exacerbate each other, and relieving symptoms of one often reduces the severity of the other. Some herbs have been clinically shown to have antidepressant as well as anxiolytic effects in humans. Among those herbs are *Cinnamomum zeylanicum, Crocus sativus, Hypericum perforatum, Lavandula angustifolia, Matricaria recutita, Rhodiola rosea,* and *Rosmarinus officinalis.* For full discussion, see Mendelson.[36]

The addition of the essential oil of *Cinnamomum zeylanicum* in individuals who had not responded to fluoxetine alone significantly improved response to treatment.[37] Enough clinical studies of the antidepressant effect of *Crocus sativus* in human subjects have been performed to warrant reviews of this effect. The conclusions have been that supplementation with the herb can significantly improve symptoms of depression in adults with major depression.[38–40]

Hypericum perforatum is perhaps the most thoroughly researched herbal treatment of MDD. In a 2008 review written for the well-respected Cochrane Review, authors analyzed the results of 29 studies, including comparisons with placebo and comparisons with standard antidepressant medications in adults suffering from mild to moderately severe symptoms. It was concluded that "*Hypericum* extracts tested in the included trials are superior to placebo in patients with MDD; are similarly effective as standard antidepressants; and have fewer side effects than standard antidepressants."[41]

In a 70-day, randomized, placebo-controlled study of mixed anxiety and depressive disorder, Silexan (a proprietary preparation of *Lavandula angustifolia*) significantly reduced scores on the Montgomery Åsberg Depression Rating Scale. It also significantly reduced anxiety per the Hamilton Anxiety Rating Scale. Compared to placebo, the patients treated with Silexan had a better overall clinical outcome and showed more pronounced improvements of impaired daily living skills and health-related quality of life.[42]

A 2012 study evaluated effects of *Matricaria recutita* in subjects that comorbidly suffered anxiety and depression. The analysis of results performed with the use of the Hamilton Depression Rating Scale revealed a slight but significant decrease in depression symptoms in the *Matricaria recutita* group in comparison with the control group.[43]

Studies on the effects of *Rhodiola rosea* on MDD in humans are few and inconsistent. In a head-to-head comparison with sertraline, *Rhodiola rosea* did not exhibit significant antidepressant effect.[44] However, in subjects with mild to moderate degrees of MDD, daily dosing of extract of *Rhodiola rosea* significantly relieved symptoms of depression, insomnia, emotional instability, and somatization.[45] The most important contribution of *Rhodiola rosea* may be its actions as an adaptogen. Daily dosing of extract of the herb produced a significant lessening in symptoms of "burnout" as measured by the Pines Burnout Measure.[46]

Numerous studies have shown antidepressant-like effects of *Rosmarinus officinalis* in rodents. In a study of the effects of *Rosmarinus officinalis* on mood in humans, treatment with *Rosmarinus officinalis* twice a day for 1 month improved anxiety and, albeit to a lesser degree, mood.[47]

Three of the traditional Chinese herbal combinations that have been found to successfully treat anxiety, *ban xia hou pu*, *gui pi*, and *xiao yao san*, are also among the most commonly used herbal treatments for depression in traditional Chinese medicine.[48] *Ban xia hou pu* was significantly more effective than an active control treatment in treating symptoms of anxiety and depression in a group of subjects with globus hystericus.[49] *Gui pi* was as effective in treating depression and insomnia as was the combination of zolpidem, flupentixol, and the tricyclic antidepressant melitracen.[50] In evaluation of 50 patients with depressive disorders treated with *xiao yao san*, 26 showed marked improvement, 17 enjoyed modest improvement, and only 7 patients experienced no improvement.[51]

Similar to traditional Chinese medicine, Ayurvedic medicine does not recognize a specific pathological entity analogous to major depression. Rather, Ayurvedic philosophy sees a variety of imbalances of *vata*, *pitta*, and *kapha doshas* that might be diagnosed as the single diagnosis of major depression by Western diagnostic protocols. Among these disorders in Ayurvedic medicine are *avasada*, *manodhukhaja unmada*, *visadam*, and *kapha unmada*. Of those, *visadam* and *kapha unmada* are said to most closely resemble the classical Western illness of major depression, with *kapha unmada* being the most severe psychically and vegetatively.[52] Some of the anxiolytic herbs discussed in this volume are among the herbs commonly used by Ayurvedic practitioners to alleviate the symptoms of the depression-like syndromes. Those herbs include *Bacopa monnieri*, *Centella asiatica*, *Convolvulus pleuricaulis*, *Nardostachys jatamansi*, *Tinospora cordifolia*, *Valeriana jatamansi*, and *Withania somnifera*.[53]

Three of the above herbs have been shown in clinical studies to possess anti-depressant effects. *Bacopa monnieri* alleviated symptoms of depression in elderly subjects.[54] A clinical trial of *Centella asiatica* showed it to reduce symptoms of depression, though the study had no control group.[55] A study published in a journal of Ayurvedic medicine found that *Withania somnifera* plus *shirodhara* therapy significantly relieved symptoms of major depression in a manner similar to the active control treatment of fluoxetine 40mg a day.[56]

11.5.2 Insomnia

Insomnia, anxiety, and depression are common comorbidities. In one study, 40% of those presenting for treatment of anxiety or depression also met criteria to diagnose insomnia per the Insomnia Severity Index.[57] Almost all herbs that are helpful for rapid relief of anxiety are also helpful for insomnia. It is generally a matter of dose, with slightly higher doses being more effective in getting a person to sleep. Nonetheless, among the anxiolytic herbs that have been clinically proven effective for treating insomnia are *Cannabis sativa*, *Eschscholzia californica*, *Humulus lupulus*, *Lavandula angustifolia*, *Matricaria recutita*, *Melissa officinalis*, *Nardostachys jatamansi*, *Passiflora incarnata*, *Piper methysticum*, *Valeriana officinalis*, *Withania somnifera*, and *Zizyphus jujuba*.

A recent review found that species of *Cannabis* can be helpful in aiding sleep in those suffering insomnia. However, the authors note inconsistencies in the literature. It was suggested that cannabidiol may have therapeutic potential for the treatment of insomnia, whereas while delta-9-tetrahydrocannabinol may decrease sleep latency, it may go on to impair sleep quality long-term.[58] Interestingly, a survey of *Cannabis* users found that people preferred *Cannabis indica*—often richer in cannabidiol than delta-9-tetrahydrocannabinol—over *Cannabis sativa* in its helpfulness for insomnia, anxiety, and pain management.[59]

In a study of subjects complaining of insomnia, *Eschscholzia californica* was significantly more effective than the well-known sleep-inducing herb *Passiflora incarnata* in increasing duration of sleep. Unfortunately, there was no placebo control.[60] When *Eschscholzia californica* was combined with *Valeriana officinalis*, there were significant improvements in various components of the Insomnia Severity Index, although, surprisingly, this did not include shortening of sleep latency.[61]

Humulus lupulus, or hops, has a reputation for improving sleep, but the existing data is not strong. A study evaluating the combination of *Humulus lupulus* and *Valeriana officinalis* found the combination significantly superior to the placebo in reducing the sleep latency while the *Valeriana officinalis* extract alone was not.[62] Others saw this effect as well.[63] Thus, *Humulus lupulus* might at least be seen as useful in combination with other herbs in treating insomnia. If other comorbidities are present, such as menopausal symptoms (see the following), it might be an even more reasonable addition.

There are studies showing *Lavandula angustifolia* to be effective in improving sleep parameters when inhaled or massaged into the body using techniques of aromatherapy.[64–65] There is also at least one randomized, double-blinded study of the effects of orally administered essential oil of *Lavandula angustifolia* on sleep. Sleep was significantly improved per the Pittsburgh Sleep Quality Index. Moreover, as expected, anxiety was also reduced per the Hamilton Anxiety Rating Scale.[66]

Chamomile tea, from decoction of *Matricaria recutita*, is an ancient folk remedy for insomnia. Thankfully, its soporific effects have been established in clinical trials. In a study of patients suffering heart disease, 3 days of treatment with extract of *Matricaria recutita* significantly improved sleep per the St. Mary's Hospital Sleep Questionnaire.[67] Similar benefits, using that same sleep questionnaire, were observed in elderly patients newly admitted to a nursing home.[68] One randomized, placebo-controlled study of subjects suffering primary insomnia showed only modest, non-significant effects of *Matricaria recutita*.[69]

Melissa officinalis has long been thought helpful for insomnia. A study found that twice daily oral dosing of a hydroalcoholic extract of *Melissa officinalis* significantly improved both anxiety and sleep in subjects chosen for suffering a psychiatrically diagnosed anxiety disorder as well as a sleep disorder.[70] Dried extract of *Melissa officinalis* also improved both anxiety and sleep parameters in patients diagnosed with chronic angina pectoris, a particularly stressful condition.[71]

Nardostachys jatamansi has long been valued by practitioners of Ayurvedic medicine for its sedative and soporific effects.[72] However, true to Ayurvedic tradition, *Nardostachys jatamansi* is rarely used alone for such purpose. Rather, it tends to be used in combination with other herbs. Nonetheless, one study showed that, on its own, powdered *jatamansi* three times a day for 1 month significantly improved latency to sleep and sleep duration while reducing sleep disturbances in individuals diagnosed with primary insomnia.[73] A similar study found *Nardostachys jatamansi* effective in improving sleep parameters in patients suffering anxiety, fatigue, and insomnia.[74]

Passiflora incarnata is yet another time-honored remedy for anxiety and sleep disturbance. The *British Herbal Compendium* recommends its use for sleep disorders.[75] Unfortunately, there are few formal studies of such effects. In a double-blind, randomized, placebo-controlled, polysomnographic study of patients diagnosed with primary insomnia, treatment with extract of *Passiflora incarnata* for 2 weeks increased sleep duration.[76]

Along with reports of *Piper methysticum* relieving anxiety and depression, it is also frequently recommended for sleep disorders. In a large, randomized, placebo-controlled, double-blinded study of individuals with sleep disturbances associated with anxiety, a standardized extract of *Piper methysticum*, WS 1490, was found to both relieve anxiety, per the Hamilton Anxiety Rating Scale and Clinical Global Impression scale, and also improve sleep. Treatment with the extract for 4 weeks significantly improved quality of sleep and recuperative effect after sleep, per the German sleep questionnaire B.[77]

Although *Valeriana officinalis* has a strong reputation for helping resolve insomnia, the results of studies are less compelling. Some studies do demonstrate benefits for sleep. For example, in one study, extract of *Valeriana officinalis* significantly decreased subjective reports of sleep latency while significantly increasing sleep quality.[78] On the other hand, another randomized, placebo-controlled, double-blind study found no improvements in the sleep of cancer patients undergoing chemotherapy.[79] A large review and meta-analysis found some reports of improvement of sleep but other reports of ineffectiveness. The rather unenthusiastic conclusion was that "valerian might improve sleep quality without producing side effects."[80] As noted previously, two studies showed *Valeriana officinalis* combined with *Humulus lupulus* to be an effective sleep aid.

Withania somnifera is a staple of Ayurvedic herbal medicine, in which it is known as *ashwagandha*. It is considered a *rasayana*, or rejuvenating herb, but appears to both strengthen and calm. Of note, the species name, *somnifera*, itself means sleep inducing. Although often used in Ayurvedic medicine as part of a combination of herbs, there are studies showing *Withania somnifera* to improve sleep on its own. One randomized, double-blind, placebo-controlled study evaluated the effects of *Withania somnifera* in subjects who complained of frequent, non-restorative sleep but were otherwise healthy. Based on activity monitoring data, 6 weeks of treatment with *Withania somnifera* significantly improved sleep efficiency, total sleep time, sleep latency, and awakening after sleep onset in comparison to placebo after 6 weeks.[81] In a similar study, subjects diagnosed with insomnia by *DSM* standards also enjoyed significant improvements in sleep latency, sleep efficiency, and sleep quality after 10 weeks of treatment with *Withania somnifera*. The fact that chronic treatment improves sleep is important, but many would like an immediate effect to end a sleepless night. There is evidence from animal studies that acute treatment with *Withania somnifera* has sleep-inducing effects.[82]

Zizyphus jujuba is a staple in traditional Chinese medicine, and it is often included in treatments of insomnia. The seed of *Zizyphus jujuba* is called *suanzaoren*, and it lends its name to the formula called *suanzaoren* used in traditional Chinese medicine for treatment of anxiety and insomnia. However, both the seed and fruit (known as *dazao*) are used to relieve insomnia. On its own, the seed of *Zizyphus jujuba* significantly improves sleep.[83] A review of clinical studies of the use of the *suanzaoren* formulas strongly suggests its effectiveness in treating insomnia.[84] The anxiolytic combinations *xiao yao*[85] and *gui pi tang*[86] are commonly used to treat insomnia as well as anxiety. Those combinations are discussed in Chapter 7.

11.5.3 MENOPAUSE AND DYSMENORRHEA

A review and meta-analysis of treatment with *Trifolium pratense* led to the conclusion that the herb can relieve distressing symptoms of menopause, particularly vasomotor symptoms such as night sweats and hot flashes. These benefits are likely due to the isoflavones—formononetin, biochanin A, diadzen, and genistein—that act as phytoestrogens.[87] At the same time, the herb relieves symptoms of anxiety in menopausal women.[88] These benefits may be due in part to relief from physical distress of menopausal but also to additional anxiolytic effects of some of its constituent flavonoids. *Foeniculum vulgare*[89] and *Vitex agnus-castus*[90] may also be helpful in treating anxiety in the context of menopause, as both are known to contain phytoestrogens and to relieve not only emotional but some of the physical manifestations of menopause. *Lepidium meyenii* has been found not only to relieve the anxiety and depression of menopause but to increase sex drive in postmenopausal women as well.[91] *Humulus lupulus* has also been found to relieve physical symptoms of menopause.[92] It has not been evaluated specifically for anxiety and irritability of menopause, but having been shown to have more general anxiolytic effects, it would appear to be a good candidate for such use.

Primary dysmenorrhea, or menstrual pain, is a common condition. It is thought to be due to myometrium contractions induced by prostaglandins in the second half of the menstrual cycle. Many women experience primary dysmenorrhea, and it can occur in up to half of their menstrual cycles.[93] Anxiety and primary dysmenorrhea are commonly comorbid. While each is likely to exacerbate the other, there is suspicion of genetic links.[94] Studies have found that tea from *Matricaria recutita*, i.e., simple chamomile tea, can relieve the pain of dysmenorrhea.[95] There are also studies showing the ability of *Valeriana officinalis*,[96] *Salvia officinalis*,[97] and *Foeniculum vulgare*[98] to relieve the discomfort of menstrual cramps. *Vitex agnus-castus* can relieve discomfort of mastalgia and menstrual cramps.[99]

11.5.4 Pain

Many of the herbs that are useful for anxiety have also been found to help relieve various types of pain. Anxiety and pain tend to aggravate each other, and both can prevent restful, restorative sleep. Thus, the treatment of comorbid pain is an important consideration in choosing herbs to treat anxiety.

Although seen primarily as a *rasayana* herb to improve mood and cognitive function, Ayurvedic physicians have also long recommended *Bacopa monnieri* to treat arthritic and neuropathic pain. In a study of adults whose primary complaint was poor sleep, an extract of *Bacopa monnieri* over 4 weeks significantly reduced pain-related complaints.[100]

Boswellia is another genus known to relieve certain types of pain. A review and meta-analysis revealed that treatment with *Boswellia serrata*, which is similar to the previously discussed *Boswellia carterii* in its phytochemical composition, significantly reduced pain and inflammation associated with osteoarthritis in human subjects.[101]

Cannabis sativa is helpful in relieving migraine. This effect of cannabis was mentioned in the early 20th-century writings of William Osler, who is often considered the father of modern medicine.[102] In fact, *Cannabis sativa* has long been used to alleviate various types of pain, with reference to such use in the Chinese literature dating back several thousand years.[103] Several large reviews find that cannabis is useful for treatment of chronic pain.[104] Of particular interest is the apparent ability of cannabinoids to enhance the antinociceptive effects of opiates and to even allow the decrease in use of opiates.[105]

Eschscholzia californica is a member of the botanical family, *Papaveraceae*, and a cousin to the opium poppy, *Papaver somniferum*. Not surprisingly, it has long been found useful in treating various pain conditions. Its analgesic effects were favored by the Native Americans who inhabited what is now California.[106] One study found it effective in treating the pain of migraine.[107]

Although best known for its calming, anxiolytic effects, *Matricaria recutita* has also long been prized for anti-inflammatory and analgesic effects.[108] Interestingly, topical application of the essential oil of *Matricaria recutita* has been reported to relieve pain of migraine[109] and osteoarthritis of the knee.[110]

Tinospora cordifolia, a mainstay of Ayurvedic medicine, has anxiolytic effects along with significant anti-inflammatory and pain-relieving effects.[111] It has been found to be particularly useful in providing relief from diabetic nerve pain.[112]

Ingestion of *Withania somnifera* over 4 weeks was found to significantly reduce arthritic knee pain, and this was attributed to an anti-inflammatory effect.[113] However, a single dose of extract of *Withania somnifera* raised pain threshold and improved pain tolerance in human subjects in a model of mechanically induced pain. Thus, *Withania somnifera* may also offer some degree of acute pain relief.[114]

Many members of the *Lamiaceae* family of plants have reputations for anti-inflammatory and analgesic effects. They have been used in folk medicines around the world for such purposes.[115] Of the species in *Lamiaceae* that have been shown to have anxiolytic effects, there is clinical evidence of additional analgesic effects for only a few.

Lavandula angustifolia has long been used in traditional and herbal medicine for relief from inflammation and pain. Several studies have shown that application of essential oil of *Lavandula angustifolia* by massage can help relieve the pain of active labor in childbirth[116] as well as pain following cesarean surgery.[117]

Several studies have revealed analgesic effects of *Melissa officinalis*. In one impressive study, drinking tea made with *Melissa officinalis* significantly reduced pain and inflammation in patients who had undergone orthopedic procedures in their lower limbs.[118] In another study, ingestion of capsules containing powdered dried leaves of *Melissa officinalis* significantly reduced postpartum pain.[119]

Salvia officinalis has been found to be helpful in the relief of a variety of different types of pain in human subjects. It was shown to relieve the pain of acute pharyngitis[120] and, when added to treatment with an NSAID, to further reduce the pharyngeal pain after tonsillectomy.[121]

11.5.5 INFLAMMATION

Many pathophysiological circumstances can trigger the inflammatory response, including infection, injury, and even psychic stress. Once triggered, the response follows a typical course with the release of a variety of chemical messengers that can produce tissue damage and pain. It has only recently been appreciated that inflammation can also exacerbate psychiatric illness, including anxiety and depression,[122] and further neurodegenerative process, such as Alzheimer's and Parkinson's disease.[123]

Almost all the herbs discussed in this book as having anxiolytic effects in human subjects have also been found to offer significant anti-inflammatory effects. They can be useful in alleviating some of the symptoms of rheumatoid arthritis, various connective tissue diseases, and various autoimmune disorders, all of which involve abnormal inflammatory responses. Some of these effects are likely due to the actions of flavonoids. Among the best-established anti-inflammatory flavonoids are rutin, hesperidin, epigallocatechin-3-gallate, apigerin, diosmin, vitexin, quercetin, and naringenin. Interestingly, these substances can act at different stages of the inflammatory response and thus likely interact to reduce resulting inflammation.[124] Terpenes contained in herbs are also capable of significant anti-inflammatory effects. Notable among those anti-inflammatory terpenes—including some that have been mentioned in this text—are boswellic acid, celastrol, crocin, emodinol, geniposide, maslinic acid, torilin, and ursolic acid.[125]

A wide variety of phytochemicals, particularly the flavonoids that are ubiquitous in herbs, have been found to exhibit anti-inflammatory effects. Accordingly, many herbs offer some anti-inflammatory benefits. However, a recent review discussed herbs that have most convincingly been shown to exhibit anti-inflammatory effects for treatment of inflammatory conditions such as rheumatoid arthritis, osteoarthritis, fibromyalgia, inflammatory bowel disease, and uveitis.[126] Among those anti-inflammatory herbs that also offer anxiolytic effects—either when tested alone or when evaluated in commonly used anxiolytic combinations of Chinese or Ayurvedic herbal medicine—are *Curcuma longa, Zingiber officinale, Rosmarinus officinalis, Boswellia serrata*, and *Salvia officinalis*.

There are additional reports of anxiolytic herbs offering anti-inflammatory benefits. Daily consumption of green tea (*Camellia sinensis*) lessens pain and improves mobility in human subjects with osteoarthritis.[127] *Centella asiatica*, which has a reputation for healing inflammatory skin disease, was case reported to significantly improve psoriasis in a patient.[128] A review found *Crocus sativus* to provide patients significant relief from symptoms of rheumatic disease.[129] The combination of *Lippia citriodora* and fish oil significantly improved pain and immobility in human patients with inflamed joints.[130] Reviewers concluded that *Matricaria recutita* significantly improves a variety of inflammatory illnesses in human subjects.[131] *Tinospora cordifolia* reduced pain and inflammation in sufferers of rheumatoid arthritis.[132]

11.5.6 Irritable Bowel Syndrome

Anxiety and irritable bowel syndrome (IBS) are often found to be comorbid.[133] It is unclear if they are connected in some fundamental physiological or even genetic basis. Nonetheless, it is certainly the case that they exacerbate each other and that relief from one will ease the other. Several herbs with anxiolytic effects have been tested in clinical trials and found also to be helpful for treatment of IBS.

One or two tablets of dried standardized extract of *Curcuma longa* over 8 weeks was found to significantly improve the abdominal pain and discomfort from IBS.[134] In a randomized, double-blind, placebo-controlled trial, extract of *Hypericum perforatum* taken twice a day over 12 weeks significantly reduced symptoms of IBS and improved quality of life.[135] One capsule of peppermint oil (*Menthe piperita*) three times a day for 8 weeks also significantly improved pain and other symptoms of irritable bowel syndrome, as well as enhanced general quality of life.[136]

11.5.7 Diabetes

Many herbs with anxiolytic effects also have been shown to have beneficial effects in individuals suffering diabetes, specifically type II diabetes. Studies over the last 40 years have shown *Panax ginseng* to have hypoglycemic effects in animals and humans.[137] A recent review and metanalysis showed that supplementation with *Panax ginseng* in patients diagnosed with diabetes type 2 improved fasting glucose, postprandial insulin, and insulin sensitivity as measured by the Homeostatic Model

Assessment for Insulin Resistance. There were also significant improvements in serum triglycerides, total cholesterol, and LDL levels, though no differences were seen in HDL.[138]

Cinnamomum species have also been found to improve glucose regulation in diabetics. A review and meta-analysis revealed that supplementation with cinnamon was associated with statistically significant decreases in levels of fasting plasma glucose, total cholesterol, LDL-C, and triglycerides and an increase in HDL levels. Curiously, no significant effects on hemoglobin A1c were found. There was noted to be a high degree of heterogeneity in results, which authors believed may limit generalizability.[139]

Two months of treatment with *Ginkgo biloba* reduced serum markers of inflammation and reduced insulin resistance in human subjects.[140] A review of the benefits of *Humulus lupulus* showed the herb reduced systemic inflammation and improved metabolic syndrome in human subjects.[141] A recent study in humans suffering type 2 diabetes suggested impressive effects of tea made from *Matricaria recutita* on indexes of glycemic control. Consumption of chamomile tea three times a day for 8 weeks resulted in significant improvements in fasting insulin levels, insulin resistance, and HgA1c levels.[142] Reviews also show antidiabetic effects of *Rosmarinus officinalis*[143] and *Crocus sativus*.[144]

Scutellaria baicalensis extract inhibits the enzyme glucosidase,[145] whereas extract of *Rhodiola rosea* inhibits α-amylase.[146] Each of those effects would slow down the digestion of starch and in turn the absorption of sugar into the bloodstream. Thus, daily intake of one or more of these herbs can improve blood sugars in people with diabetes. Of course, since increased serum levels of glucocorticoids induced by anxiety and stress can raise serum glucose, the anxiolytic effects themselves can be helpful in managing diabetes.

11.5.8 DEMENTIA

Anxiety and agitation are common issues among the elderly suffering dementia. However, several herbs with anxiolytic effects have also been found to be helpful in slowing the relentless progression of dementia. *Ginkgo biloba* is one of the herbs that has gained a reputation for improving cognitive function and perhaps helping prevent dementia. Many studies and subsequent reviews and meta-analysis have tended to support the notion that the herb can be helpful in this regard. A review from 2015 that was consistent with the rigor of the Cochrane Library concluded that daily treatment with the standardized *Ginkgo biloba* extract, EGb761, at 240mg/day was able to stabilize or slow decline in cognition, function, behavior, and global change at 22–26 weeks. This was seen to be especially apparent in patients with neuropsychiatric symptoms.[147] These effects were attributed to ability to reduce amyloid aggregation and toxicity,[148] protect against oxidative damage,[149] and improve blood viscosity and microperfusion.[150] Indeed, there is evidence of efficacy in both Alzheimer's and vascular forms of dementia.[151]

Like *Ginkgo biloba*, *Bacopa monnieri* has been regarded as helpful in maintaining and improving cognitive function. A well-performed meta-analysis, which included studies of normal subjects as well as some with Alzheimer's dementia, demonstrated that *Bacopa monnieri* can improve cognitive function across a range of patients and conditions.[152] Among the mechanisms by which *Bacopa monnieri* might enhance cognition and slow the degenerative processes of Alzheimer's disease are antioxidant effects, enhancement of cholinergic activity, and reduction of amyloid deposition.[153]

Other anxiolytic herbs have also been evaluated for ability to enhance cognition and possibly impede the development of dementia. In a review and meta-analysis of *Withania somnifera*, with standards consistent with those of the Cochrane Library, the herb was found to improve performance in cognitive tasks, executive function, attention, and reaction time. It was noted, however, that the studies were quite heterogenous and the results difficult to extrapolate.[154]

Crocus sativus, which exhibits anxiolytic and antidepressant effects, has also been found to improve cognitive function in patients suffering Alzheimer's disease. A review of four randomized, controlled studies found that it significantly improved cognitive function measured by the Alzheimer's Disease Assessment Scale–Cognitive Subscale and Clinical Dementia Rating Scale–Sums of Boxes compared to placebo. It also appeared to perform as well as standard, prescribed anticholinesterase medications.[155]

In a large review of the literature, again using quality standards of the Cochrane Library, it was concluded that *Salvia officinalis*, *Rosmarinus officinalis*, and *Melissa officinalis* were each able to improve components of cognitive function in healthy adults, as well as in those suffering some degree of Alzheimer's disease, though the latter results were less consistent. The benefits of those herbs were largely attributed to the effects of rosmarinic acid. That substance, which is present in significant amounts in all three of these herbs, is known to exhibit anticholinesterase activity.[156]

Tinospora cordifolia, or *guduchi*, has long been considered a tonic and *rasayana* in Ayurvedic medicine and is considered an adaptogen in the Western perspective. It is often recommended by Ayurvedic practitioners to strengthen and restore the mind. There are data from animal studies to support the use of *Tinospora cordifolia* to treat and possibly prevent dementia but no compelling human studies.[157] *Rhodiola rosea* is another herb recognized as an adaptogen and possibly an enhancer of cognitive function. In healthy volunteers, it was found to enhance short-term memory and psychomotor vigilance.[158] In animal studies, *Rhodiola rosea* has shown promise for preventing progression of Alzheimer's disease.[159] However, there are no studies in humans suffering Alzheimer's disease.

Ganoderma lucidum, the revered *reishi* of traditional Chinese medicine, has long had a reputation as being a tonic and restorative herb. It has showed promise in studies utilizing animal models of Alzheimer's disease. Unfortunately, in the first human trial of *Ganoderma lucidum* as a treatment for Alzheimer's disease, it was found to be ineffective in improving cognitive deficits.[160]

11.6 SAFETY

Last but not least in considering which herb or herbs to use for treatment of anxiety is concern for safety. One major safety concern is the purity of the herbs to be used. Most people will not forage for their own herbs. Indeed, except for the most common and easily identified herbs, collecting herbs is another task best left to the experts.

Most people will buy the herbs they intend to use for treatment of anxiety. There are many herbal products available to purchase in stores and online. However, the usual protections in place to ensure our food and medicines are safe and reliable do not always apply to herbal treatments. The FDA classifies medicinal herbs as mere "dietary supplements" and does not evaluate their safety or efficacy. The only requirement is that manufacturers of herbal products follow standard manufacturing practices and that supplements meet basic quality standards. These regulations are intended to keep the wrong ingredients and contaminants out of supplements and to make sure that the right ingredients are included in appropriate amounts. If the FDA finds reason to declare a product unsafe, it can take action. However, whereas pharmaceutical manufacturers must provide the FDA with proof of efficacy for a prescription drug to enter the market, the FDA must establish proof of toxicity for a supplement to be removed from public sale. That process can take a long time. Thus, it is prudent to obtain herbs or herbal preparations from trusted sources.

Another safety issue to overcome is the common belief that since herbs are natural, they are naturally safe. This is not true. There is wisdom in the old saying that "anything strong enough to help you is also strong enough to hurt you." If used improperly, any herb can be dangerous. In most cases, the safety of an herb is simply a matter of dose. If used within a moderate dose range, most herbs will have no major adverse effects. On the other hand, some herbs are so dangerous that use even in small doses is inadvisable unless guided by an expert. *Aconitum carmichaelii*, known in Chinese as *fuzi* and in English as monkshood, has been used for centuries in traditional Chinese medicine for treatment of malaise, general weakness, poor circulation, cancer, and heart disease. In China, it has at times been referred to as "the king of all herbs." However, there is a very low margin of safety between therapeutic and toxic doses of the herb. *Aconitum carmichaelii* contains a deadly poison, aconitine, and none but experts are confident in preparing and prescribing it.[161] Another example is *Acorus calamus*, or sweet flag. That herb has long been used in Ayurvedic medicine, with little evidence of significant or widespread harm. However, the herb has been banned for use in the United States due to concern over the risk of liver cancer. For all herbs, caution is imperative and guidance advisable.

What must also be considered is the condition under which an herb is being used. For example, an herb generally safe for any woman to use may not be suitable for use during pregnancy. Other herbs may be safe for most people but not safe for individuals with certain medical conditions such as liver, heart, or kidney problems. For example, *Piper methysticum* can be hepatotoxic, and individuals with liver disease should not use it.[162] Whereas *Piper methysticum* has been the most publicized for its potential for liver damage, such hepatotoxicity has also been seen with use of *Echinacea angustifolia*, *Hypericum perforatum*, *Scutellaria baicalensis*, *Valeriana officinalis*, and even concentrated preparations of extracts of *Camellia sinensis*— that is, common green tea. Though the product of millennia of use, experience, and care, Chinese and Ayurvedic herbal treatments may also produce liver damage.[163–165] It should be noted that many prescribed psychiatric medications have been case reported to produce hepatotoxic effects, and some such medications, including valproate, carbamazepine, and nefazodone, should be strictly avoided in individuals with liver disease.[166] Great caution should be exercised in starting herbal treatment in anyone with chronic medical issues, and, in every case, some wariness should be exercised.

A final cause for safety concerns involves possible interactions of herbs with prescribed medications. Some phytochemicals can compete with prescribed medications as substrates for cytochrome P450 enzymes that break down such substances. This may cause the blood level of a medication to rise above its therapeutic level. On rare occasions, a phytochemical may increase the activity on an enzyme and thus lower the concentration of a medication below its therapeutic level. For most herbs used in prudent fashion, effects on liver enzymes and resulting effects on blood levels of prescribed medications are inconsequential. However, there are some notable exceptions. For an in-depth review of herb-drug interactions, see Posadzki et al.[167]

Some of the herbs discussed in this book are mentioned in the Posadzki review. He notes potential issues with *Curcuma longa*, as it has been reported to interact with beta-blockers or anticoagulants. They also allude to potential drug interactions with *Crocus sativus*, *Lavandula angustifolia*, *Ganoderma lucidum*, *Rosmarinus officinalis*, *Echinacea angustifolia*, and *Cinnamomum spp*. Nonetheless, all those potential interactions were described as being only minor concerns. The *Botanical Safety Handbook* voiced no concerns over any of them. Other potential interactions were seen as more significant. *Cannabis sativa*, *Matricaria recutita*, *Ginkgo biloba*, *Trifolium pratense*, and *Hypericum perforatum* have all been found to have interactions with the blood-thinning medication warfarin. Interestingly, warfarin itself was discovered as a natural substance in spoiled sweet clover hay when animals feeding on it developed fatal bleeding disorders.[168]

Ginkgo biloba has been suspected of potentially dangerous interactions with medications that have included not only anticoagulants but also anticonvulsants, MAO inhibitors, alprazolam, and haloperidol. Indeed, extract of *Ginkgo biloba* can either dampen or induce the activities of catabolic enzymes. Some authors suggest that reports of dangerous interactions of *Ginkgo biloba* with medications are misleading, as standard dosages of the herb tend not show such effects in vivo in human subjects.[169] On the other hand, one study discussed the ability of *Ginkgo biloba* to enhance the activity of the liver enzyme CYP2C19, and this has resulted in subtherapeutic blood levels of depakote and dilantin. These effects have resulted in relapse into seizures.[170]

Clinically significant interactions have been identified between *Hypericum perforatum* and prescribed medicines, including warfarin, phenprocoumon, cyclosporin, HIV protease inhibitors, theophylline, digoxin, and oral contraceptives. These interactions with *Hypericum perforatum* have resulted in decreases in concentrations and effects of those medicines. *Hypericum perforatum* may also increase blood levels of some psychiatric medications. There have even been reports of serotonin syndrome in geriatric patients after adding the herb to prescribed antidepressants.[171]

Although green tea, prepared from *Camellia sinensis*, is relatively innocuous, large doses of epigallocatechin-3-gallate extracted from the plant have potential for concerning interactions.[172] Caffeine from *Camellia sinensis* is metabolized by CYP1A2. Other medications largely metabolized by CYP1A2 include mexiletine, clozapine, psoralens, idrocilamide, phenylpropanolamine, furafylline, theophylline, and quinolones.[173] *Piper methysticum* can interfere with activity of CYP2E1. Among the drugs metabolized in part by CYP2E1 are ethanol, nicotine, acetaminophen, acetone, aspartame, chloroform, chlorzoxazone, and some antiepileptic drugs like phenobarbital.[174] It is suggested that anesthesiologists be aware of a patient taking *Piper methysticum* before any surgeries.[175]

With so many specialists now involved in each individual's health care, it is not uncommon for a physician to prescribe a medication for a skin condition without being aware of some other doctor, perhaps a cardiologist or gastroenterologist, having prescribed yet another medication for an ailing heart or stomach. It is often the pharmacist dispensing these various medications who sounds the alarm for potential dangers of interactions the patient's doctors may not even know are occurring. Pharmacists are well positioned to have such overview and are well equipped with computer systems and databases to point out not only interactions of drugs but also interactions between medications and herbs that patients may be taking with or without their doctors' knowledge. Their skill set should be used to best advantage.

11.7 FINAL CONSIDERATIONS ABOUT THE PRACTICAL USE OF HERBS

There are issues in medicine that arise regardless of whether one recommends herbs or prescribes more standard medications. Those include how one goes about starting, maintaining, changing, adjusting, and eventually stopping treatment. Although critical, how to address these concerns is rarely taught to physicians. It sometimes becomes a matter of guess work. Indeed, it is distressingly common to encounter patients who have been taking a medication for years because it was started but never stopped, even after it was no longer necessary. On the other hand, one wants to avoid the mistake that patients themselves sometimes make—that is, to arbitrarily stop a medication because they feel well and come to believe they no longer need it. That not uncommonly results in relapse, as it was likely the medicine that was helping them feel better.

Unfortunately, there are no hard and fast rules for treatment with medication, herbal or otherwise. There are "rules of thumb" that are wise to heed. For example, the old maxim "start low and go slow" is often prudent, though the severity of illness may demand more aggressive measures. In the treatment of major depression with antidepressants, it is often suggested (though I don't recall by whom) that patients started for the first time on an antidepressant should remain on it for 8 to 10 months, and, if they have consistently felt well, it is recommended to taper it off and see how they do. If, due to relapse, the medication needs to be started a second time, it should be continued a bit longer—perhaps a year or so—before tapering off can again be considered. If the antidepressant needs to be started a third time, it may be wise to simply continue it. In this regard, there have also recently been discussions among psychiatrists about how rapidly a patient should be tapered off a psychoactive medication. Many now suspect that patients are taken off such medications too rapidly.

It is also common for a patient to not respond well to a specific treatment. At some point, one must consider increasing the dose, changing the treatment altogether, or augmenting the less than effective medication. In psychiatry, various algorithms have been formulated to address treatment-resistant major depression and move on to other more potent and hopefully more effective medications or combinations. These algorithms come and go and are constantly being adjusted and improved. Nonetheless, there continues to be a percentage of patients who do not respond. All these issues make one aware of the fact that medicine is indeed an art and not merely applied science.

For those first wading into the use of herbs as treatment for anxiety and other psychiatric conditions, it might be comforting to know that they will encounter the same challenges and uncertainties in managing herbal medications that they are accustomed to in their use of more standard, pharmaceutically produced medications. In their very useful book, *Commonly Used Chinese Herbal Formulas*, Hsu and Hsu address some practical issues in the use of Chinese herbal treatments.[176] They recommend starting with traditional doses, which they say rarely need to be altered for individuals. This, they imply, may come later. However, this is not unlike standard starting doses of prescribed medications that come in specific, regimented doses. They add that if symptoms persist or new symptoms appear, the dosage may be adjusted. They suggest increasing the taking of medication from twice to three times daily. For ongoing treatment after stabilization, they recommend reducing dosage by half. These recommendations should not appear odd, for they address the same problems one is likely to encounter using more ordinary allopathic medications.

Hsu and Hsu do not give general advice on when or how to stop herbal treatments. However, this leaves the same challenge that practitioners face when treating patients with medications not sprung from the earth but rather manufactured in laboratories. Few studies of herbal treatments discussed in this book offer any direction in this regard, as most take place over several weeks to months with no further observations or adjustments in treatment conveyed. Of note, in the discussions of the herbal combinations *kami-shoyo-san* and *hange-koboku-to*, found in Chapter 7 of this book, the authors noted that several weeks after ending the successful herbal treatment, the symptoms of anxiety and panic returned, and the treatment was restarted with subsequent remission of symptoms. This is common in typical psychiatric practice. The message to be distilled from these bits of advice about the management of herbal treatment is that it is quite the same as any other medicinal treatment. After all, herbs act not through magic but molecules.

REFERENCES

1. Sacketts DL, Straus SE, Richardson WS, Rosenberg W, Haynes RB. *Evidence-Based Medicine: How to Practice and Teach EBM*, 2nd edition. New York: Churchill Livingstone; 2000.
2. Einerson LS. *A Delphi Study on Herbs Used to Address Depression and Anxiety According to Master Herbalists.* Lubbock: Texas Tech University; 2017.
3. Ceremuga TE, Valdivieso D, Kenner C, et al. Evaluation of the anxiolytic and antidepressant effects of asiatic acid, a compound from gotu kola or *Centella asiatica*, in the male Sprague Dawley rat. *AANA J.* 2015;83(2):91–98.
4. Pitsikas N, Tarantilis PA. The GABAA-benzodiazepine receptor antagonist flumazenil. Abolishes the anxiolytic effects of the active constituents of *Crocus sativus* L. Crocins in rats. *Molecules.* 2020;25:564.
5. Ishola IO, Katola FO, Adeyemi OO. Involvement of GABAergic and nitrergic systems in the anxiolytic and hypnotic effects of *Curcuma longa*: Its interaction with anxiolytic-hypnotics. *DMPT.* 2021;36(2):135–143.

6. Liu Y, Wang Z, Wang C, et al. Comprehensive phytochemical analysis and sedative-hypnotic activity of two *Acanthopanax* species leaves. *Food Function.* 2021;12(5):2292–2311.

7. Vandenbogaerde A, Zandi P, Puia G, et al. Evidence that the total extract of *Hypericum perforatum* affects exploratory behaviour and exerts anxiolytic effects in rats. *Pharmacol Biochem Behav.* 2000;65:627–633.

8. Grundmann O, Wang J, McGregor GP, et al. Anxiolytic activity of a phytochemically characterized *Passiflora incarnata* extract is mediated via the GABAergic system. *Planta Medica.* 2008;74(15):1769–1773.

9. Kuribara H, Weintraub ST, Yoshihama T, et al. An anxiolytic-like effect of *Ginkgo biloba* extract and its constituent, ginkgolide-A, in mice. *J Nat Prod.* 2003;66(10):1333–1337.

10. Hoffmann KM, Beltrán L, Ziemba PM, et al. Potentiating effect of glabridin from *Glycyrrhiza glabra* on GABAA receptors. *Biochem Biophys Rep.* 2016;6:197–202.

11. Fierascu RC, Fierascu I, Ortan A, et al. *Leonurus cardiaca* L. as a source of bioactive compounds: An update of the european medicines agency assessment report (2010). *Biomed Res Int.* 2019:4303215.

12. Cayer C, Ahmed F, Filion V, et al. Characterization of the anxiolytic activity of Nunavik *Rhodiola rosea. Planta Medica.* 2013;79(15):1385–1391.

13. Kumar A, Kalonia H. Effect of *Withania somnifera* on sleep-wake cycle in sleep-disturbed rats: Possible GABAergic mechanism. *Indian J Pharm Sci.* 2008;70(6):806–810.

14. Abdelhalim A, Karim N, Chebib M, et al. Antidepressant, anxiolytic and antinociceptive activities of constituents from *Rosmarinus officinalis. J Pharm Pharm Sci.* 2015;18(4):448–459.

15. Tabari MA, Tehrani MAB. Evidence for the involvement of the GABAergic, but not serotonergic transmission in the anxiolytic-like effect of bisabolol in the mouse elevated plus maze. *N-S Arch Pharmacol.* 2017;390:1041–1046.

16. Granger RE, Campbell EL, Johnston GAR. (+)- and (–)-borneol: Efficacious positive modulators of GABA action at human recombinant α1β2γ2L GABAA receptors. *Biochem Pharmacol.* 2005;69(7):1101–1111.

17. Hui KM, Huen MS, Wang HY, et al. Anxiolytic effect of wogonin, a benzodiazepine receptor ligand isolated from *Scutellaria baicalensis* Georgi. *Biochem Pharmacol.* 2002;64:1415–1424.

18. de Carvalho RSM, Duarte FS, de Lima TCM. Involvement of GABAergic non-benzodiazepine sites in the anxiolytic-like and sedative effects of the flavonoid baicalein in mice. *Behav Brain Res.* 2011;221(1):75–82.

19. Takemoto H, Ito M, Asada Y. Inhalation administration of the sesquiterpenoid aristolen-1 (10)-en-9-ol from *Nardostachys chinensis* has a sedative effect via the GABAergic system. *Planta Medica.* 2015;81(5):343–347.

20. Garrett KM, Basmadjian G, Khan IA, et al. Extracts of kava (*Piper methysticum*) induce acute anxiolytic-like behavioral changes in mice. *Psychopharmacology.* 2003;170:33–41.

21. Gao Y, Yan H, Jin R, Lei P. Antiepileptic activity of total triterpenes isolated from *Poria cocos* is mediated by suppression of aspartic and glutamic acids in the brain. *Pharm Biol.* 2016;54(11):2528–2535.

22. Sharma A, Kalotra S, Bajaj P, et al. Butanol extract of *Tinospora cordifolia* ameliorates cognitive deficits associated with glutamate-induced excitotoxicity: A mechanistic study using hippocampal neurons. *Neuromolecular Med.* 2020;22(1):81–99.

23. Han HS, Ma YA, Eun JS, et al. Anxiolytic-like effects of methanol extract of *Zizyphi Spinosi Semen* in mice. *Biomol Ther.* 2007;15(3):175–181.

24. Zhang M, Ning G, Shou C, et al. Inhibitory effect of jujuboside A on glutamate-mediated excitatory signal pathway in hippocampus. *Planta Medica.* 2003;69(08):692–695.

25. Heidari MR, Azad EM, Mehrabani M. Evaluation of the analgesic effect of *Echium amoenum* Fisch & C.A. Mey. extract in mice: Possible mechanism involved. *J Ethnopharmacol.* 2006;103(3):345–349.

26. Nissan HP, Lu J, Booth NL, et al. A red clover (*Trifolium pratense*) phase II clinical extract possesses opiate activity. J Ethnopharmacol. 2007;112(1):207–210.

27. Kumarihamy M, Leon F, Pettaway S, et al. Cannabinoid and opioid receptor displacement affinities of *Eschscholzia californica*. *Planta Medica.* 2015;81(05):PC18.

28. Garige BSR, Keshetti S, Vattikuti UMR. Assessment of antinociceptive and anti-inflammatory activities of *Galphimia glauca* stem methanol extract on noxious provocation induced pain and inflammation in in-vivo models. *J Chem Pharm Res.* 2016;8(4):1282–1289.

29. Sharma A, Angulo-Bejarano PI, Madariaga-Navarrete A, et al. Multidisciplinary investigations on galphimia glauca: A Mexican medicinal plant with pharmacological potential. *Molecules.* 2018;23(11):2985–3007.

30. Borgonetti V, Governa P, Biagi M, et al. Novel therapeutic approach for the management of mood disorders: In vivo and in vitro effect of a combination of l-theanine, *Melissa officinalis* L. And *Magnolia officinalis* Rehder & EH Wilson. *Nutrients.* 2020;12(6):1803–1818.

31. Ligresti A, Villano R, Allarà M, et al. Kavalactones and the endocannabinoid system: The plant-derived yangonin is a novel CB1 receptor ligand. *Pharmacol Res.* 2012;66(2):163–169.

32. Hecksel R, LaVigne J, Streicher JM. In defense of the "entourage effect": Terpenes found in *Cannabis sativa* activate the cannabinoid receptor 1 in vitro. *FASEB* 2020; 34(Suppl 1):1.

33. Guimarães AG, Quintans JSS, Quintans-Júnior LJ. Monoterpenes with analgesic activity—a systematic review. *Phytother Res.* 2013;27:1–15.

34. Blumenthal M, Busse WR, Goldberg A, et al. *The Complete German Commission E Monographs.* Austin, TX: American Botanical Council; 1998.

35. Huppert JD. Anxiety disorders and depression comorbidity. In: MM Antony, MB Stein (Eds.), *Oxford Handbook of Anxiety and Related Disorders.* Oxford: Oxford University Press; 2008. pp. 576–584.

36. Mendelson S. *Herbal Treatment of Major Depression: Scientific Basis and Practical Use.* Boca Raton, FL: CRC Press; 2019.

37. Ghaderi H, Nikan R, Rafieian-Kopaei M, et al. The effect of *Cinnamon zeylanicum* essential oil on treatment of patients with unipolar nonpsychotic major depression disorder treated with fluoxetine. *Pharmacophore.* 2017;8(3):24–31.

38. Hausenblas HA, Saha D, Dubyak PJ, et al. Saffron (*Crocus sativus* L.) and major depressive disorder: A meta-analysis of randomized clinical trials. *J Integr Med.* 2013;11(6):377–383.

39. Lopresti AL, Drummond PD. Saffron (*Crocus sativus*) for depression: A systematic review of clinical studies and examination of underlying antidepressant mechanisms of action. *Hum Psychopharmacol.* 2014;29(6):517–527.

40. Kamalipour M, Jamshidi AH, Akhondzadeh S. Antidepressant effect of *Crocus sativus*: An evidence-based review. *J Med Plant.* 2010;9(6):35–38.

41. Linde K, Berner MM, Kriston L. St John's wort for major depression. *Cochrane DB Syst Rev.* 2008;4: CD000448.

42. Kasper S, Volz HP, Dienel A, et al. Efficacy of Silexan in mixed anxiety-depression—a randomized, placebo-controlled trial. *Eur Neuropsychopharm.* 2016;26(2):331–340.

43. Amsterdam JD, Shults J, Soeller I, et al. Chamomile (*Matricaria recutita*) may provide antidepressant activity in anxious, depressed humans: An exploratory study. *Altern Ther Health Med.* 2012;18(5):44–49.

44. Mao JJ, Xie SX, Zee J, et al. *Rhodiola rosea* versus sertraline for major depressive disorder: A randomized placebo-controlled trial. *Phytomedicine.* 2015;22(3):394–399.
45. Darbinyan V, Aslanyan G, Amroyan E, et al. Clinical trial of *Rhodiola rosea* L. extract SHR-5 in the treatment of mild to moderate depression. *Nord J Psychiat.* 2007;61(6):343–348.
46. Olsson EMG, von Schéele B, Panossian AG. A randomized, double-blind, placebo-controlled, parallel-group study of the standardized extract SHR-5 of the roots of *Rhodiola rosea* in the treatment of subjects with stress-related fatigue. *Planta Med.* 2009;75:1–5–112.
47. Nematolahia P, Mehrabani M, Karami-Mohajer S, et al. Effects of *Rosmarinus officinalis* L. on memory performance, anxiety, depression, and sleep quality in university students: A randomized clinical trial. *Complement Ther Clin.* 2018;30:24–28.
48. Yeung W-F, Chung KF, Ng KY, et al. A systematic review on the efficacy, safety and types of Chinese herbal medicine for depression. *J Psychiat Res.* 2014;57:165–175.
49. Guo Y, Kong L, Wang Y, et al. Antidepressant evaluation of polysaccharides from a Chinese herbal medicine *banxia-houpu* decoction. *Phytother Res.* 2004;18(3):204–207.
50. Chen H. *Guipi* and *Ganmai* Chinese date decoction treat depressed disordered concerned insomnia. *J Tradit Chin Med.* 2010;2010:3.
51. Zhang LD. Traditional Chinese medicine typing of affective disorders and treatment. *Am J Chin Med.* 1994;22(3–4):321–327.
52. Steer E. A cross comparison between Ayurvedic etiology of major depressive disorder and bidirectional effect of gut dysregulation. *J Ayurveda Integr Med.* 2019;10(1):59–66.
53. Bishnoi S, Prajapat P, Mishra PK, et al. An Ayurvedic management of *manoavasada* depression: A review article. *World J Pharm Res.* 2021;10(2):494–508.
54. Hingorani L, Patel S, Ebersole B. Sustained cognitive effects and safety of HPLC-standardized *Bacopa Monnieri* extract: A randomized, placebo controlled clinical trial. *Planta Med.* 2012;78–PH22.
55. Jana U, Sur TK, Maity LN, et al. A clinical study on the management of generalized anxiety disorder with *Centella asiatica. Nepal Med Coll J.* 2010;12(1):8–11.
56. Fulzele A, Hudda N. Selective Ayurvedic therapy for the management of major depressive disorder: A randomized control trial. *Anc Sci Life.* 2012;32(Suppl 1): S41.
57. Mason EC, Harvey AG. Insomnia before and after treatment for anxiety and depression. *J Affect Dis.* 2014;168:415–421.
58. Babson KA, Sottile J, Morabito D. Cannabis, cannabinoids, and sleep: A review of the literature. *Curr Psychiatry Rep.* 2017;19(4):1–12.
59. Pearce DD, Mitsouras K, Irizarry KJ. Discriminating the effects of *Cannabis sativa* and *Cannabis indica*: A web survey of medical cannabis users. *J Altern Complement Med.* 2014;20(10):787–791.
60. Arora A. A study to compare the efficacy of *Eschscholzia californica* MT and *Passiflora incarnata* MT in insomnia. *Int J Hom Sci.* 2019;3(03):18–22.
61. Abdellah SA, Berlin A, Blondeau C, et al. A combination of *Eschscholzia californica* Cham. and *Valeriana officinalis* L. Extracts for adjustment insomnia: A prospective observational study. *J Tradit Complement Med.* 2020;10(2):116–123.
62. Koetter U, Schrader E, Käufeler R, et al. A randomized, double blind, placebo-controlled, prospective clinical study to demonstrate clinical efficacy of a fixed valerian hops extract combination (Ze 91019) in patients suffering from non-organic sleep disorder. *Phytother Res.* 2007;21(9):847–851.
63. Morin CM, Koetter U, Bastien C, et al. Valerian-hops combination and diphenhydramine for treating insomnia: A randomized placebo-controlled clinical trial. *Sleep.* 2005;28(11):1465–1471.
64. Jung HN, Choi HJ. Effects of *Lavandula angustifolia* aroma on electroencephalograms in female adults with sleep disorders. *J Life Sci.* 2012;22(2):192–199.

65. Lewith GT, Godfrey AD, Prescott P. A single-blinded, randomized pilot study evaluating the aroma of *Lavandula augustifolia* as a treatment for mild insomnia. *J Altern Complement Med.* 2005;11(4):631–637.
66. Kasper S, Anghelescu I, Dienel A. Efficacy of orally administered Silexan in patients with anxiety-related restlessness and disturbed sleep—a randomized, placebo-controlled trial. *Eur Neuropsychopharmacol.* 2015;25(11):1960–1967.
67. Rashidi S, Shafie D, Mazaheri M, et al. Effect of *Matricaria Recutita* drop on sleep quality in patients with chronic heart disease: A randomized controlled trial. *Arch Pharm Prac.* 2020;1:162–167.
68. Abdullahzadeh M, Naji SA. The effect of *Matricaria chamomilla* on sleep quality of elderly people admitted to nursing homes. *Iran J Nurs.* 2014;27(89):69–79.
69. Zick SM, Wright BD, Sen A, et al. Preliminary examination of the efficacy and safety of a standardized chamomile extract for chronic primary insomnia: A randomized placebo-controlled pilot study. *BMC Complement Altern Med.* 2011;11(1):1–8.
70. Cases J, Ibarra A, Feuillère N, et al. Pilot trial of *Melissa officinalis* L. Leaf extract in the treatment of volunteers suffering from mild-to-moderate anxiety disorders and sleep disturbances. *Med J Nutrition Metab.* 2011;4(3):211–218.
71. Haybar H, Javid AZ, Haghighizadeh MH, et al. The effects of *Melissa officinalis* supplementation on depression, anxiety, stress, and sleep disorder in patients with chronic stable angina. *Clin Nutr ESPEN.* 2018;26:47–52.
72. Pandey MM, Katara A, Pandey G, et al. An important Indian traditional drug of ayurveda *jatamansi* and its substitute *bhootkeshi*: Chemical profiling and antioxidant activity. *eCAM.* 2013;2013: Article ID 142517.
73. Toolika E, Bhat NP, Shetty SK. A comparative clinical study on the effect of *Tagara* (*Valeriana wallichii* DC.) and *Jatamansi* (*Nardostachys jatamansi* DC.) in the management of *Anidra* (primary insomnia). *Ayu.* 2015;36(1):46–49.
74. Misar SD, Kuchewar V. A comparative study of efficacy of *jatmansi vati* and *abhyanga* in management of *andira* with special reference to insomnia. *IAMJ.* 2016;4(7):1102–1111.
75. Bergner P. Passionflower. *Med Herbal.* 1995;7(12):13–14.
76. Lee J, Jung HY, Lee SI, et al. Effects of *Passiflora incarnata* Linnaeus on polysomnographic sleep parameters in subjects with insomnia disorder: A double-blind randomized placebo-controlled study. *Int Clin Psychopharmacol.* 2020;35(1):29–35.
77. Lehrl S. Clinical efficacy of kava extract WS® 1490 in sleep disturbances associated with anxiety disorders: Results of a multicenter, placebo-controlled, double-blind clinical trial. *J Affect Dis.* 2004;78(2):101–110.
78. Leathwood PD, Chauffard F, Heck E, et al. Aqueous extract of valerian root (*Valeriana officinalis* L.) improves sleep quality in man. *Pharmacol Biochem Behav.* 1982;17(1):65–71.
79. Barton DL, Atherton PJ, Bauer BA, et al. The use of *valeriana officinalis* (valerian) in improving sleep in patients who are undergoing treatment for cancer: A phase III randomized, placebo-controlled, double-blind study: NCCTG Trial, N01C5. *J Support Oncol.* 2011;9(1):24–31.
80. Bent S, Padula A, Moore D, et al. Valerian for sleep: A systematic review and meta-analysis. *Am J Med.* 2006;119(12):1005–1012.
81. Deshpande A, Irani N, Balkrishnan R, et al. A randomized, double blind, placebo-controlled study to evaluate the effects of *ashwagandha* (*Withania somnifera*) extract on sleep quality in healthy adults. *Sleep Med.* 2020;72:28–36.
82. Kumar A, Kalonia H. Effect of *Withania somnifera* on sleep-wake cycle in sleep-disturbed rats: Possible GABAergic mechanism. *Indian J Pharm Sci.* 2008;70(6):806–810.
83. Shergis JL, Hyde A, Meaklim H, et al. Medicinal seeds *Zizyphus spinosa* for insomnia: A randomized, placebo-controlled, cross-over, feasibility clinical trial. *Complement Ther Med.* 2021;57:102657.

84. Zhou QH, Zhou XL, Xu MB, et al. *Suanzaoren* formulae for insomnia: Updated clinical evidence and possible mechanisms. *Front Pharmacol.* 2018;9: Article 76.
85. Wing YK. Herbal treatment of insomnia. *Hong Kong Med J.* 2001;7(4):392–402.
86. Yeung WF, Chung KF, Poon MM, et al. Chinese herbal medicine for insomnia: A systematic review of randomized controlled trials. *Sleep Med Rev.* 2012;16(6):497–507.
87. Myers SP, Vigar V. Effects of a standardized extract of *Trifolium pratense* (Promensil) at a dosage of 80 mg in the treatment of menopausal hot flushes: A systematic review and meta-analysis. *Phytomedicine.* 2017;15(24):141–147.
88. Lipovac M, Chedraui P, Gruenhut C, et al. Improvement of postmenopausal depressive and anxiety symptoms after treatment with isoflavones derived from red clover extracts. *Maturitas.* 2010;65(3):258–261.
89. Rahimikian F, Rahimi R, Golzareh P, et al. Effect of *Foeniculum vulgare* mill. (fennel) on menopausal symptoms in postmenopausal women: A randomized, triple-blind, placebo-controlled trial. *Menopause.* 2017;24(9):1017–1021.
90. Van Die MD, Burger HG, Teede HJ, et al. *Vitex agnus-castus* (Chaste-Tree/Berry) in the treatment of menopause-related complaints. *J Altern Complement Med.* 2009;15(8):853–862.
91. Brooks NA, Wilcox G, Walker KZ, et al. Beneficial effects of *Lepidium meyenii* (Maca) on psychological symptoms and measures of sexual dysfunction in postmenopausal women are not related to estrogen or androgen content. *Menopause.* 2008;15(6):1157–1162.
92. Aghamiri V, Mirghafourvand M, Mohammad-Alizadeh-Charandabi S, et al. The effect of Hop (*Humulus lupulus* L.) on early menopausal symptoms and hot flashes: A randomized placebo-controlled trial. *Complement Ther Clin Pract.* 2016;23:130–135.
93. Dawood MY. Primary dysmenorrhea: Advances in pathogenesis and management. *Obstet Gynecol.* 2006;108:428–441.
94. Silberg JL, Martin NG, Heath AC. Genetic and environmental factors in primary dysmenorrhea and its relationship to anxiety, depression, and neuroticism. *Behav Genet.* 1987;17(4):363–383.
95. Jenabi E, Ebrahimzadeh S. Chamomile tea for relief of primary dysmenorrhea. *Iran J Obstet Gynecol Infertil.* 2010;13(1):39–42.
96. Kazemian A, Parvin N, Delaram M, et al. Comparison of analgesic effect of *Valeriana officinalis* and mefenamic acid on primary dysmenorrhea. *J Med Plant.* 2017;16(64):153–159.
97. Kalvandi R, Alimohammadi S, Pashmakian Z, et al. The effects of medicinal plants of *melissa officinalis* and *salvia officinalis* on primary dysmenorrhea. *Avicenna J Clin Med.* 2014;21(2):105–111.
98. Bokaie M, Farajkhoda T, Enjezab B, et al. Oral fennel (*Foeniculum vulgare*) drop effect on primary dysmenorrhea: Effectiveness of herbal drug. *Iran J Nurs Midwifery Res.* 2013;18(2):128–132.
99. Niroumand M, Heydarpour F, Farzaei M. Pharmacological and therapeutic effects of *Vitex agnus-castus* L.: A review. *Pharmacogn Rev.* 2018;12(23):103–114.
100. Lopresti AL, Smith SJ, Ali S, et al. Effects of a *Bacopa monnieri* extract (Bacognize®) on stress, fatigue, quality of life and sleep in adults with self-reported poor sleep: A randomised, double-blind, placebo-controlled study. *J Funct Foods.* 2021;85:104671.
101. Yu G, Xiang W, Zhang T, et al. Effectiveness of *Boswellia* and *Boswellia* extract for osteoarthritis patients: A systematic review and meta-analysis. *BMC Complement Med Ther.* 2020;20(1):1–6.
102. Boes CJ. Osler on migraine. *Can J Neurol Sci.* 2015;42(2):144–147.
103. Touw M. The religious and medicinal uses of cannabis in China, India and Tibet. *J Psychoactive Drugs.* 1981;13:23–34.
104. Aviram J, Samuelly-Leichtag G. Efficacy of cannabis-based medicines for pain management: A systematic review and meta-analysis of randomized controlled trials. *Pain Physician.* 2017;20(6):E755–796.

105. Boehnke KF, Litinas E, Clauw DJ. Medical cannabis use is associated with decreased opiate medication use in a retrospective cross-sectional survey of patients with chronic pain. *J Pain.* 2016;17(6):739–744.
106. Rolland A, Fleurentin J, Lanhers MC, et al. Behavioural effects of the American traditional plant *Eschscholzia californica*: Sedative and anxiolytic properties. *Planta Medica.* 1991;57(03):212–216.
107. Kaushik A, Arora P, Arora A. To study efficacy of *Eschscholzia californica* mother tincture (California poppy) in treatment of migraine headaches. *Int J Hom Sci.* 2019;3(3):62–68.
108. McKay DL, Blumberg JB. A review of the bioactivity and potential health benefits of chamomile tea (*Matricaria recutita* L.). *Phytother Res.* 2006;20:519–530.
109. Zargaran A, Borhani-Haghighi A, Salehi-Marzijarani M, et al. Evaluation of the effect of topical chamomile (*Matricaria chamomilla* L.) oleogel as pain relief in migraine without aura: A randomized, double-blind, placebo-controlled, crossover study. *Neurol Sci.* 2018;39(8):1345–1353.
110. Shoara R, Hashempur MH, Ashraf A. Efficacy and safety of topical *Matricaria chamomilla* L.(chamomile) oil for knee osteoarthritis: A randomized controlled clinical trial. *Complement Ther Clin Prac.* 2015;21(3):181–187.
111. Jahan R, Khatun A, Nahar N, et al. Use of *Menispermaceae* family plants in folk medicine of Bangladesh. *Adv Nat Appl Sci.* 2011;4(6):1779–1780.
112. Chavan SP, Kadlaskar BB, Gholap A, et al. Literary review article on efficacy of *Guduchi* in diabetic peripheral neuropathy. *IJAR.* 2017;3(2):200–203.
113. Ramakanth GS, Kumar CU, Kishan PV, et al. A randomized, double blind placebo controlled study of efficacy and tolerability of *Withaina somnifera* extracts in knee joint pain. *J Ayurveda Integr Med.* 2016;7(3):151–157.
114. Murthy MN, Gundagani S, Nutalapati C, et al. Evaluation of analgesic activity of standardized aqueous extract of *Withania somnifera* in healthy human volunteers using mechanical pain model. *J Clin Diagn Res.* 2019;13(1).
115. Uritu CM, Mihai CT, Stanciu GD, et al. Medicinal plants of the family *Lamiaceae* in pain therapy: A review. *Pain Res Manag.* 2018;2018: Article ID 7801543.
116. Mohammadkhani SL, Abbaspour Z, Aghel N, et al. Effect of massage aromatherapy with lavender oil on pain intensity of active phase of labor in nulliparous women. *J Med Plant.* 2012;11(Suppl 9):167–176.
117. Hosseini SE, Keramaty F, Naeiny KS. A comparative study of massage with lavender (*Lavandula*) essential oil and almond oil on pain relief after cesarean operation in primiparous women. *Med J Tabriz Univ Med Sci Health Serv.* 2016;38(2):22–27.
118. Saidi R, Heidari H, Sedehi M, et al. Evaluating the effect of *Matricaria chamomilla* and *Melissa officinalis* on pain intensity and satisfaction with pain management in patients after orthopedic surgery. *J Herbmed Pharmacol.* 2020;9(4):339–345.
119. Dastjerdi MN, Darooneh T, Nasiri M, et al. Investigating the effect of *Melissa officinalis* on after-pains: A randomized single-blind clinical trial. *J Caring Sci.* 2019;8(3):129–138.
120. Hubbert M, Sievers H, Lehnfeld R, et al. Efficacy and tolerability of a spray with *Salvia officinalis* in the treatment of acute pharyngitis-a randomised, double-blind, placebo-controlled study with adaptive design and interim analysis. *Eur J Med Res.* 2006;11(1):20–26.
121. Lalićević S, Djordjević I. Comparison of benzydamine hydrochloride and *Salvia officinalis* as an adjuvant local treatment to systemic nonsteroidal anti-inflammatory drug in controlling pain after tonsillectomy, adenoidectomy, or both: An open-label, single-blind, randomized clinical trial. *Curr Ther Res.* 2004;65(4):360–372.
122. Salim S, Chugh G, Asghar M. Inflammation in anxiety. *Adv Protein Chem Struct Biol.* 2012;88:1–25.
123. Wyss-Coray T, Mucke L. Inflammation in neurodegenerative disease—a double-edged sword. *Neuron.* 2002;35(3):419–432.

124. Ferraz CR, Carvalho TT, Manchope MF, et al. Therapeutic potential of flavonoids in pain and inflammation: Mechanisms of action, pre-clinical and clinical data, and pharmaceutical development. *Molecules*. 2020;25(3):762797.

125. Carvalho AMS, Heimfarth L, Santos KA, et al. Terpenes as possible drugs for the mitigation of arthritic symptoms—a systematic review. *Phytomedicine*. 2019;57:137–147.

126. Ghasemian M, Owlia S, Owlia MB. Review of anti-inflammatory herbal medicines. *Adv Pharmacol Sci*. 2016;2016.

127. Hashempur MH, Sadrneshin S, Mosavat SH, et al. Green tea (*Camellia sinensis*) for patients with knee osteoarthritis: A randomized open-label active-controlled clinical trial. *Clin Nutr*. 2018;37(1):85–90.

128. Sinimol TP, Surendran E, Meghna PP. Ayurvedic management of plaque psoriasis-a case study. *Int J Ayurveda Pharma Res*. 2019 Dec 25:41–46.

129. Tsiogkas SG, Grammatikopoulou MG, Gkiouras K, et al. Effect of *Crocus sativus* (Saffron) intake on top of standard treatment, on disease outcomes and comorbidities in patients with rheumatic diseases: Synthesis without meta-analysis (SWiM) and level of adherence to the CONSORT statement for randomized controlled trials delivering herbal medicine interventions. *Nutrients*. 2021;13(12):4274.

130. Caturla N, Funes L, Pérez-Fons L, et al. A randomized, double-blinded, placebo-controlled study of the effect of a combination of lemon verbena extract and fish oil omega-3 fatty acid on joint management. *J Altern Complement Med*. 2011;17(11):1051–1063.

131. Gupta V, Mittal P, Bansal P, et al. Pharmacological potential of *Matricaria recutita*-A review. *Int J Pharm Sci Drug Res*. 2010;2(1):12–16.

132. Gulati OD. Clinical trial of *Tinospora cordifolia* in rheumatoid arthritis. *Rheum*. 1980;15:143–148.

133. Fond G, Loundou A, Hamdani N, et al. Anxiety and depression comorbidities in irritable bowel syndrome (IBS): A systematic review and meta-analysis. *Eur Arch Psychiatry Clin Neurosci*. 2014;264:651–660.

134. Bundy R, Walker AF, Middleton RW, et al. Turmeric extract may improve irritable bowel syndrome symptomology in otherwise healthy adults: A pilot study. *J Altern Complement Med*. 2004;10:1015–1018.

135. Saito YA, Rey E, Almazar-Elder AE, et al. A randomized, double-blind, placebo-controlled trial of St John's wort for treating irritable bowel syndrome. *Am J Gastroenterol*. 2010;105:170–177.

136. Cappello G, Spezzaferro M, Grossi L, et al. Peppermint oil (Mintoil) in the treatment of irritable bowel syndrome: A prospective double blind placebo-controlled randomized trial. *Dig Liver Dis*. 2007;39:530–536.

137. Konno C, Sugiyama K, Kano M, et al. Isolation and hypoglycaemic activity of panaxans A, B, C, D and E, glycans of *Panax ginseng* roots. *Planta Med*. 1984;50(5):434–436.

138. Gui QF, Xu ZR, Xu KY, et al. The efficacy of ginseng-related therapies in type 2 diabetes mellitus: An updated systematic review and meta-analysis. *Medicine*. 2016;95(6):1–10.

139. Allen RW, Schwartzman E, Baker WL, et al. Cinnamon use in type 2 diabetes: An updated systematic review and meta-analysis. *Ann Fam Med*. 2013;11(5):452–459.

140. Siegel G, Ermilov E, Knes O, et al. Combined lowering of low grade systemic inflammation and insulin resistance in metabolic syndrome patients treated with *Ginkgo biloba*. *Atherosclerosis*. 2014;237(2):584–588.

141. Ponticelli M, Russo D, Faraone I, et al. The promising ability of *Humulus lupulus* L. Iso-α-acids vs. diabetes, inflammation, and metabolic syndrome: A systematic review. *Molecules*. 2021;26(4):954–986.

142. Zemestani M, Rafraf M, Asghari-Jafarabadi M. Chamomile tea improves glycemic indices and antioxidants status in patients with type 2 diabetes mellitus. *Nutrition*. 2016;32(1):66–72.

143. Selmi S, Rtibi K, Grami D, et al. Rosemary (*Rosmarinus officinalis*) essential oil components exhibit anti-hyperglycemic, anti-hyperlipidemic and antioxidant effects in experimental diabetes. *Pathophysiology*. 2017;24(4):297–303.

144. Farkhondeh T, Samarghandian S. The effect of saffron (*Crocus sativus* L.) and its ingredients on the management of diabetes mellitus and dislipidemia. *Afr J Pharmacy Pharmacol*. 2014;8(20):541–549.

145. Park JH, Kim RY, Park E. Antioxidant and α-glucosidase inhibitory activities of different solvent extracts of skullcap (*Scutellaria baicalensis*). *Food Sci Biotechnol*. 2011;20(4):1107–1112.

146. Kwon YI, Jang HD, Shetty K. Evaluation of *Rhodiola crenulata* and *Rhodiola rosea* for management of type II diabetes and hypertension. *Asia Pac J Clin Nutr*. 2006;15(3):425–432.

147. Tan MS, Yu JT, Tan CC, et al. Efficacy and adverse effects of *ginkgo biloba* for cognitive impairment and dementia: A systematic review and meta-analysis. *J Alzheimer's Dis*. 2015;43(2):589–603.

148. Ramassamy C, Longpre F, Christen Y. *Ginkgo biloba* extract (EGb 761) in Alzheimer's disease: Is there any evidence? *Curr Alzheimer Res*. 2007;4:253–262.

149. Kampkotter A, Pielarski T, Rohrig R, et al. The *Ginkgo biloba* extract EGb761 reduces stress sensitivity, ROS accumulation and expression of catalase and glutathione S-transferase 4 in *Caenorhabditis elegans*. *Pharmacol Res*. 2007;55:139–147.

150. Koltringer P, Langsteger W, Eber O. Dose-dependent hemorheological effects and microcirculatory modifications following intravenous administration of *Ginkgo biloba* special extract EGb 761. *Clin Hemorheol*. 1995;15:649–656.

151. Hashiguchi M, Ohta Y, Shimizu M, et al. Meta-analysis of the efficacy and safety of *Ginkgo biloba* extract for the treatment of dementia. *J Pharm Health Care Sci*. 2015;1(1):1–12.

152. Kongkeaw C, Dilokthornsakul P, Thanarangsarit P, et al. Meta-analysis of randomized controlled trials on cognitive effects of *Bacopa monnieri* extract. *J Ethnopharmacol*. 2014;151(1):528–535.

153. Chaudhari KS, Tiwari NR, Tiwari RR. Neurocognitive effect of nootropic drug *Brahmi* (*Bacopa monnieri*) in Alzheimer's disease. *Ann Neurosci*. 2017;24:111–122.

154. Ng QX, Loke W, Foo NX, et al. A systematic review of the clinical use of *Withania somnifera* (*Ashwagandha*) to ameliorate cognitive dysfunction. *Phytother Res*. 2020;34(3):583–590.

155. Ayati Z, Yang G, Ayati MH, et al. Saffron for mild cognitive impairment and dementia: A systematic review and meta-analysis of randomized clinical trials. *BMC Complement Med Ther*. 2020;20(1):1–10.

156. Shinjyo N, Green J. Are sage, rosemary and lemon balm effective interventions in dementia? A narrative review of the clinical evidence. *Eur J Integr Med*. 2017;15:83–96.

157. Mutalik M, Mutalik M. *Tinospora cordifolia*: Role in depression, cognition and memory. *Aust J Herb Med*. 2011;23(4):168–173.

158. Al-Kuraishy HM. Central additive effect of *Ginkgo biloba* and *Rhodiola rosea* on psychomotor vigilance task and short-term working memory accuracy. *J Intercult Ethnopharmacol*. 2016;5(1):7–13.

159. Tang H, Wang J, Zhao L, et al. *Rhodiola rosea* L extract shows protective activity against Alzheimer's disease in 3xTg-AD mice. *Trop J Pharm Res*. 2017 Apr 4;16(3):509–514.

160. Wang GH, Wang LH, Wang C, et al. Spore powder of *Ganoderma lucidum* for the treatment of alzheimer disease: A pilot study. *Medicine*. 2018;97(19):e0636.

161. Fruehauf H. The flagship remedy of Chinese medicine: Reflections on the toxicity and safety of aconite. *J Chinese Med*. 2012;100:36–41.

162. Ernst E. A re-evaluation of kava (*Piper methysticum*). *Brit J Clin Pharmacol*. 2007;64(4):415–417.

163. Licata A, Macaluso FS, Craxì A. Herbal hepatotoxicity: A hidden epidemic. *Intern Emerg Med.* 2013;8(1):13–22.

164. Abdualmjid RJ, Sergi C. Hepatotoxic botanicals-an evidence-based systematic review. *J Pharm Pharm Sci.* 2013;16(3):376–404.

165. Teschke R, Bahre R. Severe hepatotoxicity by Indian Ayurvedic herbal products: A structured causality assessment. *Ann Hepatol.* 2009;8(3):258–266.

166. Sedky K, Nazir R, Joshi A, Kaur G, Lippmann S. Which psychotropic medications induce hepatotoxicity? *Gen Hosp Psychiatry.* 2012;34(1):53–61.

167. Posadzki P, Watson L, Ernst E. Herb—drug interactions: An overview of systematic reviews. *Brit J Clin Pharmacol.* 2013;75(3):603–618.

168. Heck AM, DeWitt BA, Lukes AL. Potential interactions between alternative therapies and warfarin. *Am J Health Syst Pharm.* 2000;57(13):1221–1227.

169. Unger M. Pharmacokinetic drug interactions involving *Ginkgo biloba. Drug Metab Rev.* 2013;45(3):353–385.

170. Kupiec T, Raj V. Fatal seizures due to potential herb-drug interactions with *Ginkgo biloba. J Anal Toxicol.* 2005;29(7):755–758.

171. Russo E, Scicchitano F, Whalley BJ, et al. *Hypericum perforatum*: Pharmacokinetic, mechanism of action, tolerability, and clinical drug—drug interactions. *Phytother Res.* 2014;28(5):643–655.

172. Basch E, Conquer J, Culwell S, et al. *Green Tea (Camellia sinensis)*. Natural Standard Professional Monograph. www.naturalstandard.com.

173. Carrillo JA, Benitez J. Clinically significant pharmacokinetic interactions between dietary caffeine and medications. *Clin Pharmacokinet.* 2000;39(2):127–153.

174. García-Suástegui WA, Ramos-Chávez LA, Rubio-Osornio M, et al. The role of CYP2E1 in the drug metabolism or bioactivation in the brain. *Oxi Med Cell Longev.* 2017;2017: Article ID 4680732.

175. Ulbricht C, Basch E, Boon H, et al. Safety review of kava (*Piper methysticum*) by the natural standard research collaboration. *Expert Opin Drug Saf.* 2005;4:779–794.

176. Hsu HY, Hsu CS. *Commonly Used Chinese Herb Formulas Companion Handbook.* Long Beach, CA: Oriental Healing Arts Institute; 1997.

Index

Page numbers in *italic* indicate a figure, and page numbers in **bold** indicate a table on the corresponding page.

NUMBERS

1,8-cineol, 240
1H-MRI studies, 13
3,'4',5,7-tetrahydroxyflavone, 44
3-carene, 39
5,7-dihydroxy-8-methoxyflavone, 47
5,7-dihydroxyflavone, 39–40
5-alpha-reductase inhibitors, 4
7,8,dihydroxyflavone, 40

A

Abies pindrow, 39
abnormal heart rhythms, 3
Acanthaceae, 36
Acanthopanax senticosus, 76
acetylcholine, 14
acne, 132
Aconitum carmichaelii, 274
Acorus calamus, 55–56, 215, 216, 274
Acorus gramineus, 191
acupuncture, 183
adaptogens, 35, 231–234
    in chronic treatments, 263–264
    Crocus sativus, 70
    Echinacea angustifolia, 73
    Eleutherococcus senticosus, 231
    Schisandra chinensis, 122
    Tinospora cordifolia, 127
    Withania somnifera, 134
ADHD, 60
adjustment disorder, 134
aftimooni, 219
aging, 122
agitation, 90
Aglaomorpha quercifolia, 45
agoraphobia, 181–182
akashvalli, 219
akathisia, 4
Albizia julibrissin, 191–192
Albizzia lebbeck, 217
alcohol dependence, 42
Alexander, F. Matthias, 8
Alexander Technique, 8
alkaloids, 35–36
allergies, 87

Allium cepa, 45, 217
Allium sativum, 45
allopregnanolone, 28
Aloysia citrodora, 47, 96
alpha-2-receptor antagonists, 4
alpha-pinene, 241
alprazolam, 88, 183
Alstonia scholaris, 36
alstonine, 36
alterative herbs, 73
Alzheimer's disease
    Crocus sativus and, 273
    galantamine and, 36
    Ganoderma lucidum and, 86
    nobiletin and, 46
    yi gan san and, 186
AM630, 38
amenorrhea, 101
amentoflavone, 34, 37
American ginseng, 107
American skullcap, 124–125
amygdala, 11
Anacyclus pyrethrum, 217
Andrographis paniculata, 47
Anemarrhena asphodeloides, 44
anemia, 101, 222
Angelicae gigantis, 192
Angelica sinensis, 192, 193
angina, 186
Anodendron affine, 47
anorexia, 140
anthocyanidins, 33
antibiotics, 4
antidepressants *see* depression
antiseizure effects, 46, 84; *see also* convulsions
anxiety, explained, 1–4
anxiolytic drug action, 28–29
anxiolytic phytochemicals, 33–48
    3-carene, 39
    7,8,dihydroxyflavone, 40
    alkaloids, 35–36
    amentoflavone, 37
    for anxiety relief, 36–48
    apigenin, 37
    baicalein, 38
    bisabolol, 38
    caffeic acid, 38

carvacrol, 39
chrysin, 39
ellagic acid, 40
epigallocatechin gallate, 40–41
eugenol, 41
ferulic acid, 41
flavonoids, 33–34
hispidulin, 42
hyperoside, 42
icariin, 42–43
isopulegol, 43
kaempferol, 43
limonene, 43
linalool, 43–44
luteolin, 44
mangiferin, 44–45
menthol, 44
myricetin, 45
naringin, 45
nerolidol, 45
nobiletin, 45–46
pinene, 46
quercetin, 46–47
resveratrol, 46
rosmarinic acid, 47
ß-caryophyllene, 38
terpenes, 34–35
ursolic acid, 47
wogonin, 47–48
aphrodisiacs, 70, 94, 139
apigenin, 34, 37
Apium graveolens, 34, 37
apple skins, 40
Arisaema heterophyllum, 190
aromatherapy, 237–253
    in animals, 237–238
    Boswellia carterii, 241–242, 252
    Cananga odorata, 250, 252
    Chamaemelum nobile, 250, 252
    Cinnamomum camphora, 252
    Citrus aurantium, 242, 250, 252
    Citrus bergamia, 250
    Citrus reticulata, 251
    Citrus sinensis, 242
    Cymbopogon citratus, 242–243, 250
    efficacy of, 252
    Eucalyptus, 250
    Eugenia aromaticum, 242
    herbal combinations, 249–251
    herbs utilized in, 241–249
    Jasminum officinale, 243
    Jasminum spp, 252
    Juniperus communis, 252
    Lavandula angustifolia, 252
    Lavandula officinalis, 250, 251, 252
    Lavandula spp, 244–245
    Matricaria recutita, 245

Melissa officinalis, 245
Mentha piperita, 245–246
Nardostachys jatamansi, 246
neroli oil, 246
Ocimum basilicum, 252
Origanum majorana, 252
Ormenis multicaulis and, 252
overview, 237–241
Pelargonium graveolens, 246–247, 251
Pogostemon cablin and, 252
Rosa damascena, 247–248, 251, 252
Rosmarinus officinalis, 248
Salvia officinalis, 248–249
Santallum spp, 249
Santalum album, 251
shirodhara, 237
sleep and, 251–252
Vetiveria zizanoides and, 252
Artemisia, 42
arthritis, 91, 105, 242, 269, 270, 271
asanas, 8
ashwagandha, 134, 208–209, 212, 225
Asparagus racemosus, 218
Asplenium montanum, 44
Asteraceae, 140
asthma, 4
    Boswellia carterii and, 242
    Galphimia glauca and, 84
    Ganoderma lucidum and, 85
    Ginkgo biloba and, 87
    Melissa officinalis and, 101
    Ocimum sanctum and, 105
    Salvia officinalis and, 121
    Trifolium pratense and, 128
Atharva Veda, 61–62
Avena sativa, 41, 44, 57–58
Awareness Through Movement, 8
ayahuasca, 113
Ayurvedic medicine, 205–225
    Acorus calamus, 216
    Albizzia lebbeck, 217
    Allium cepa, 217
    Anacyclus pyrethrum, 217
    ashwagandha, 208
    Asparagus racemosus, 209, 218
    bach, 55–56
    Bacopa monnieri, 58, 218
    Benincasa hispida, 218–219
    blood pressure, 213–214, 215
    Brahmi gritha, 209
    cannabis, 61–62
    Cannabis sativa, 219
    Centella asiatica, 64, 219
    cinnamon, 66
    compared to traditional Chinese medicine, 206
    Convolvulus pluricaulis, 69–70, 219
    Cuscuta reflexa, 219–220

Cynodon dactylon, 220
depression, 265–266
Evolvulus alsinoides, 81, 220
Ficus religiosa, 220–221
Geriforte, 209–210
Glycyrrhiza glabra, 209, 221
Guduchi, 126–128
guduchyadi medhya rasayana, 210
herbal treatments, 207–225
Hyoscyamus niger, 221–222
Jasminum officinale, 243
Juglans regia, 222
Kushmandadi ghrita, 210–211
Lawsonia inermis, 222
literature, 207
mainstays of, 216–225
mandookaparni, 208–209
mansyadi kwatha, 214–215
Medhyarasayana ghrita, 211
Mentat, 211–212
Moringa oleifera, 223
Nardostachys jatamansi, 104, 223
Ocimum sanctum, 105
OCTA, 212
overview, 205–206
Piper nigrum, 223
Punica granatum, 224
Rauwolfia serpentina, 213–214
sarasvata choorna, 212–213
Saussurea lappa, 224
Schisandra chinensis, 122
shankhapushpi, 215
shankhapushpi panak, 214–215
shirodhara, 214–215
Tinospora cordifolia, 224–225
Trifolium pratense, 128
vacha, 55–56
vacha brahmi ghan, 216
vachadi ghrita, 211
Valeriana jatamansi, 225
Valeriana jatamansi Jones, 130
Vitex negundo, 225
Withania somnifera, 134, 135, 225
Worry Free, 216

B

Bacopa monnieri, 58–59, 212, 218, 232, 269, 272–273
bacosides, 58
baicalein, 36, 38
bai he, 95–96
bai zi yang xin tang, 178–179
Ballota nigra, 79
banhabakchulchunma, 188
Banisteriopsis caapi, 36, 113
ban xia hou pu, 98, 179, 265

bao shen, 180
basswood, 140
Benincasa hispida, 211, 218–219
Benson, Herbert, 8
benzodiazepine receptors, 262
benzodiazepines, xx, 12, 23–25
    concerns with, 24–25
    flavonoids and, 34
bergamot oil, 67, 250
Bermuda grass, 220
beta-blockers, 27–28
Betonica officinalis, 38
Betula, 42
Betula pendula, 45
bicyclic monoterpene, 46
biflavonoids, 37
bisabolol, 38
bis-apigenin, 37
bitter orange, 67–68, 242, 246
blood, 185, 187
blood pressure, 66, 87, 213–214, 215
blood sugar, 66
bo he, 102
Bombax ceiba, 44
borage, 74
Borago officinalis, 74
Borago officinalis, 138
borderline personality disorder, 187
Boswellia, 269
Boswellia carterii, 252, 269
Boswellia sacra, 43, 47
Boswellia serrata, 269, 271
brahmi, 58
Brahmi gritha, 209
brain; *see also* cognitive function, Western medicine understanding of, 175
brain circuitry of anxiety, 11
breastfeeding, 65
brexanolone, 28
bronchitis, 101, 121, 128, 222
Bryonia alba, 232
Bupleurum chinense, 185, 192
Bupleurum falcatum, 192
Bupleurum scorzonerifolium, 192
Bupleurum yinchowense, 192
bupropion, 4
bu shen yang xue wan, 180
buspirone, 25

C

caffeic acid, 38
caffeine, 60
calderona amarilla, 84
calor, 16
Camellia sinensis, 33, 38, 40, 42, 45, 46, 59–61, 80, 271, 274, 275

Camptotheca acuminate, 42
Cananga odorata, 250, 252
cancer, 128, 216, 224, 251, 274
cannabidiol (CBD), 62
cannabigerol, 35
cannabinoid receptors, 14, 262–263
cannabinoids, 35
cannabis, 14
Cannabis indica, 61, 266
Cannabis ruderalis, 61
Cannabis sativa, 34, 35, 38, 39, 43, 45, 46, 61, 75,
    219, 266, 269, 275
Canscora decussata, 81
cardiovascular insufficiency, 87
carob powder, 40
carvacrol, 39
catechin, 33
catnip, 139
CBD *see* cannabidiol (CBD)
Celsus, Aulus Cornelius, 16
Centella asiatica, 64–65, 208–209, 216, 219, 271
cerebrovascular insufficiency, 87
chaihu, 192
chai hu jia long gu mu li, 124
chai hu jia long gu mu li tang, 189
chalcones, 34
Chamaecyparis obtusa, 37
Chamaemelum nobile, 245, 250, 252
chamomile, 99–101, 269
chaste tree, 132–134, 225
childbirth, 242, 243, 244, 246, 247, 248, 270
China root, 112
Chinese cinnamon, 66
Chinese date, 136
Chinese Herbal Medicine (Scheid et al.), 189
Chinese herbal treatment *see* traditional Chinese
    medicine
Chinese licorice, 194
Chinese skullcap, 124–125
chittodvega, 55, 69, 208, 211, 212–213, 215;
    see also generalized anxiety disorder
    (GAD)
chlordiazepoxide, 23
chlorogenic acid, 38
cholesterol, 35
choosing herbal treatment, 259–277
    anxiety type, 261
    chronic anxiety disorders, 263–264
    comorbidities, 264–273
    efficacy, 259–260
    safety, 273–276
    single herbs or combinations, 261–263
chronic anxiety disorders, 263–264
chronic stress, 15–16, 17
chrysin, 39–40
cicadas, 184
cinnabar, 190

cinnamaldehyde, 66
Cinnamomum, 272
Cinnamomum camphora, 252
Cinnamomum cassia, 66
Cinnamomum spp, 66–67, 275
Cinnamomum verum, 41, 43
Cinnamomum zeylanicum, 66
cinnamyl alcohol glycoside, 37
cintronella grass, 242
citrus, 37, 43, 45
Citrus aurantium, 43, 67–68, 242, 246, 250, 252
Citrus bergamia, 250
Citrus reticulata, 251
Citrus sinensis, 242
Citrus spp, 45, 46
ciwujia, 76
clarithromycin, 4
Classic of Poetry, 136
Claviceps purpurea, 36
"clinically anxious," 11
Clitorea ternatea, 81
clonidine, 28
cloves, 41, 242
Cnidium officinale, 193
Coffea arabica, 44
cognitive behavioral therapy, 7
cognitive function
    Asparagus racemosus and, 209, 218
    Bacopa monnieri and, 58
    caffeine and, 60
    Evolvulus alsinoides and, 81
    Lavandula angustifolia and, 240
    Mentat and, 211–212
    Rosmarinus officinalis and, 240
Cola acuminata, 79
Cola nitida, 80
colds, 105, 121
colic, 101
colorectal cancer, 44
common liverwort, 35
Commonly Used Chinese Herbal Formulas
    (Hsu and Hsu), 188, 277
comorbid bipolar affective disorder, 42
comorbidities, 264–273
    dementia, 272–273
    diabetes, 271–272
    dysmenorrhea, 269
    inflammation, 270–271
    insomnia, 266–268
    irritable bowel syndrome, 271
    major depression, 264–266
    menopause, 268–269
    pain, 269–270
Convolvulaceae, 81
Convolvulus pluricaulis, 69–70, 81, 82, 215, 219
convulsions, 105, 196, 198; *see also* antiseizure
    effects

COPD, 4, 184
Coptis chinensis, 193
cortisol, 87, 231–232
Corydalis yanhusuo, 78
cough, 105, 112
coumarin, 66
Crassulaceae, 117
Crataegus oxyacantha, 78, 79, 80
Crocus sativus, 70–71, 271, 272, 273, 275
Crossostephium chinense, 42
Curcuma longa, 71–73, 194, 232, 271, 275
Curcuma wenyujin, 194
Curcuma zedoria, 72, 73
curcumin, 232
Cuscuta chinensis, 42
Cuscuta reflexa, 219–220
CY1A2, 67
CY2E1, 67
CY3A4, 84
cyclopeptide alkaloids, 36
Cyclopia, 44
Cymbopogon citratus, 43, 45, 46, 242–243, 250
Cynodon dactylon, 220
Cynomorium songaricum, 194
CYP1A2, 73, 89, 91, 93, 99, 131
CYP2A, 71
CYP2B, 71
CYP2B6, 73
CYP2C8, 89
CYP2C9, 64, 73, 89, 91, 93
CYP2C11, 71
CYP2C19, 64, 88, 89, 91, 93
CYP2D6, 56, 65, 73, 78, 91, 93, 125, 131
CYP2E1, 111, 131, 276
CYP3A, 71, 108
CYP3A4, 56, 64, 65, 68, 73, 78, 91, 93, 110,
        119, 131
cytochrome P450 enzymes, 58
cytokine IL-6, 41

D

daidzein, 34
dandelion, 140
Datura stramonium, 36
Daucus carota, 39–40
DBI *see* diazepam binding inhibitor (DBI)
Deanxit, 112, 186
dehydroepiandrosterone sulfate (DHEAS), 38
delta-9-tetrahydrocannabinol (THC), 62
dementia, 87, 186
    comorbidities, 272–273
    Lavendula and, 244–245
    Medhyarasayana ghrita and, 211
    Melissa officinalis and, 245
dental anxiety, 247, 249
depression, 4, 25–26

Albizia julibrissin and, 191
alkaloids and, 36
Anacyclus pyrethrum and, 217
Asparagus racemosus and, 218
in Ayurvedic medicine, 265–266
Bacopa monnieri and, 58
ban xia hou pu and, 265
caffeine and, 60
Cinnamomum zeylanicum and, 264
cormobidities and, 264–266
Crocus sativus and, 70, 264
Curcuma wenyujin and, 194
Cynodon dactylon and, 220
Ginkgo biloba and, 87
Glycyrrhiza uralensis and, 195
guduchyadi medhya rasayana and, 210
gui pi and, 265
Humulus lupulus and, 88
Hypericum perforatum and, 89–90, 264
Lavandula angustifolia and, 264
Leonurus cardiaca and, 93
Magnolia officinalis and, 98
Matricaria recutita and, 100, 264, 265
Melissa officinalis and, 101
monoamine oxidase inhibitors and, 102
naringin and, 45
Piper methysticum and, 111
Psilocybe spp and, 114
Rehmannia glutinosa and, 198
Rhodiola rosea and, 118, 264, 265
Rosmarinus officinalis and, 264, 265
sarasvata choorna and, 213
Schisandra chinensis and, 122
Scutellaria baicalensis and, 124
Tinospora cordifolia and, 127
ursolic acid and, 47
Withania somnifera and, 134
xiao yao san and, 185, 265
xin wei tang and, 185
DHEAS *see* dehydroepiandrosterone sulfate
        (DHEAS)
diabetes, 197, 212, 271–272
diagnosis, 190
Diagnostic and Statistical Manual, 1, 3
diarrhea, 84, 105, 112, 224
diazepam binding inhibitor (DBI), 24
digestive system
    Ban xia hou pu and, 179
    Boswellia carterii and, 242
    Curcuma wenyujin and, 194
    Mentha piperita and, 103
    Poria cocos and, 112
    rikkunshinto and, 182
    Scutellaria baicalensis and, 124
    Taraxacum officinale and, 140
    vacha brahmi ghan and, 216
    xin wei tang and, 185

yukgunja and, 188
dimethyltryptamine, 36, 113
ding zhi wan, 189
Dioscorea villosa, 35
diosgenin, 35
dizziness, 85, 87, 112, 182
dl-p-chlorophenilalanine ethyl ester, 38
Doctrine of Signatures, 177
dolor, 16
dong quai, 192
doob, 220
dopamine, 14
doshas, 205–206, 224, 265
"Dragon Tooth Powder to Clear the Ethereal
    Soul," 189
Drosera rotundifolia, 42
drumstick tree, 223
*DSM-III-R see Diagnostic and
    Statistical Manual*
dwarf morning glory, 69, 81, 219, 220
dysentery, 105, 222, 224
dysmenorrhea, 269

E

Earl Grey tea, 67
ECGC *see* epigallocatechin gallate (EGCG)
Echinacea, 35
Echinacea angustifolia, 38, 73–74, 274, 275
Echinacea purpurea, 38
Echium amoenum, 47, 74–76
efficacy, 252, 259–260
electroacupuncture, 183
Eleutherococcus senticosus, 36, 46, 76–78,
    89, 107
eleutherosides, 36
ellagic acid, 40
"Emperor of Heaven's Special Pill to Tonify
    the Heart," 189
endocannabinoids, 14
endocannabinoids, 35
endorphins, 14–15
"entourage effect," 35
Ephedra sinica, 36
ephedrine, 36
epigallocatechin gallate (EGCG), 33, 34, 40–41
epilepsy, 101, 217, 223, 224
Epimedium grandiflorum, 42
Eschscholzia californica, 78–79, 80, 266, 269
essential oils, 35, 252; *see also* aromatherapy
Eucalyptus, 43, 240, 250
Eugenia aromaticum, 242
eugenol, 41
Euphytose, 79–81
European borage, 74
Evolvulus alsinoides, 69

Evolvulus alsinoides, 38, 81, 81–82, 208, 215,
    219, 220
exercise, benefits of, 9

F

fatigue, 112
fear, 1, 127, 182, 210
Feldenkrais, Moshe, 8
fertility, 132, 209
ferulic acid, 41
fever, 84, 105
fibromyalgia, 86
fibrositis, 90
Ficus religiosa, 220–221
finasteride, 4
five elements, 177, 205
Five Spirits, 175–176, 177
flatulence, 101, 103
flavanone-7-O-glycoside, 45
flavanones, 34
flavonoids, xix, 33–34
flavonols, 33
flax, 35
Florida fishpoison tree, 140
fluid retention, 112
flumazenil, 37, 38, 262
Foeniculum vulgare, 41, 43, 44, 46, 47, 82–84,
    268, 269
forgetfulness *see* memory enhancement
frankincense, 241–242
"free and easy wanderer," 185
Fridericia chica, 42
fu ling, 112
fuzi, 274

G

GABA *see* gamma amino butyric acid (GABA)
GABA-A, 12, 24, 34, 37
GABA-B, 12
gabapentin, 26
GABA receptor complex, 12
GAD *see* generalized anxiety disorder (GAD)
Galantamine, 36
Galanthus caucasicus, 36
gallbladder, 103
Galphimia glauca, 84–85
gamma amino butyric acid (GABA), 4, 12–13, 36
ganaxolone, 28
gan cao tang, 188
gan mai da zao tang, 188
Ganoderma lingzhi, 38, 41, 46
Ganoderma lucidum, 85–86, 194, 273, 275
gansong, 104
Gardenia jasminoides, 184
gastrointestinal disorders *see* digestive system

generalization, 2
generalized anxiety disorder (GAD), 2–3
   Acorus calamus and, 55–56
   ashwagandha churna and, 208
   banhabakchulchunma and, 188
   bao shen, 180
   Brahmi gritha and, 209
   Centella asiatica and, 64
   Convolvulus pluricaulis and, 69, 219
   cortisol and, 231
   Crocus sativus and, 70
   Echium amoenum and, 75–76
   Eschscholzia californica and, 78
   Euphytose and, 80
   Galphimia glauca and, 84
   Hypericum perforatum and, 90
   jiu wei zhen xin and, 181
   Kushmandadi ghrita, 211
   Lilium brownii and, 96
   Matricaria recutita and, 100, 245
   Ocimum sanctum and, 105–106
   Passiflora incarnata and, 109
   Poria cocos and, 112, 197
   psychotherapy and, 7
   sarasvata choorna and, 212–213
   shunkhapushpi panak and, 215
   suan zao ren tang and, 184
   in traditional Chinese medicine, 176
   Withania somnifera and, 134, 225
   yang xin tang and, 186
   yi qi yang xin and, 187
   yukgunja and, 188
   Zizyphus jujuba and, 198
geng ni an chun, 112, 180
genistein, 34
geranium, 246–247
Geriforte, 209–210
German chamomile, 99, 245
Ginkgo biloba, 37, 43, 44, 46, 87–88, 232, 272, 275
Ginkgophyta, 87
ginseng, 35, 76, 106–108, 195–196, 232, 272
   American, 107
   Chinese, 107
   Korean, 106
   Siberian, 36, 76, 107
globus hystericus, 179
glutamate, 13, 60
glutamic acid decarboxylase, 4
glycine, 15
Glycine max, 34
glycyrrhetic acid, 35
Glycyrrhiza glabra, 35, 194, 208, 209, 210–211, 221
Glycyrrhiza uralensis, 194–195, 221
Godmania aesculifolia, 40
gotu kola, 64–65, 219

"Grand Communication Pill," 189–190
green tea, 40, 59–61, 271
Grindelia squarrosa, 42
guan ye lian qiao, 89
guarana, 80
guduchi, 126–128, 224, 273
guduchyadi medhya rasayana, 210
gui pi, 265
gui pi tang, 180–181
gui zhi jia long gu mu li tang, 189
gui zhi qu shao yao jia shu qi long gu mu li tang, 189
Gyorgi, Albert Szent, xix

H

haloperidol, 88
Hamilton's Brief Psychiatric Rating Scale, 56, 64
hange-koboku-to, 181–182, 277
harmala alkaloids, 36
hay fever, 84
hazelnuts, 40
headaches
   Melissa officinalis and, 101
   Saussurea lappa and, 224
   vacha brahmi ghan and, 216
heart, 105, 186
heart-leaved moonseed, 126
Helichrysum, 35
henbane, 214–215
hepatitis, 140
Herbal Treatment of Major Depression (Mendelson), 111
hesperidin, 24, 34
Hibiscus, 45
hispidulin, 42
histamine, 15
hoelen, 112
hops, 88
Humulus, 35
Humulus lupulus, 41, 88–89, 266, 268, 272
Hun, 175, 176
hydroxyzine, 27
Hyoscyamus niger, 221–222
Hypericum perforatum, 37, 42, 43, 46, 89–91, 271, 274, 275
hyperoside, 42
hysteria, 101, 224

I

icariin, 42–43
immunity, 218
Indian Ayurvedic medicine *see* Ayurvedic medicine
Indian pennywort, 64
Indian snakeroot, 213

indigestion, 91, 101; *see also* digestive system
infertility *see* fertility
inflammation, 16, 231–232
    Boswellia carterii and, 242
    comorbidities, 270–271
    Ginkgo biloba and, 87
    Lavandula angustifolia and, 91
    Lawsonia inermis and, 222
    tetrad of, 16
    Trifolium pratense and, 128
insomnia *see* sleep
insulin resistance, 16
Iranian borage, 74
Iris unguicularis, 44
iron filings, 190
irritable bowel syndrome, 182, 242, 271
isoflavones, 34, 129
isopulegol, 43

J

Jacobson, Edmund, 8
jaladhara, 69
jalbrahmi, 64
Jamaican dogwood, 140
JAMA Psychiatry, 8
James, William, 27
Japan, 182, 186
jasmine, 243
Jasminum officinale, 240, 243
Jasminum spp, 45, 252
jatamansi, 104
jatipushpa, 243
jiao tai wan, 189–190
jiu wei zhen xin, 181
Juglans regia, 222
jujuba, 136
jujubogenins, 58
jun chen zuo shi, 178
Juniperus communis, 252

K

kaempferol, 33, 43
kami-shoyo-san, 181–182, 277
Kampo medicine, 182, 186
kaphas, 205, 206, 265
karpooravalli, 121
kavalactones/kavapyrones, 110
kidneys, 180, 184, 197, 248
kola nut, 80
k-opioid antagonists, 37
Korean traditional medicine, 190–191
kreteks, 242
Kundalini yoga, 8
Kushmandadi ghrita, 210–211

L

Lactuca vurosa, 140
Lamiaceae, 119, 139, 270
Lamiaceae Stachys, 42
Laserpitium latifolium, 38
Lavandula angustifolia, 34, 39, 43, 45, 46,
    67, 91–93, 240–241, 252, 266, 270, 275
Lavandula officinalis, 250, 251, 252
Lavandula spp, 91–93, 244–245, 247–248
Lawsonia inermis, 222
lemon balm, 101
lemongrass, 242
lemon verbena, 96
Leonurus cardiaca, 38, 41, 93–94
Lepidium meyenii, 43, 94–95, 268
Lepidium sativum, 39
"lettuce opium," 138
Librium, 23
licorice root, 209, 210, 221
lignans, 123
Lilium brownii, 95–96
limbic system, 11
limonene, 39, 43
linalool, 43–44, 92
linden, 140
lingzhi, 85
Linum usitatissimum, 35
Linus Pauling Institute, 33
Lippia citriodora, 96–98, 271
Lippia triphylla, 96
Littorina littorea, 36
liver
    Acorus calamus and, 216, 274
    Mentha haplocalyx and, 102
    Ocimum sanctum and, 105
    Piper methysticum and, 111
    Polygonum multiflorum and, 197
    Silybum marianum and, 125
    suan zao ren tang and, 184
    Taraxacum officinale and, 140
    Xiao yao san and, 185
long chi qing hun san, 189
longevity, 134, 218, 225
Lophophora williamsii, 36
LSD *see* Lysergic acid diethylamide (LSD)
L-theanine, 60
luteolin, 34, 44
Lysergic acid diethylamide (LSD), 36, 113

M

maca, 94
Magnolia officinalis, 98–99
magnolia vine, 122
maidenhair tree, 87
malaise, 101

malaria, 105, 223
Malvaceae, 36
mandookaparni, 208–209
mandowega, 208; *see also* generalized anxiety
    disorder (GAD)
mandukparni, 64
Mangifera indica, 44, 45
mangiferin, 44–45
mango tree, 44
mansyadi kwatha, 214–215
Marchantia polymorpha, 35
"Marvelously Fragrant Powder," 189
Massa Medicata Fermentata, 188
Matricaria chamomilla, 34, 37, 38, 39–40, 43,
    44, 46
Matricaria recutita, 99–101, 127, 245, 266, 267,
    269, 271, 272, 275
medhya rasayana, 58
Medhyarasayana ghrita, 211
medical conditions causing anxiety, 3–4
Medical Herbalism (Hoffmann), 233
medications for anxiety, 23–29
    antidepressants, 25–26
    benzodiazepines, 23–25
    buspirone, 25
    clonidine, 28
    gabapentin, 26
    hydroxyzine, 27
    mechanisms of, 28–29
    neurosteroids, 28
    pregabalin, 27
    propranolol, 27–28
meditation, 9
Melaleuca alternifolia, 45
Melissa officinalis, 37, 38, 41, 43, 44, 47,
    101–102, 245, 266, 267, 270, 273
memory enhancement
    Asparagus racemosus and, 209
    Bacopa monnieri and, 58
    cinnamon and, 66
    Ginkgo biloba and, 87
    Lavandula angustifolia and, 240
    Mentat and, 212
    naringin and, 45
    Poria cocos and, 112
    Rosmarinus officinalis and, 240
    Zizyphus jujuba and, 136
menopause
    Asparagus racemosus and, 209, 218
    comorbidities, 268–269
    Foeniculum vulgare and, 83, 268
    geng ni an chun and, 112, 180
    Glycyrrhiza glabra and, 209
    Humulus lupulus and, 268
    Hypericum perforatum and, 90
    Lepidium meyenii and, 94–95, 268
    Panax ginseng and, 107

    Poria cocos and, 112, 197
    Salvia officinalis and, 121
    Trifolium pratense and, 128, 268
    Vitex agnus-castus and, 132–133, 225, 268
    Zingiber officinale and, 218
menstruation, 132, 209, 247, 269; *see also*
    premenstrual syndrome
Mentat, 211–212
Mentha, 43, 44
Mentha aquatica, 45
Mentha haplocalyx, 102
Mentha piperita, 38, 43, 46, 102–104, 242,
    245–246
Mentha suaveolens, 43
Menthe piperita, 271
menthol, 44
mescaline, 36, 113
metabolic syndrome, 16–17
Mexican folk medicine *see* traditional Mexican
    folk medicine
miao xiang san, 189
mifepristone, 28
migraine, 87, 121, 269
milk thistle, 125
mindfulness, 9
mitochondria, 17
mitral valve prolapse, 3
Modern Herbal, A (Grieve), 101
mo li hua, 243
"monarch, minister, assistant and envoy" 178
monkshood, 274
monoamine oxidase, 41
monoamines, 13–14
Moringa oleifera, 223
morning glory, 215, 219
Moroccan folk medicine, 217
morphine, 36
"Mother of Pearl Pill," 190
motherwort, 93
multiple sclerosis, 242
myalgia, 103
myocardial infarction, 41
myricetin, 45
Myrtaceae, 242

N

Nardostachys chinensis, 104
Nardostachys grandiflora, 104
Nardostachys jatamansi, 47, 104–105, 223, 246,
    266, 267
naringenin, 34
naringin, 45
naturopathic medicine, 212
nausea, 101, 182
Nepeta cataria, 139
nerolidol, 45

neroli oil, 246
nervines, 233
nervios, 66
nervous exhaustion, 134
neuralgia, 90, 103
neurobiology of anxiety, 11–18
    brain circuitry of anxiety, 11
    inflammation, 16
    metabolic syndrome, 16–17
    neurochemistry, 12–15
    stress, 15–16
neurochemistry, 12–15
    acetylcholine, 14
    endocannabinoids, 14
    endorphins, 14–15
    gamma amino butyric acid, 12–13
    glutamate, 13
    glycine, 15
    histamine, 15
    monoamines, 13–14
neuroinflammation, 41
neurological conditions, 124
neurosis, 76
neurosteroids, 13, 28
Nicotiana tabacum, 35
nicotine, 14, 35
nightshade, 225
nirgundi, 225
nitrosative damage, 17
nobiletin, 45–46
non-pharmacological treatments, 7–9
norepinephrine, 13
"Nourish the Heart Decoction,"
    185–186, 189
Nux vomica, 15

O

oats, 41, 57
obsessive compulsive disorder
    Echium amoenum and, 75
    Silybum marianum and, 125–126
    Valeriana officinalis and, 131
Ocimum basilicum, 37, 39, 41, 105, 252
Ocimum sanctum, 43, 44, 47, 105–106
Ocimum tenuiflorum, 38, 105
OCTA, 212
olfactory system, 238–239
O-methylated flavone, 46, 47
onions, 40
opiate crisis, xx
opiate receptors, 262
Orchidaceae, 45
Origanum majorana, 39, 252
Origanum vulgare, 39, 45
Ormenis multicaulis, 252

Oroxylum indicum, 38, 39–40
oxidative damage, 87
oxidative stress, 17

P

P450 enzymes, 59, 67, 89, 91, 92–93, 108
Paeonia lactiflora, 195
pain
    Cannabis sativa and, 64
    Cnidium officinale and, 193
    comorbidities, 269–270
    Piscidia piscipula and, 140
    Salvia officinalis and, 121
    vacha brahmi ghan and, 216
palmatine, 127
palpitations, 85, 127, 182, 216
Panax ginseng, 35, 76, 106–108, 195–196,
    232, 272
Panax notoginseng, 106, 107
Panax quinquefolius, 107
Panax spp, 107
panic attacks, 3, 134, 181–182
Papaveraceae, 269
Papaver somniferum, 36, 269
parasika yavani, 221
parasites, 224
Parkinson's disease, 46, 241
paroxetine, 180, 184, 187
Passiflora incarnata, 36, 38, 39–40, 44, 79, 80,
    108–110, 127, 266, 267
Paullinia cupana, 79, 80
pecans, 40
Pelargonium, 43
Pelargonium graveolens, 41, 246–247, 251
pentylenetetrazol, 38
peppermint, 102, 271
Pericarpium zanthoxyli, 15
perrottetinene, 35
Petroselinum crispum, 46
peyote cactus Lophophora williamsii, 113
P-glycoprotein, 91, 119
Phellodendron amurense, 98
pheochromocytoma, 3
pheromones, 239, 240
phobias, 2
Phyllanthaceae, 36
physical exercise, 9
phytochemicals, xix
phytoestrogens, 123, 129
Phytonoxon, 78
Pinaceae species, 39
Pinellia ternata, 196
pinene, 39, 46
pine tree, 46

Piper methysticum, 110–112, 266, 267, 274, 275–276
Piper nigrum, 39, 223
Piscidia piscipula, 140
pittas, 205, 206, 265
plums, 40
Po, 175
Pogostemon cablin, 252
Polygala tenuifolia, 196–197
Polygonum multiflorum, 197
polyphenols, 33
pomegranate, 224
Poria cocos, 112–113, 197
postmenopause *see* menopause
postpartum, 209, 251, 270
posttraumatic stress disorder (PTSD), 1
practical considerations, 276–277
pranayama techniques, 8
pregabalin, 27
pregnancy, 55, 251
premenstrual syndrome, 83, 132–133, 195;
    see also menstruation
Primula vulgaris, 40
progressive relaxation, 8
propranolol, 27–28
Prunella vulgaris, 42
Prunus avium, 45
pseudojujubogenins, 58
Psilocybe mushrooms, 36
Psilocybe spp, 113–117
psilocybin, 36, 113–117
psychodynamic therapy, 7
psychosis, 101
psychosomatic medicine, 182
psychotherapy, 7–8
PTSD *see* posttraumatic stress disorder (PTSD)
public speaking, 62
Punica granatum, 224

Q

Qi, 85, 102, 175, 190, 243
quercetin, 33, 34, 46–47

R

Radix Bupleuri chinense, 192–193
Rauwolfia serpentina, 213–214
red clover, 128
red date, 136
Rehmannia glutinosa, 197–198
reishi, 85
reishi fungus, 194
restlessness, 112, 221
resveratrol, xix, 46
retinal light sensitivity, 93

rheumatism, 101
Rhodiola rosea, 37, 117–119, 232, 272, 273
rikkunshinto, 182
rimonabant, 14
Roman chamomile, 99, 245
Rosa damascena, 247–248, 251, 252
Rosa species, 41, 43
Rosa spp, 43
rosavin, 37
Rose geranium, 246–247
rosemary *see Rosmarinus officinalis*
rosmarinic acid, 47
Rosmarinus officinalis, 38, 39, 43, 46, 47, 119–120, 240, 248, 271, 272, 273, 275
Rubiaceae, 36
rubor, 16
Rumex acetosella, 42
Rutaceae family, 37

S

safety, 273–276
saffron, 70
sage, 120, 248–249
Salacia, 44
Salvia, 38, 42
Salvia lavandulaefolia, 121
Salvia officinalis, 38, 43, 46, 47, 120–122, 248–249, 269, 270, 271, 273
Salvia osmarinus, 119
san, 178
sanjoinine, 36
sankhaholi, 81
Santallum spp, 249
Santalum album, 241, 251
sarasvata choorna, 212–213
sarpagandha, 213
Saussurea involucrata, 42
Saussurea lappa, 224
Schisandra chinensis, 46, 122–124, 198, 232
Schisandra chinensiss, 38
schizandra, 122
Schizandra chinensis, 232
schizophrenia, 184
sciatica, 90
scopolamine, 36
Scrophularia, 38
Scutellaria, 38, 47
Scutellaria baicalensis, 36, 37, 39–40, 45, 124–125, 192, 272, 274
Scutellaria lateriflora, 124–125
seasonal affective disorder, 93
secondary disorder, 3
sedative formulas, 188
seizures *see* antiseizure effects

selective serotonin reuptake inhibitors (SSRIs), 26
semen Zizyphus jujuba, 183
sensitivity plant, 139
serotonin, 13
serotonin/norepinephrine reuptake inhibitors (SNRIs), 26
sertraline, 84
sexual energy, 134
shankhapushpi, 69, 81, 208, 215, 219
shankhapushpi panak, 214–215
shankpushpi, 81
shatavari, 209
Shen, 175–176
Shennong Bencao Jing, 136, 192
shen qi wu wei zi, 182–183, 183
shen song yang xin, 183
shevga, 223
shirodhara, 69, 214–215, 237, 246
shortness of breath, 85
shuganjieyu, 89–90
shu gan ning shen san, 179
Siberian ginseng, 36, 76, 107
Silexan, 264
Silybum marianum, 125–126
Sinclair, David, xix
skin conditions, 128, 222, 224
skullcap, 36, 124–125
sleep
    3-carene and, 39
    Albizia julibrissin and, 191
    Angelicae gigantis and, 192
    aromatherapy and, 251–252
    Boswellia carterii and, 252
    Cananga odorata and, 252
    cannabis and, 62
    Cannabis indica and, 266
    Cannabis sativa and, 266
    Chamaemelum nobile and, 252
    Cinnamomum camphora and, 252
    Citrus aurantium and, 252
    comorbidities, 266–268
    Cuscuta reflexa and, 219–220
    Eschscholzia californica and, 78, 266
    Ganoderma lucidum and, 85
    guduchyadi medhya rasayana and, 210
    gui pi and, 265
    gui pi tang and, 181
    Humulus lupulus and, 88, 266
    Hyoscyamus niger and, 221
    isopulegol and, 43
    Jasminum spp and, 252
    Juniperus communis and, 252
    Lactuca virosa and, 138
    Lavandula angustifolia and, 91, 252, 266
    Lavandula officinalis and, 252
    Lippia citriodora and, 97
    Matricaria recutita and, 266, 267
    Melissa officinalis and, 101, 266, 267
    Nardostachys jatamansi and, 266, 267
    Ocimum basilicum and, 252
    Origanum majorana and, 252
    Ormenis multicaulis and, 252
    Passiflora incarnata and, 266, 267
    Pinellia ternata and, 196
    pinene and, 46
    Piper methysticum and, 266, 267
    Piscidia piscipula and, 140
    Pogostemon cablin and, 252
    Polygonum multiflorum and, 197
    Poria cocos and, 112
    Rosa damascena and, 252
    Santallum spp and, 249
    suan zao ren tang and, 183, 184
    Tinospora cordifolia and, 127
    ursolic acid and, 47
    vacha brahmi ghan and, 216
    Valeriana officinalis and, 131, 266, 267–268
    Vetiveria zizanoides and, 252
    Withania somnifera and, 134, 135, 225, 266, 268
    xiao yao san and, 185
    yi gan san and, 186
    zhi zi chi tang and, 183, 184
    Zizyphus jujuba, 266, 268
    Zizyphus jujuba and, 136
SNRIs see serotonin/norepinephrine reuptake inhibitors (SNRIs)
social anxiety disorder, 2, 7, 62, 84
Solanaceae, 225
Solanum lycopersicum, 45
soybean, fermented, 184
spiced apple, 240
spikenard, 104
spirit, 177
spleen, 140, 185, 187
spontaneous abortion, 65
srotas, 206
ß-asarone, 56
ß-caryophyllene, 38, 75
SSRIs see selective serotonin reuptake inhibitors (SSRIs)
stamina, 193
State-Trait Anxiety Inventory, 41, 58
Sternbach, Leo, 23
steroids, 13, 35
St. John's wort, 89
stress, 15–16, 17
strychnine, 15
suan zao ren tang, 180, 183–184
Sushruta Samhita, 64, 219
sweet basil, 105
sweet flag, 55, 274
sweet orange, 242

syncope, 101
Synopsis of Prescriptions of the Golden Chamber, 183
Syzygium aromaticum, 38, 41, 242
Szent-Györgyi, Albert, xix, 24

T

Tagetes, 42, 45
talk therapy *see* psychotherapy
tang, 178
tea, 59
    Earl Grey, 67
    green, 40, 59–61, 67, 271
terpenes, 34–35
THC *see* delta-9-tetrahydrocannabinol (THC)
Theobroma cacao, 33, 45
thryallis, 84
Thymus vulgaris, 39
tian wang bu xin dan, 189
tiao qi, 124
Tilia, 43
Tilia spp, 140–141
Tinospora cordifolia, 126–128, 224–225, 270, 271, 273
tinosporicide, 127
touch-me-not, 139
traditional Chinese medicine
    Acorus, 55
    Acorus gramineus, 191
    adaptogens in, 233
    Albizia julibrissin, 191–192
    Anemarrhena asphodeloides, 44
    Angelicae gigantis, 192
    anxiety treatments, 177
    bai zi yang xin tang, 178–179
    banhabakchulchunma, 188
    ban xia hou pu, 179, 265
    bao shen, 180
    Centella asiatica, 64
    cinnamon, 67
    Cnidium officinale, 193
    Coptis chinensis, 193
    Curcuma wenyujin, 194
    Curcuma zedoria, 72
    Cynomorium songaricum, 194
    dan shen, 121
    diagnosis in, 190
    Eleutherococcus senticosus, 76, 89
    explained, 175–176
    Ganoderma lucidum, 194
    geng ni an chun, 180
    Glycyrrhiza uralensis, 194–195
    gui pi, 265
    gui pi tang, 180–181
    hange-koboku-to, 181–182
    herbal treatments, 177–188

Hypericum perforatum, 89
Jasminum officinale, 243
jiu wei zhen xin, 181
kami-shoyo-san, 181–182
Lilium rythro, 95–96
Magnolia officinalis, 98–99
mainstays of, 190–198
Paeonia lactiflora, 195
Panax ginseng, 195–196
Panax spp, 107
philosophy of, 177–178
Pinellia ternata, 196
Polygala tenuifolia, 196–197
Polygonum multiflorum, 197
Poria cocos, 112, 197
Qi, 175
Radix Bupleuri chinense, 192–193
Rehmannia glutinosa, 197–198
rikkunshinto, 182
Schisandra chinensis, 122, 198
Scutellaria baicalensis, 124–125
shen qi wu wei zi, 182–183
shen song yang xin, 183
suan zao ren tang, 183–184
untested, 188–190
Valeriana jatamansi Jones, 130
wen dan tang, 184–185
xiao yao san, 185, 265
xin wei tang, 185
yang xin tang, 185–186
yi gan san, 186–187
yi qi yang xin, 187
yukgunja, 187–188
zhi zi chi tang, 183–184
Zizyphus jujuba, 36, 58, 136–137, 198
traditional Mexican folk medicine, 66
trauma and stressor-related disorder, 1–2
Tridax procumbens, 40
Trifolium pratense, 43, 46, 128–130, 268, 275
triptan medications, 4
triterpenoids, 58
TrkB *see* tropomyosin receptor kinase B (TrkB)
tropomyosin receptor kinase B (TrkB), 40
"true cinnamon," 66
tulsi, 105
tumor, 16, 112
turmeric, 71

U

ulcers, 101
Umbellifere, 64
Unani medicine, 72, 138, 217
untested herbal treatments, Chinese, 188–190
    chai hu jia long gu mu li tang, 189
    ding zhi wan, 189
    gan cao tang, 188

gan mai da zao tang, 188
gui zhi jia long gu mu li tang, 189
gui zhi qu shao yao jia shu qi long gu mu li
    tang, 189
tian wang bu xin dan, 189
zhen jing ji, 188
untested herbal treatments, Western
    Borago officinalis, 138
    jiao tai wan, 189–190
    Lactuca virosa, 138
    long chi qing hun san, 189
    miao xiang san, 189
    Mimosa pudica, 139
    Nepeta cataria, 139
    Piscidia piscipula, 140
    Taraxacum officinale, 140
    Tilia spp, 140–141
    zhen zhu mu wan, 190
urination, 112
ursolic acid, 47
US National Center for Health Statistics, 23

V

vacha brahmi ghan, 216
valerian, 104
Valeriana jatamansi, 104, 225
Valeriana jatamansi Jones, 130–131
Valeriana officinalis, 79, 80, 130, 131–132, 266,
    267–268, 269, 274
Valeriana wallichii, 130
vatas, 205, 206, 265
vertigo, 101
Vetiveria zizanoides, 252
visceral fat, 17
vitamin P, xix, 24
Vitex agnus-castus, 37, 43, 46, 132–134, 225,
    268, 269
vitexin, 37
Vitex negundo, 225
Vitis vinifera, 33
vomeronasal organ, 239–240
vomiting, 105, 224

W

wan, 178
warfarin, 275
warm gallbladder decoction, 184
water hyssop, 58
weakness, 122, 134
wen dan tang, 184–185
Western herbalism, 55–141
    Acorus calamus, 55–56
    Avena sativa, 57–58
    Bacopa monnieri, 58–59

Camellia sinensis, 59–61
Cannabis sativa, 61
Centella asiatica, 64–65
chamomile, 99–101
Cinnamomum spp, 66–67
Citrus aurantium, 67–68
Convolvulus pluricaulis, 69–70
Crocus sativus, 70–71
Curcuma longa, 71–73
Echinacea angustifolia, 73–74
Echium amoenum, 74–76
Eleutherococcus senticosus, 76–78
Eschscholzia californica, 78–79
Euphytose, 79–81
Evolvulus alsinoides, 81–82
Foeniculum vulgare, 82–84
Galphimia glauca, 84–85
Ganoderma lucidum, 85–86
Ginkgo biloba, 87–88
Guduchi, 126–128
Humulus lupulus, 88–89
Hypericum perforatum, 89–91
Lavandula angustifolia, 91–93
Leonurus cardiaca, 93–94
Lepidium meyenii, 94–95
Lilium rythro, 95–96
Lippia citriodora, 96–98
Magnolia officinalis, 98–99
Matricaria recutita, 99–101
Melissa officinalis, 101–102
Mentha piperita, 102–104
Nardostachys jatamansi, 104–105
Ocimum sanctum, 105–106
Panax ginseng, 106–108
Passiflora incarnata, 108–110
Piper methysticum, 110–112
Poria cocos, 112–113
Psilocybe spp, 113–117
Rhodiola rosea, 117–119
Rosmarinus officinalis, 119–120
Salvia officinalis, 120–122
Schisandra chinensis, 122–124
Scutellaria baicalensis, 124–125
Silybum marianum, 125–126
Tinospora cordifolia, 126–128
Trifolium pratense, 128–130
untested, 137–141
Valeriana jatamansi Jones, 130–131
Valeriana officinalis, 131–132
Vitex agnus-castus, 132–134
Withania somnifera, 134–136
Zizyphus jujuba, 136–137
wild lettuce, 138
wine, 45
winter melon, 211
Withania somnifera, 35, 134–136, 225, 231, 266,
    268, 270, 273

wogonin, 47–48
Wolfiporia extensa, 112
Worry Free, 216
wounds, 101
wuling, 112
wu wei zi, 122

X

Xanax, 183
xenohormesis, xix–xx
Xerophyta, 37
xiao yao san, 185, 265
xin wei tang, 185

Y

yang, 176
yang xin tang, 185–186, 189
Yao's Collection of Effective Prescriptions, 184
yastimadhu, 208
Yi, 175, 176

yi gan san, 186–187
yin, 176
yi qi yang xin, 187
ylang ylang, 250
yoga, 8
yoga nidra, 8
yohimbine, 4
yokukansan, 186
yukgunja, 187–188

Z

zhen jing ji, 188
zhen zhu mu wan, 190
Zhi, 175
zhi zi chi tang, 183–184
zi hou po, 98
Zingiber officinale, 45, 218, 271
Zizyphus fructus, 198
Zizyphus jujuba, 36, 37, 44, 58, 136–137, 183, 198, 266, 268
Zizyphus spinosa, 198

Printed in the United States
by Baker & Taylor Publisher Services